Conciliation in Healthcare

Conciliation in Healthcare
Managing and resolving complaints and conflict

ANNE WARD PLATT BA(Hons), PGCE
Director, AWP Associates

Foreword by
SIR LIAM DONALDSON
Chief Medical Officer

Radcliffe Publishing
Oxford • New York

Radcliffe Publishing Ltd
18 Marcham Road
Abingdon
Oxon OX14 1AA
United Kingdom

www.radcliffe-oxford.com
Electronic catalogue and worldwide online ordering facility.

British Library Cataloguing in Publication Data

A catalogue record for this book is available from the British Library.

ISBN-13: 978 184619 085 8

Typeset by Pindar New Zealand (Egan Reid), Auckland, New Zealand
Printed and bound by Hobbs the Printers Ltd, Southampton, Hampshire, UK

Contents

To Martin

Foreword

Complaints about healthcare arise when treatment has not matched the expectations of patients, carers or relatives. Sometimes, the outcome may have been a patient damaged by a safety failure, perhaps seriously or fatally. Sometimes, diagnosis and treatment may not have improved the patient's condition in the way hoped for and expected. More often, care will have been given safely and effectively, but in a way that was considered too slow, or took place in poor surroundings, or – especially – was inadequately communicated.

Those making a complaint have varying hopes. They may seek redress, either financial or perhaps just in the form of an apology. They may wish to see those they consider responsible held visibly to account. They may simply be seeking further information about what happened and why, and regard a complaint as the best way to achieve this. Very commonly, they perceive that something has gone wrong and wish to protect future patients from a recurrence.

The response to complaints has often been problematic for the National Health Service. Staff may feel that they have already given all of the explanation that they have, and may not know what more they can do. None of us likes to revisit emotionally painful episodes, and the effects of failures of care on staff who were trying to do their best may be underestimated. Staff may feel that individuals, society and the mass media have unrealistic expectations of what health services can achieve that make disappointment more likely or sometimes inevitable. They may consider responding to complaints to be a distraction from pressing clinical duties.

While from the different perspectives of patients, carers, relatives, staff and managers these disparate and sometimes conflicting reactions are very understandable, the result of their interaction is all too often unhelpful. It is rare in the NHS for complaints to be considered a valuable resource to improve the match between expectation and delivery, as many commercial organisations have learned to see them. Responses may be defensive, argumentative or uncommunicative, meetings frosty or hostile. Too often, the effect is a widening gap of understanding between the parties, which obfuscates and confuses rather than revealing what happened and why, and that inevitably and progressively frustrates the participants. Anyone who considers this description overstated need only consider the number and frequency of attempts to reform or reconfigure NHS complaints procedures and redefine the role of organisations involved in resolving complaints to realise the difficulty of the area, as well as its importance.

Conciliation offers a significant opportunity. It can re-establish stalled dialogue. It can help participants to understand that there are other valid points of view, and narrow the gap between differing expectations. The potential benefits are considerable, both for those who can feel that their voice has been heeded and their understanding improved, and for those who have the opportunity to help make the services they provide safer, more effective and better matched with expectations.

For conciliation to help achieve this worthwhile prize, it must be readily available, carried out well, and focused on outcomes. This book explains how and why, clearly and effectively.

Sir Liam Donaldson
Chief Medical Officer
Department of Health
November 2007

About the author

Anne Ward Platt has been involved in healthcare conciliation since 1997 when she was appointed an independent conciliator to the former Newcastle and North Tyneside Health Authority. She has subsequently acted in this capacity for Newcastle, North Tyneside and Gateshead Primary Care Trusts. Widely experienced as a conciliator in relation to both primary and secondary healthcare, she is director of a management consultancy specialising in conciliation, complaints and conflict management. She is a graduate of Bristol University where she also trained as a teacher. She has undertaken health and social care research, health-related project management in the voluntary sector, and from 1998 she has served as a Non-Executive Director in the NHS. She is currently a Non-Executive Director of Northumberland, Tyne and Wear NHS Trust.

Acknowledgements

I would like to thank all those who have contributed to my understanding and experience of conciliation, including those who have appointed and trained me, staff involved in complaints handling, fellow conciliators and mediators, and especially those who have entrusted me with the task of helping them to resolve issues of complaint, concern or conflict.

I would also like to thank my wonderful family, friends and colleagues for their interest, encouragement and support.

Anne Ward Platt

Introduction

This book sets out to be a comprehensive guide to the use of conciliation in the context of healthcare complaints and other situations of conflict or dispute. It relates this to existing procedures both in the United Kingdom (UK) and other countries, exploring the rationale for its use, and the situations in which it can be helpful. Practical advice is also given about the conduct of the conciliation process, highlighting the importance of appropriate support for both complainants and staff, and considering its relationship with other aspects of clinical and organisational governance. Many of the points made are generic, and will have relevance in any context in which the effective handling of complaints is seen as both a priority and a learning opportunity.

'Conciliation' is the term used in the National Health Service (NHS) to describe a particular form of dispute resolution that is used in relation to the complaints process. The 1996 complaints procedure included the requirement that conciliation services should be provided in relation to primary care complaints. No such requirement was made in relation to secondary care. As a result, conciliation has been an important tool in relation to the resolution of primary care complaints, but has not been widely used in NHS organisations providing secondary care.

In 2004, however, revised complaints procedures were introduced, and included the requirement for all NHS organisations in England to ensure the availability of conciliation in relation to healthcare complaints. Although NHS Foundation Trusts may follow their own local resolution procedures, the proven value of conciliation should ensure that it is not overlooked. Countries beyond the UK also recognise the effectiveness of conciliation, and it is of significance in relation to the healthcare complaints procedures currently operative, for example, in Australia, New Zealand and Canada.

In writing this book, I have considered the implications of implementing the conciliation process more widely in the UK, and I have drawn on my own experiences as a conciliator in relation to both the primary and secondary healthcare sectors, in the context of complaints covering a wide range of issues, relating to children and adults of all ages. From my perspective as a Non-Executive Director in the NHS, I am also aware not only of the importance of effective complaints handling in terms of its impact on the individual's experience of their healthcare, but also as an essential component of clinical and organisational governance.

This book is designed primarily for those concerned with complaints in the NHS and private providers of NHS care. This includes conciliators themselves and those involved in their training, as well as staff responsible for implementing the complaints procedure, and those involved directly in handling healthcare complaints. I hope it will also be a useful resource for those organisations whose staff provide advocacy and other forms of support for complainants, and for those against whom complaints have been made.

My contact with healthcare staff has highlighted the lack of practical guidance relating to conciliation, and the need for clear information to dispel misconceptions and misunderstandings about the process. Apart from its use in relation to complaints, conciliation can also be of value in situations where there has been a serious deterioration, or breakdown, in the clinical relationship or engagement between staff and patients, or their relatives and carers. The points raised will have similar relevance for those considering the use of conciliation for resolving conflicts or concerns arising in the workplace.

There is also general acknowledgement in the UK, as well as in other countries, that there is a need to improve complaints handling across all government departments. This encompasses a recognition of the benefits of providing a range of dispute resolution services, including conciliation, in relation to complex complaints and disputes. These alternatives have the advantage of being more accessible and cost-effective than some of the processes currently in use. Aspects of this book should, therefore, be of relevance to those organisations where there is a commitment to improving the management of complaints through a range of measures.

I hope that this book will make a significant contribution towards raising the profile of conciliation as an important means of resolving complaints, as well as highlighting the value of conciliation in other situations of conflict or dispute, both within the NHS and beyond the field of healthcare.

CHAPTER 1

Conciliation and complaints

- → Context and meaning of 'conciliation' and other forms of dispute resolution.
- → Mediation and conciliation.
- → What constitutes a complaint?
- → Aspects of effective complaints management.
- → Why do people complain?
- → Complaints made by, or on behalf of, patients or service users.
- → Complaints made in relation to, or by, children and young people.
- → Obstacles that prevent people complaining.

Context and meaning of 'conciliation' and other forms of dispute resolution

'Conciliation' is the term used in the National Health Service (NHS) in England to describe a particular form of dispute resolution that is used in relation to the complaints process.

> 'NHS Conciliation is a method of facilitating a dialogue to resolve an issue. It is an intervention whereby a third party helps the parties to reach a common understanding. It gives space to resolve issues, preserve on-going relationships and time to defuse or calm heightened situations.'

Department of Health. *Handling complaints in the NHS – good practice toolkit for local resolution.* Department of Health, 2005. Accessible at: http://www.dh.gov. uk/en/Publicationsandstatistics/Publications/PublicationsPolicyAndGuidance/ Browsable/DH_4108465 accessed August 2007.

Conciliation has been an important tool in relation to the resolution of primary care complaints in the NHS since its inclusion in the 1996 complaints procedure.

However, the *National Health Service (Complaints) Regulations 2004* now give conciliation prominence as a tool for the resolution of complaints in both primary and secondary care.

> 'The complaints manager may, in any case where he thinks it would be appropriate to do so and with the agreement of the complainant, make arrangements for conciliation, mediation or other assistance for the purposes of resolving the complaint, and in any such case the NHS body must ensure that appropriate conciliation or mediation services are available.'

> Statutory Instrument 2004 No. 1768. *The National Health Service (Complaints) Regulations 2004*. London: HMSO, 2004. Regulation 12 (2).

Conciliation is also of significance in relation to the healthcare complaints procedures currently operative in Scotland, Wales and Northern Ireland, as well as in countries beyond the UK; for instance, Australia, New Zealand, parts of the USA, Canada and parts of mainland Europe, where it is also recognised as providing an additional resource for those involved in handling healthcare complaints.

> 'A range of options will be available to the authority for dealing with the complaint (eg, review competence, counselling, conciliation, or taking no further action).'

> Minister of Health. *Improving quality (IQ): a systems approach for the New Zealand health and disability sector*. Wellington: Ministry of Health, 2003.

The closest similarities exist between the complaints procedures in the UK and Australia, which promote informal resolution of complaints, wherever possible, at the earliest opportunity by the organisation or practitioner involved, before formal procedures are initiated. They also emphasise the value of conciliation where appropriate.

There is information about conciliation in *Handling complaints in the NHS – good practice toolkit for local resolution* which can be found on the Department of Health website. While this demonstrates the principles of conciliation, it does not address all the practical issues that arise when staff are required to implement the process. This has resulted in locally agreed procedures, and the use, practice, quality and evaluation of conciliation is consequently variable in different parts of the UK. The absence of a prescriptive approach does, however, have advantages in terms of flexibility and the opportunities it provides for local innovation and improvement. This point is emphasised in the guidance that supports the complaints regulations.

'The Guidance expands on the statutory framework set out in the Regulations. It is not meant to be all-embracing or to cover every contingency, but is a guide to the mandatory aspects of the complaints procedure. It should be supported by locally developed guidance, allowing bodies to approach management of the complaints procedure in the way that best meets local circumstances.'

Department of Health. *Guidance to support implementation of the National Health Service (Complaints) Regulations.* Department of Health, 2004. Paragraph 1.9.

Ideally, complaints should be managed and resolved as early as possible at a local level. This is the first stage of the complaints procedure and is known as 'Local Resolution'.

'Local Resolution seeks to provide prompt investigation and resolution of the complaint at a local level aiming to satisfy the complainant whilst being fair to staff.'

Department of Health. *Guidance to support implementation of the National Health Service (Complaints) Regulations.* Department of Health, 2004. Paragraph 1.2.

Where there has been a failure to achieve resolution at a local level, the second stage of the procedure is handled in England by The Commission for Healthcare Audit and Inspection (commonly known as The Healthcare Commission). It includes referral of unresolved complaints for mediation or conciliation as a possible outcome of its initial review of a complaint.

'At the initial review stage, we can decide to either:
- ➡ take no further action
- ➡ refer the complaint back to the NHS organisation, in order for them to try to resolve the issues
- ➡ carry out a full investigation
- ➡ refer your case to an independent panel
- ➡ refer your case to mediation or conciliation.'

Healthcare Commission. *Complaints* (leaflet). Commission for Healthcare Audit and Inspection, 2007. www.healthcarecommission.org.uk (Based on: Statutory Instrument 2004 No. 1768. *The National Health Service (Complaints) Regulations 2004.* London: HMSO, 2004. Regulation 16)

This function of second-stage complaints review is performed in Wales by the Healthcare Inspectorate Wales, in Scotland by NHS Quality Improvement Scotland, and in Northern Ireland by the Health and Personal Social Services

Regulation and Improvement Authority. Similar bodies also exist in the different jurisdictions in Australia which may also determine that conciliation is the most appropriate means of dealing with complaints that have not been resolved at an earlier stage.

Legislation in Australia which relates to healthcare complaints also extends to details of the conciliation process itself. In New South Wales, for example, the Health Conciliation Registry was established as a result of the *Health Care Complaints Act 1993*, and from 2005 it was integrated with the New South Wales Health Care Complaints Commission.

> 'The function of a conciliator is:
> a. to bring the parties to the complaint together for the purpose of promoting the discussion, negotiation and settlement of the complaint, and
> b. to undertake any activity for the purpose of promoting that discussion, negotiation and settlement, and
> c. if possible, to assist the parties to the complaint to reach agreement.'
>
> New South Wales Consolidated Acts. *Health Care Complaints Act 1993.*
> Section 49, 'Role of conciliator'.

It is not only the statutory bodies responsible for health in the UK that recognise the need to ensure effective and efficient complaints handling using the most appropriate means to achieve this. There is also widespread recognition among other government departments, both in the UK and elsewhere, of the benefits of providing a range of dispute resolution services. These can be a speedier and more cost-effective way of achieving resolution, particularly in relation to complex and emotionally charged disputes, and can also provide greater flexibility and accessibility than some of the procedures currently in use.

> 'Conciliation involves an impartial third party helping the parties to resolve their dispute by hearing both sides and offering an opinion on settlement. It requires both parties' willing and informed consent to participate. The parties determine the outcome, usually with advice from the conciliator.'
>
> Secretary of State for Constitutional Affairs and Lord Chancellor. *Transforming public services: complaints, redress and tribunals.* (Command Paper: Cm 6243.)
> London: HMSO, 2004.

Conciliation has uses beyond the resolution of complaints. It can be of value in any situation where the clinical relationship has broken down. I co-authored a paper considering this issue in relation to two high-profile cases in the UK involving disputes between the parents of premature babies with severe disabilities and the clinical teams involved. In both cases the situation escalated to the point where legal intervention was requested by the healthcare providers concerned in order to obtain a ruling in relation to the options for treatment. It is not known publicly whether or not conciliation was considered at any stage. Equally, conciliation may be used in an attempt to restore relationships as part of conflict management, either within the NHS or in other organisations where conflict or disagreement exists (*see* Chapter 5).

> 'There is general agreement that courts are not the places where it is optimal to define clinical management, and that every avenue should be explored to obtain resolution of differences without recourse to judicial input.'
>
> Ward Platt M, Ward Platt A. Conflicts of care. *Archives of Disease in Childhood.* 2005; 90: 331.

Mediation and conciliation

'Mediation' is the term used to describe the process by which an intermediary, the mediator, attempts to facilitate the resolution of differences or disputes between individuals or organisations. The process can be applied to a wide range of situations in both formal and informal settings. The context and situation in which the terms 'mediation' and 'conciliation' are used will indicate the particular model of the process to which reference is being made. In the UK the Department of Health uses the word 'mediation' primarily in relation to clinical litigation and personal injury claims. In contrast, the term 'conciliation' tends to be reserved for the process used in relation to the complaints procedure.

At the present time, healthcare complaints in England are handled separately from claims and clinical litigation cases (which are handled by the NHS Litigation Authority), although consideration has been given to the implications of promoting a more integrated approach (Department of Health. *Making amends: a consultation paper setting out proposals for reforming the approach to clinical negligence in the NHS. A report by the Chief Medical Officer*, June 2003). However, in 2006 the *NHS Redress Act* was passed, reflecting recommendation 1 from *Making amends*, and enabling changes in the way the NHS handles some incidents of clinical negligence in relation to hospital care in England and Wales. Compensation may be awarded up to a maximum of £20,000 and the Act also provides for non-monetary forms of redress. It is intended that claims which fall within the remit of the redress scheme will be settled without recourse to civil court proceedings.

> 'An NHS Redress Scheme should be introduced to provide investigations when things go wrong; remedial treatment, rehabilitation and care where

needed; explanations and apologies; and financial compensation in certain circumstances.'

Department of Health. *Making amends: a consultation paper setting out proposals for reforming the approach to clinical negligence in the NHS. A report by the Chief Medical Officer*. Department of Health, 2003. Recommendation 1.

There is clearly potential within the NHS Redress Scheme for conciliation and mediation to be used to facilitate agreement in relation to the exact forms of redress that will produce a satisfactory outcome for the parties involved.

In contrast, financial outcomes in relation to the complaints procedures are limited and likely to involve small amounts. The resolution of dental complaints occasionally includes a financial component relating to dental charges, and *ex gratia* payments are sometimes made as a result of certain claims, particularly if a patient has suffered loss or damage to property, for example. The Annual Report of the Parliamentary and Health Service Ombudsman for 2005–06 promoted wider use of financial redress as a possible outcome for some complaints.

'We have argued for some time that it is an essential part of good complaints handling to put a complainant back in the position they would have been in if the failing had not occurred.'

Parliamentary and Health Service Ombudsman. *Making a difference: Annual Report 2005–6*. (HC 1363). London: The Stationery Office, 2006.

It is a feature of the conciliation process as it is applied in relation to healthcare complaints in some jurisdictions in Australia that financial settlements may be made as part of the agreed outcome.

'Issues which have been managed in Conciliation include . . . complaints where medical negligence and liability have been explored and compensation negotiated.'

Health Rights Commission, Queensland. *Annual Report 2005–6*. Queensland: HRCQ, 2006.

The terms 'mediation' and 'conciliation' are often used synonymously both in this country and overseas. In certain contexts they are used to signify an internationally recognised method of Alternative Dispute Resolution (ADR). This is the model that is used in relation to civil litigation claims as a means of avoiding expensive and lengthy court proceedings. It also has other advantages beyond the purely financial: a range of outcomes is possible, including the restoration of working relationships. This can have significant implications in a commercial context where goodwill may be regarded as a very valuable commodity. It also provides an opportunity for apologies and explanations to be given which may be particularly significant for some claimants; for example, in relation to clinical negligence claims.

Although there are some variations in the models used in different contexts, conciliation and mediation share these characteristics:

- the use of a neutral intermediary who acts as an impartial and independent facilitator using specific skills aimed at bringing about a resolution of the dispute to the satisfaction of the parties concerned
- the process is based on an agreed framework or code of conduct
- any information that is disclosed during the process is 'without prejudice', which means that it cannot normally be used in any subsequent court proceedings
- the parties agree to take part in the process voluntarily
- the parties can withdraw at any time
- the mediator or conciliator does not impose a solution on the parties
- the private sessions between the mediator or conciliator and each party are confidential (within certain limits, discussed in Chapter 3), and only such information as is agreed is passed on to the other party
- there is opportunity for joint sessions involving both parties
- the process provides a 'safe' environment in which the participants can express their feelings and emotions
- the outcome may include apologies; explanations; evidence of organisational change (for example, action plans); evidence of individual change (for example, learning or re-training); or restoration of relationships between parties; as well as financial settlements where provision is made for this
- the outcome is not legally binding, but where the process is being used as an alternative to a court hearing, the parties may agree subsequently to a legally binding contract.

> 'The key to effective mediation is to:
> - offer it as early as possible before positions become entrenched;
> - promote an understanding of the benefits of mediation and conciliation among staff who may find themselves the subject of complaint; and
> - be clear that this is a confidential process.'
>
> Department of Health. *Learning from complaints: social services complaints procedure for adults.* Department of Health, 2006. Paragraph 6.2.4.

Where mediation is used as an alternative to judicial proceedings, the process tends to be conducted within a tightly managed time frame, which will have been agreed in advance with the parties concerned. Depending on the issues to be covered, it is possible for the entire mediation process to be concluded in a single day. In some cases the time factor may be crucial, not only in reducing any financial impact relating to the dispute, but also in restoring important working relationships between individuals and organisations.

In contrast, healthcare conciliations tend to be conducted over a longer period of time. This will be influenced by considerations such as the complainant's health or other personal circumstances. With these caveats in mind, however, it is clearly in everyone's interest for the process to maintain a sense of momentum and for unnecessary delays to be avoided. Although health service providers within the NHS are expected to adhere to the timescales set out in the NHS Complaints Regulations as closely as possible, there is provision for these to be extended in specific circumstances.

A further difference is that where mediation is used specifically as an alternative to a civil Court hearing, a key part of the process usually involves a joint session, or sessions, with all parties present. This is by no means an essential part of the conciliation model used in the healthcare situation. It is possible for a healthcare complaint to be resolved satisfactorily without the need for the parties to meet.

The role of the conciliator is sometimes described as being more proactive or interventionist than that of the mediator in relation to some conciliation models. In both cases, the skill of the mediator or conciliator relates strongly to their abilities in facilitating agreement effectively between the parties. However, it is worth noting that in the 1998 guidance produced by the Department of Health in relation to the use of conciliation for primary care complaints, the conciliator is not constrained by any particular approach.

'The conciliator may adopt such procedures as he determines are most appropriate for conducting the conciliation process.'

Department of Health. *Directions to health authorities on dealing with complaints about family health services practitioners and providers of personal medical services.* Department of Health, 1998.

Healthcare staff sometimes comment that they feel as though the complaints procedures are weighted in favour of the complainant. This often demonstrates a lack of understanding both about the procedures themselves and also about the principles of good customer care. While complaints handling in any organisation should be scrupulously fair to the staff involved, the aim of the procedures should be to resolve the complaint to the satisfaction of the customer or client. The process should be viewed as a positive opportunity for the organisation to improve its complaints handling, and to learn from the complainant's perspective about the treatment or care they received.

'Rights based conciliation' is the term sometimes used to refer to the conciliation process adopted when the individual or organisation against which the complaint is being made has specific obligations towards the complainant. In the context of the Disability Conciliation Service, for example, the conciliator has to ensure that the resolution of the disputed issues is commensurate with the service user's rights, which are non-negotiable. This particular conciliation model, therefore, differs from those where the parties are viewed as having equal rights by the conciliator or mediator.

Another area in which conciliation or mediation is widely used is in the field of family law in relation to separation or divorce, where conflicts frequently arise over a range of issues including, crucially, those between parents in relation to their children. In such circumstances the importance of maintaining communication, and achieving resolution of emotionally charged issues between the parties, is self-evident.

When referring to conciliation, people sometimes ask how it compares with two other forms of alternative dispute resolution, namely 'arbitration' and 'adjudication'. These differ radically from 'mediation' and 'conciliation' in that neither of the processes involves negotiation between the parties. Instead, the processes may involve a hearing or may be based solely on the submission of written documentation in which the parties provide the evidence and arguments relating to their dispute. The decision, or 'determination', as it is sometimes called, is made either by a single adjudicator or arbitrator, or in some circumstances by a panel, and it may be legally binding (*see* Glossary for further details).

What constitutes a complaint?

In considering the value of conciliation in relation to complaints resolution, it is useful at this stage to explore what actually constitutes a complaint and how it may be defined. Health service providers should ensure that staff have not only training in relation to complaints procedures and processes (*see* Chapter 5), but also an understanding of the organisation's definition of what constitutes a complaint.

The NHS Complaints Toolkit gives the succinct definition of a complaint used in *The Citizen's Charter Complaints Task Force. Information note: accessible complaints policies 2003*, quoting the Cabinet Office (1997), as 'any expression of dissatisfaction that needs a response'.

At one time, the British Standards Institute gave a fuller definition (BS 8600:1999) as follows: 'Any expression of dissatisfaction by a customer, with a product or service, however small, whether considered justified or not.' The latter part of this statement highlights two important points. Complaints which may appear trivial and insignificant to staff are not viewed in this light by the complainant. If staff adjust the quality of their response in such situations, there is not only a risk that further complaints will follow as the situation escalates, but also that the overall standard of complaints handling within that service will be compromised.

> 'A Complaint is "an expression of dissatisfaction made to an organization, related to its products, or the complaints handling process itself, where a response or resolution is explicitly or implicitly expected".'
>
> International Organization for Standardization. *ISO 10002: 2004* (Note: supersedes BS 8600: 1999). Geneva: ISO, 2004.

This point is made very effectively by the Treasury Board of Canada Secretariat (*Quality Service – Effective Complaint Management (Guide XI)*) which has adapted their definition of a complaint from Sydney Electric in Australia as follows: 'An expression of dissatisfaction with the organization's procedures, charges, employees, agents or quality of service.' This is supplemented by the advice that: 'A good way to determine if an expression of dissatisfaction is a complaint is to ask, "Does the client's dissatisfaction require the organization to take some action to resolve the matter, other than providing routine services, information or explanations, or processing an appeal under standard policy?"' The concluding statement emphasises the value of screening complaints at the outset to ensure that they are dealt with appropriately and expeditiously (*see* Chapter 2).

In England, the *National Health Service (Complaints) Regulations 2004* (Statutory Instrument 2004 No. 1768, Regulation 6) provides the context in which a healthcare complaint may be made:

> '. . . a complaint to an NHS body may be about any matter reasonably connected with the exercise of its functions including in particular, in the case of an NHS trust or Primary Care Trust, any matter reasonably connected with –
>
> a. its provision of health care or any other services, including in the case of a Primary Care Trust, its provision of primary medical services under section 16CC of the 1977 Act; and
>
> b. the function of commissioning health care or other services under an NHS contract or making arrangements for the provision of such care or other services with an independent provider or with an NHS foundation trust.'

Aspects of effective complaints management

There is general acknowledgement across both the public and private sectors of the importance of effective and efficient complaints handling. Commercially successful companies are those that put the customer or client at the centre of their operations, ensuring that they are responsive to feedback whether received through market research or complaints.

'... businesses tend to see complaints as vitally important feedback that provides the opportunity for the business to improve ...'

Chief Medical Officer. *Good doctors, safer patients: proposals to strengthen the system to assure and improve the performance of doctors and to protect the safety of patients.* Chief Medical Officer, 2006.

In a competitive retail environment, staff training is seen as a crucial investment in promoting a culture where the customer is valued and every effort is made to retain their loyalty. As with retail and commercial sectors, there are many contacts between clients and patients and healthcare and social care professionals every day, and most are satisfactory for both parties. However, consumer expectations are rising, attitudes are changing, and the paternalistic approaches still evident in some places are not universally welcomed by patients or clients. Complaints can sometimes be seen as an effect of relatively disempowered people who find a voice for themselves through the complaints system.

The way in which an organisation responds to concerns or complaints is a reflection of the value given to customer satisfaction and feedback. Whether the complaint is in relation to a product or a service; whether it is made formally or informally; in writing, in person or by telephone; what the complainant requires is:

- an acknowledgement of their dissatisfaction
- an investigation into the circumstances which gave rise to the complaint
- an explanation of the outcome of that investigation
- an apology as appropriate, and/or other means of redress
- an assurance of the actions being taken to prevent a similar occurrence in the future.

The initial contact between the complainant and the organisation's representative (who may or may not be involved in the complaint) is crucial, and highlights the importance of staff training to ensure that a defensive or discourteous attitude does not cause a further escalation of the situation. Poor complaints handling, however, is cited frequently by complainants as an additional cause of inconvenience or distress and can seriously compromise an organisation's ability to provide a speedy and satisfactory response.

'Common themes include undue delays in responding to complainants' concerns, poor communication with complainants or between NHS staff and inadequate record keeping. After their long experience of receiving and handling complaints, we would expect NHS bodies to have improved their complaint handling in these respects, but we encounter these failings time and again . . .'

Health Service Ombudsman for England. Annual Report 2003–4. London:
The Stationery Office, 2004.

Effective complaints management includes:

- easy access to an open and transparent procedure
- effective screening of the complaint to determine how best to handle it
- good communication with the complainant, which includes keeping them informed at every stage, and especially if there are delays in the response
- careful, well-documented investigation if that is appropriate
- careful documentation of all contacts with the complainant, including telephone conversations and emails
- documentation of all communication with professional or specialist advisers
- availability of conciliation at any point
- sensitivity to any special needs of the complainant
- a formal second stage which, if handled within the organisation, involves senior management not involved previously with the complaint; or externally, as with healthcare complaints in the UK and elsewhere, to ensure independence
- a third stage which may involve an Ombudsman.

Why do people complain?

In considering this issue, it is useful to look at the breakdown of complaints recorded by different healthcare organisations. NHS bodies are required to produce this information, which is publicly available, in quarterly reports to their Boards and to summarise this in an annual report. In most cases, complaints about clinical care tend to dominate, followed by those relating to staff attitudes and behaviour. Concerns about communication and information, as well as delays and cancellations of appointments or procedures, also account for a high proportion of complaints. Table 1.1 emphasises these themes, covering over 90,000 written complaints received in England about hospital and community health services, in 2004–05. Concealed in these figures is the fact that a complaint that is apparently about quality of treatment, or about delays or cancellations, may have been precipitated by the offhand attitude of a member of staff, or a failure to communicate adequately.

TABLE 1.1 Written complaints about Hospital and Community Health Services, by main subject of complaint, England, 2004–05.

Reason for complaint	Number of complaints	% of total
Total	90,066	100
All aspects of clinical treatment	32,496	36
Attitude of staff	11,497	13
Appointments, delay/cancellations (outpatient)	10,957	12
Communication/information to patients (written and oral)	8,419	9

Source: National Health Service Health and Social Care Information Centre. Workforce publication and dissemination: dataset KO41a. NHS Health and Social Care Information Centre, 2005.

These same areas of concern are highlighted in the first annual report produced by the Independent Complaints Advocacy Service in England for the year 2003–04.

'Consistently the top three issues people are bringing to ICAS are complaints about:
➡ aspects of their clinical treatment;
➡ the attitude of staff; and
➡ communication/information to patients.'

Independent Complaints Advocacy Service. *The First Year of ICAS: 1 September 2003 to 31 August 2004*. Department of Health, 2004.

These issues also dominated the complaints received by the Healthcare Commission during 2005–06, which had not been resolved at local level by the organisations concerned.

'The key themes raised were poor communication, the quality of how complaints are handled locally, clinical practice and the experience patients have of the care they receive.'

Healthcare Commission. *Putting patients first: a better experience of health and healthcare. Annual report 2005/2006*. Commission for Healthcare Audit and Inspection, 2006.

In considering the context in which complaints are made, it is useful to note the attitudes – explicit or implicit – that a health service, or any other public service body, has towards its patients, clients, service users or customers. This issue is considered within the National Audit Office report *Citizen redress: what citizens can do if things go wrong with public services* (2005): 'Citizens are not simply customers, but are also stakeholders who are entitled to fair and equal treatment.

Citizens are the ultimate proprietors of public services – and, as taxpayers, the vital funders.' This outlook reflects the ethos of the NHS Foundation Trusts, established in England under the *Health and Social Care (Community Health and Standards) Act 2003*. Foundation Trusts are constituted as independent public benefit corporations accountable directly to local people.

Traditionally, the users of health services have all been called 'patients'. Implicit in this word is both illness, and an imbalance of knowledge and power between the patient and any professional looking after them. At its best, this can lead to acknowledgement of the needs of the patient, a respect for them as people, and an empathy with their illness and any associated indignity and distress. At its worst it leads to paternalism, disempowerment, and a loss of autonomy. With changes in culture and expectations in society these less desirable characteristics are regarded as less acceptable than in previous times, and may easily be a source of complaint.

> 'The majority of patients are satisfied with the quality of the healthcare that they receive. However around 100,000 formal complaints are made each year by people who have concerns about the treatment that they have received.'
>
> Healthcare Commission. *Spotlight on complaints: a report on second-stage complaints about the NHS in England 2007*. Commission for Healthcare Audit and Inspection, 2007

The word 'patient' also fails to capture the fact that many users of health services are not ill at all: they may have some physical or mental disability (but that does not necessarily make them 'ill'), or be the parents of ill children, women receiving antenatal care, people attending for screening tests, or the healthy carers of ill adults. They rightly expect to be treated as autonomous individuals. A failure to recognise this provides fertile ground for complaints.

In contrast, some health service providers have developed a more sophisticated philosophy of care. For these, the aim is to work in partnership with the patient, carer or family. In this context the person requiring care is no longer regarded as a passive recipient but an autonomous individual contributing to and influencing their own treatment. This is reflected in the change of language, which may replace the generic use of the word 'patient' (reserving it for the acutely ill), with the terms 'client' or 'service user'. Unfortunately, the substitution of words alone does not automatically guarantee that staff attitudes and behaviours are always more appropriate.

The concept of a 'patient-led NHS' is behind the reforms introduced in the UK in recent years to ensure that people have greater participation and involvement in relation to all aspects of their healthcare.

'Every aspect of the new system is designed to create a service which is patient-led, where:

→ people have a far greater range of choices and of information and help to make choices

→ there are stronger standards and safeguards for patients

→ NHS organisations are better at understanding patients and their needs, use new and different methodologies to do so and have better and more regular sources of information about preferences and satisfaction.'

> Department of Health. *Creating a patient-led NHS: delivering the NHS Improvement Plan*. Department of Health, 2005.

However, a substantial change in culture is still needed in some parts of the Health Service to ensure that people are involved properly in decisions affecting the health and well-being of themselves or those for whom they have caring responsibilities. This lack of involvement in some areas is highlighted in the report by the National Audit Office, *Progress in implementing clinical governance in primary care: lessons for the new primary care trusts.*

'Patients and carers reported feeling excluded from aspects of the patient's care and that better information would help improve health outcomes.'

> National Audit Office. *Progress in implementing clinical governance in primary care: lessons for the new primary care trusts*. London: The Stationery Office, 2007.

Unsolicited advice about a patient's lifestyle can sometimes result in complaints if this is given in a manner that is perceived by the patient as arrogant, offensive or intimidating. While there may be good clinical reasons for broaching such subjects as obesity or sexual behaviour, the consumption of alcohol or the use of recreational drugs, the timing and manner of such communications is crucial. What may seem routine questioning to the clinician may be interpreted as unwarranted and intrusive by the patient.

'Patients put empathy, understanding and respect as the key to them receiving good quality of care. The most frequent complaints were that clinicians were often insensitive or lacked appropriate knowledge about the condition they were dealing with and therefore tended to dispense treatment rather than care.'

> National Audit Office. *Progress in implementing clinical governance in primary care: lessons for the new primary care trusts*. London: The Stationery Office, 2007.

People are much less tolerant if they are anxious, in pain, in a situation where they feel vulnerable and unsure of themselves, or do not understand what is happening to them or to a dependent relative or child – in short, where they are outside their 'comfort zone'. They are likely to appreciate friendly, courteous staff, together with well-designed waiting areas, where thought has been given to their needs; for example, easy access to toilet facilities, refreshments, and reading material while they wait for their appointments, whether in a clinic, health centre or hospital. Consideration should also be given to ensuring that verbal or written instructions are user-friendly rather than officious, and that they meet the needs of people experiencing the particular service for the first time. These different initiatives help to create a welcoming environment and, by improving the quality of people's experience from the outset, may reduce possible grounds for complaint.

> '. . . there is now a wealth of research evidence to show the positive impact that the environment can have on health and healing.'
>
> Department of Health and King's Fund. *Improving the patient experience – celebrating achievement: enhancing the healing environment programme. Best practice guidance.* Department of Health, 2006.

Complaints made by, or on behalf of, patients or service users

Some healthcare organisations ensure that there are staff available to meet and greet users of their services and to provide advice and information when required. In NHS organisations in England, the Patient Advice and Liaison Service (PALS) also helps those raising concerns on an informal basis, often making a swift response from healthcare staff possible and thereby reducing the potential for a formal complaint. Where issues cannot be addressed informally, the PALS will ensure that appropriate information is given about the complaints procedure and the support available from the Independent Complaints Advocacy Service (ICAS).

The needs of some patients, particularly those with chronic or long-term conditions, require an integrated approach between health and social care. Such partnerships are often particularly strong in relation to mental health and disability provision, as well as in the treatment and ongoing care of those with chronic and/or complex conditions. An implication of care delivered by more than one organisation is that when problems arise, a complaint may relate to two or more agencies or institutions. In such contexts a seamless response to complaints is essential. This important issue is considered in Chapter 2.

When a complaint is made by or on behalf of someone with a mental illness or learning disability, whether in relation to that aspect of their health or in connection with some other condition, it is important that the complaint receives as much consideration as those concerning anyone else. This also includes complaints made by patients compulsorily detained under the *Mental Health Act*, or its equivalents outside England. In England, Wales and Northern Ireland, the Mental Health Act Commission provides advice on monitoring and investigating complaints made by persons detained under the Act; in Scotland there is a memorandum of agreement between the Scottish Public Services Ombudsman and the Mental Welfare Commission for Scotland that defines the Ombudsman as having the primary role in relation to complaints.

Complaints may be made on behalf of the patient or service user not only by a relative, but sometimes by a friend, carer, advocate or other person nominated by the patient to act on their behalf. Under normal circumstances where a complaint is not made by the patient in their own right, the organisation handling the complaint should ensure that the patient or client has given consent for the complaint to be made on their behalf. Circumstances in which this might be impossible or inappropriate include situations where the patient is 'without capacity' either temporarily or permanently, or in relation to children. Also, where a complaint is made by the patient's carer it is important to establish some common ground, especially if there is to be an attempt at restoring or maintaining a clinical relationship with the health professional concerned. In such situations, where conciliation is being used, it is often appropriate at the outset of the process for the conciliator to facilitate an agreement between the parties that the best interests of the patient are paramount.

'Persons who may make complaints

8. (1) A complaint may be made by –

(a) a patient; or (b) any person who is affected by or likely to be affected by the action, omission or decision of the NHS body which is the subject of the complaint.

(2) A complaint may be made by a person (in these Regulations referred to as a representative) acting on behalf of a person mentioned in paragraph (1) in any case where that person –

(a) has died; (b) is a child; (c) is unable by reason of physical or mental incapacity to make the complaint himself; or (d) has requested the representative to act on his behalf.'

Statutory Instrument 2004 No. 1768. *The National Health Service (Complaints) Regulations 2004.* London: HMSO, 2004.

Complaints made in relation to, or by, children and young people

The rights of children and young people to receive appropriate healthcare should also include making every effort to address concerns or complaints that may arise in the course of their treatment. Where a parent or guardian makes a complaint on behalf of their child, the extent to which the child or young person is involved in the process will depend on their age and ability to participate.

Young people who are 'looked after', who wish to dispute decisions being made about their care by Social Services, have access to complaints procedures which are designed to be accessible and relevant to their age and abilities. Healthcare organisations treating children or young people could give similar thought to producing clear and child-friendly information which encourages them to raise concerns with staff. In some cases, involving the child or young person in a conciliation process may be extremely beneficial, particularly if the staff concerned do not feel that they are regarded as sufficiently independent of the situation to resolve the complaint themselves. Where the relationship between the child or young person and members of staff has deteriorated, or where the parents, carer or guardian do not accept the explanations provided by the staff, a conciliator may be well placed to try to restore the relationship in the best interests of the child.

Obstacles that prevent people complaining

Complainants sometimes voice concern that their subsequent contacts with the healthcare provider will suffer as a direct consequence of their complaint, or that they will be discriminated against in some way in the future. This is a powerful deterrent to complaining and emphasises the importance of reflecting a positive attitude towards complaints, in both the written information provided for complainants, and through the training of staff in their response to complaints.

> 'Effective communication and attitudes are marked out by:
>   ... assuring complainants that care and service provision will not be affected by the fact they have made a complaint and a clearly expressed expectation of staff that this will be the case.'
>
> Healthcare Commission. *Effective responses to complaints about health services – a protocol.* Healthcare Commission, 2006.

Barriers which may prevent people from complaining include:
- staff who are defensive or obstructive
- information that is poor or inaccessible
- long and protracted stages to the complaints process.

While any of the above may deter some would-be complainants, others will be-come not only frustrated but determined to hold the organisation to account, including their poor experience of the complaints process as an additional cause for complaint.

Organisations can ensure that they do not create such obstacles themselves by:

- training staff to respond appropriately to complaints
- providing support and information for complainants in an easily accessible form
- ensuring that lengthy and unnecessary delays in the complaints process are avoided.

> 'Patients who complain about the care or treatment they have received have a right to expect a prompt, open, constructive and honest response including an explanation and, if appropriate, an apology. You must not allow a patient's complaint to affect adversely the care or treatment you provide or arrange.'
>
> General Medical Council. *Good medical practice.* General Medical Council, 2006.
> Paragraph 31.

More detail on complaints procedures, and the place of conciliation within them, is given in the next chapter. However, the use of conciliation as an effective means of resolving a complaint should be an option available to anyone managing a complaints procedure, whether operating in the public or private sector.

CHAPTER 2

When and why to use conciliation

- The place of conciliation in relation to healthcare complaints procedures.
- Initial screening of complaints: key issues.
- Timescales.
- Adverse events or patient safety incidents.
- Managing complaints that cross organisational boundaries.
- Using conciliation to clarify the issues: the hidden agenda or unacknowledged motive underlying the complaint.
- Complaints about attitude and manner.
- Using conciliation to rebuild or restore relationships.
- Conciliation following termination of the doctor–patient relationship.
- 'Vexatious' complaints and persistent complainants.

The place of conciliation in relation to healthcare complaints procedures

Although healthcare complaints procedures may vary in detail, they are similar in overall objectives and purpose: that is, to resolve the complaint at the earliest possible opportunity at a local level. This is sometimes referred to as Local Resolution. If the attempts made at this stage are unsuccessful, most formal complaints procedures have a second stage. In the UK this stage is handled outside the organisation in which the complaint was made, to provide an independent view of the process to date and to assess if more could be done at a local level. In the NHS in England, the Healthcare Commission currently handles the second stage. In 2003–04, the Department of Health reported that the NHS had received 3,700 requests for independent review of NHS complaints which had not been resolved by the health providers concerned.

Many countries, including the UK, also have a third stage, where referral may be made to an Ombudsman. As well as providing the ultimate review of a complaint and the manner in which it has been handled, an Ombudsman can also take an overview of complaints that cross the boundaries of agencies or government departments, ensuring an integrated approach. Up-to-date information in relation to the complaints procedures in different countries is accessed most easily via the relevant governmental or departmental websites, as well as via professional associations, many of which provide useful information, support and guidance.

In England, there is a significant requirement contained in the NHS complaints procedure (which came into force on 30 July 2004) that all NHS bodies (excluding Foundation Trusts) now have a legal obligation to ensure that conciliation and mediation services are available. However, whether such a requirement is mandatory or not, the fact that conciliation is a cost-effective and efficient means of complaints resolution should be reason enough for it to be considered. Indeed, conciliation has been an important tool in relation to the resolution of primary care complaints since its inclusion in the 1996 complaints procedure, but it is not yet used widely in secondary care. In some areas of England conciliation services are made available directly to both primary and secondary care providers by primary care trusts to assist in the local resolution process. Conciliation and mediation are also of significance in relation to the complaints procedures used in Scotland, Wales and Northern Ireland.

The emphasis in the UK and elsewhere is on improving the local response to complaints through a range of measures, including the use of conciliation. If a complainant remains dissatisfied with the outcome of the local resolution procedure and requests an independent review of the complaint, conciliation may be suggested (particularly if it has not already been attempted), and the complaint referred back to the healthcare provider. Clearly there will be circumstances where conciliation may not be possible, in which case this needs to be carefully documented in the complaints file.

'The [complaints] system must be kept as simple as possible. It must follow a well-established principle in handling complaints, that a complaint is best resolved as close as possible to the time and place it arose.'

Bristol Royal Infirmary Inquiry. *Learning from Bristol: the report of the public inquiry into children's heart surgery at the Bristol Royal Infirmary 1984–1995: final report.* (Command Paper: Cm 5207). Bristol Royal Infirmary Inquiry, July 2001.

Good complaints handling can help to mitigate some of the effects of the complaint in terms of restoring the complainant's relationship with the organisation. Equally, the initial problems can be compounded if the complaint is not well managed. Where the complainant threatens legal proceedings or makes contact in the first instance via a solicitor, it should not be assumed automatically that nothing short of litigation will suffice. At this stage it is important to gain a clear understanding of what the complainant hopes to achieve, and this may be explored most effectively through the conciliation process. Importantly, conciliation can also be used early in the complaints process, as discussed below.

Initial screening of complaints: key issues

Conciliation is likely to be most effective the earlier it is used in the complaints process. It is therefore advisable for the member of staff investigating the complaint, or the complaints manager, to consider this alongside the other issues which need to be determined during the initial screening of the complaint. For instance, whether or not conciliation is ultimately used, it is essential to establish if there is/are:

- a *prima facie* case of clinical negligence
- any indication of a criminal or unlawful activity
- allegations of abuse
- unprofessional conduct, including impropriety, ill treatment or neglect
- a need for any kind of serious incident review.

> '*Prima facie* evidence of negligence should not delay a full explanation of events and, if appropriate, an apology: an apology is not an admission of liability.'
>
> Department of Health. *Guidance to support implementation of the National Health Service (Complaints) Regulations.* Department of Health, 2004. Paragraph 3.15.

To ensure that complaints are dealt with in the most appropriate and effective manner, it is also helpful to determine

- whether a mistake has been made
- if there is an obvious misunderstanding
- whether there has been a system failure
- whether the complaint is vexatious.

Following acknowledgement of a letter of complaint, the complaints manager must decide on the most appropriate way to proceed and conciliation may be considered and offered at this stage. If, however, a full written response is made in the first instance, the complainant should be given the opportunity of a meeting to discuss any queries or remaining concerns.

One of the ways in which complainants may signal their dissatisfaction with the complaints handling process is illustrated by the volume of correspondence between the parties that may have been generated prior to the first conciliation meeting. In such cases there may have been no offer to meet with the complainant in the belief that the issues could be addressed solely in writing. Unfortunately, this sometimes generates a series of letters, some of which may illustrate misunderstandings in relation to the original issues by either party, as well as additional complaints or a reworking of earlier ones.

Complaints are not just made about individual healthcare staff: they may be made in relation to the organisation's procedures, or administrative failures, when these give rise to inconvenience or distress to patients. In such cases the response may be made on behalf of the organisation, and will not necessarily involve, or name, particular individuals other than the manager making the response. This does not, however, obviate the need to offer face-to-face meetings.

'Many complainants undoubtedly value the opportunity of a face to face meeting. One ICAS bureau examined this issue in more detail, in relation to one Trust. They found that only one percent of their clients expressed satisfaction with the outcome following receipt of the written letter only. However, where this was followed by a face to face meeting 83 per cent of clients considered that their complaint was at least partially resolved.'

Phelps E, Williams A. *The pain of complaining: CAB ICAS evidence of the NHS complaints procedure.* Citizens Advice Bureau, 2005. Paragraph 3.31.

Sometimes conciliators are asked to chair meetings between the complainant and the staff against whom the complaint has been made. This type of request may come from a healthcare organisation as part of the complaints handling process. It may be thought that the conciliator will enable the parties to discuss the issues in a more constructive way than might otherwise be the case.

The disadvantage of this approach is that the conciliator may have little or no opportunity to speak with the parties prior to the meeting and will have to rely solely on the documentation relating to the complaint for information about the issues. While it is not impossible for such a situation to have a successful outcome, it is advisable for the conciliator to meet separately with each of the parties beforehand so that any joint meeting is proposed only as an integral part of the conciliation process. This is covered in more detail in Chapter 4.

Timescales

A concern sometimes expressed by complaints staff who are unfamiliar with the conciliation process is that its use will impact on their ability to provide a response to the complaint within the required time frame. The NHS complaints procedure stipulates that a response to a complaint must be made within 25 working days from the receipt of the complaint. However, there is also recognition that this will not always be possible.

'. . . the response must be sent to the complainant within 25 working days beginning on the date on which the complaint was made, unless the complainant agrees to a longer period in which case the response may be sent within that longer period.'

> Statutory Instrument 2006 No. 2084. *The National Health Service (Complaints) Amendment Regulations 2006.* London: HMSO, 2006.
> Regulation 13 (3) (amended).

The 25-day target introduced in 2006 replaces the previous time limit of 20 working days. This was seen by some as too short a period for ensuring that all appropriate means were used when addressing a complaint.

'Yet it may well prove difficult if not impossible to carry out these additional measures adequately within the 20 day time limit. ICAS advisers report that frequently the consequence is that no face-to-face meetings are held, the complainant remains dissatisfied and so decides to refer the complaints on to the already overstretched Healthcare Commission.'

> Phelps E, Williams A. *The pain of complaining: CAB ICAS evidence of the NHS complaints procedure.* Citizens Advice Bureau, 2005.
> Paragraph 3.31.

Formerly, provision was made within the complaints regulations for a response to be made to the complainant 'as soon as reasonably practicable' on those occasions when it was not considered possible to meet the 20-day limit. The 2006 amendment requires that any extension to the 25-day limit is made only with express consent from the complainant. This is highlighted in the guidance accompanying the amendment.

'No pressure must be placed upon the complainant to agree the extension, but the complaints manager may, in suitable cases, consider it appropriate to explain that a comprehensive response may not be possible to achieve within twenty five days. The key considerations are whether an extension will genuinely enable local resolution of a complaint to be achieved, and that the complainant is involved in the discussion.'

Department of Health. *Supporting staff, improving services – guidance to support implementation of the National Health Service (Complaints) Amendment Regulations (SI 2006 No. 2084).* Department of Health, 2006.

It should be recognised that where complex issues are involved, conciliation can take time and should not be restricted by rigid adherence to arbitrary timescales, if this risks compromising the quality of the process. The desire to comply with the required timescales should be balanced against the need to provide a comprehensive response to the complainant that addresses all aspects of the complaint. However, the conciliator will wish to ensure that the momentum of the process is maintained while recognising that the complainant's health or other circumstances may require a flexible approach.

There is wide variation in the time the conciliation process can take. Occasionally, the conciliator may be able to facilitate resolution through telephone contact alone without the need for a meeting with either party. More commonly, the process will proceed at a pace dictated by the availability of the parties to attend the meetings. While the complainant may be restricted as a result of ill health or other circumstances, it is not helpful to the process if the healthcare staff themselves cause lengthy delays between meetings, since this can be interpreted by the complainant as a lack of interest or commitment to resolving the issues.

Under the NHS complaints procedure, complaints should be made within six months of the date on which the incident or circumstances occurred which gave rise to the complaint. However, provision for waiving this time limit is permitted in certain cases, particularly where the delay is a direct consequence of the ill health or distress suffered by the complainant. As with any other complaint, consideration should be given to the use of conciliation in these circumstances.

Conciliation should not be thought of only when all else fails. Sometimes this is unavoidable, but there are certain situations where the potential value of independent conciliation at an early opportunity should be considered. For instance, if the complaint follows an adverse incident or involves allegations of inappropriate clinical treatment, misdiagnosis or perceived negligence, conciliation may provide an important means of facilitating appropriate contact between the complainant and staff. The issues can then be addressed in a supportive environment. These may include explanations, expressions of regret, apology or acknowledgement of the complainant's distress or the outcome of a serious incident review or investigation, together with any offers of redress or proposed actions to avoid a recurrence of a similar situation in the future.

Adverse events or patient safety incidents

Occasionally patients are harmed, or die, as a direct consequence of receiving treatment, or from some other cause, while in the care of health professionals. This also includes those situations where all the correct procedures have been followed, and where the adverse outcome may have been a recognised risk or complication which had been highlighted previously. Complaints, or allegations of negligence, are sometimes made in such circumstances. Whatever the cause of the incident, the distress experienced by the patient and their family can be greatly exacerbated if they are met with a defensive reaction, little information, or a perceived lack of any real support.

Research carried out in a number of different countries, including the UK, Australia, New Zealand, Canada and the USA, has shown that people are far less likely to complain or resort to litigation if the details of medical errors or other adverse events are acknowledged openly. In the UK, the National Patient Safety Agency promotes the importance of effective communication and support for both patients and carers.

'Many patients and/or their carers will often only make a litigation claim when they have not received any information or apology from the healthcare teams or organisations following the incident.'

National Patient Safety Agency. *Being open: communicating patient safety incidents with patients and their carers.* (Safer Practice Notice 10). NPSA, 2005.

In Australia, the Australian Council for Safety and Quality in Healthcare provides detailed guidance for use in these circumstances in *Open Disclosure Standard: a national standard for open communication in public and private hospitals, following an adverse event in health care* (2003).

'The Standard aims to promote a clear and consistent approach by hospitals (and other organisations where appropriate) to open communication with patients and their nominated support person following an adverse event. This includes a discussion about what has happened, why it happened and what is being done to prevent it from happening again. It also aims to provide guidance on minimising the risk of recurrence of an adverse event through the use of information to generate systems improvement and promotion of a culture that focuses on health care safety.'

Australian Council for Safety and Quality in Health Care. *Open Disclosure Standard: a national standard for open communication in public and private hospitals, following an adverse event in health care.* Commonwealth of Australia, 2003.

It is important to bear in mind that an apology is not an admission of liability and that complaints which escalate, and occasionally result in litigation, may not have done so if the complainant had been met with a more open, honest and supportive approach.

Where the complaint has been made in relation to the death of a relative the involvement of an independent conciliator can be particularly helpful. Complaints arising from the death of a patient can be particularly distressing for staff too, and it is sometimes easier for all parties concerned to talk to an impartial conciliator. In some cases the death may have been inevitable despite any possible interventions, but that may not be how the bereaved complainant views it. There can be a number of reasons for this.

- People experiencing grief are not always receptive to explanations, or capable of appreciating them when they are coping with extreme loss.
- If the death was unexpected or the result of a late or mistaken diagnosis, the desire to blame someone may be a displacement for the natural feelings of anger and powerlessness.
- The way in which relatives are treated by staff immediately before or after the death may affect the way they view any explanations that follow.
- The complainant may have raised concerns about the deceased person's treatment or diagnosis which the relatives feel were ignored; the complaint may be, therefore, the culmination of a series of incidents which have alienated the complainant over a period of time.

This highlights the crucial importance of ongoing engagement between the clinical team and relatives or carers.

> 'You must be considerate to relatives, carers, partners and others close to the patient, and be sensitive and responsive in providing information and support, including after a patient has died.'
>
> General Medical Council. *Good medical practice*. General Medical Council, 2006.
> Paragraph 29.

Delays in responding to a complaint should be minimised wherever possible. Where a complaint relates to a deceased person, for example, delays should not occur automatically because the circumstances of the death involve notifying the Coroner's Office or because an inquest may be necessary.

> 'The fact that a death has been referred to the Coroner's Office does not mean that all investigations into a complaint need to be suspended. It is important

for NHS bodies to consult the Coroner's Office and, where appropriate, initiate proper investigations.'

Department of Health. *Guidance to support implementation of the National Health Service (Complaints) Regulations.* Department of Health, 2004.
Paragraph 2.7.

Managing complaints that cross organisational boundaries

Integrated complaints procedures can ensure that complaints that cross organisational boundaries are managed effectively. It is not uncommon for complaints to relate to more than one service or governmental department. Where possible, therefore, there should be a single point of entry to a process which can ensure that all aspects of the complaint are handled appropriately without subjecting the complainant to the lengthy and potentially frustrating task of accessing two different sets of procedures. This is particularly important in relation to health and social care.

'Sometimes a complaint crosses over boundaries between a local authority and the NHS. Where this happens, people who use services should not have to worry about who to approach with complaints about different aspects of the service that they receive. Instead, the complaint can be made in its entirety to any one of the bodies involved.'

Department of Health. *Learning from complaints: social services complaints procedure for adults.* Department of Health, 2006.

From 1 September 2006, amendments to the 2004 NHS complaints regulations were introduced and a consequence of this was to align the NHS complaints procedures more closely with the Social Care complaints procedures. In situations where a complaint relates to both Health and Social Care, each agency is required to address the aspects of the complaint that relate specifically to their own organisation, and to handle these in accordance with their own complaints procedures. In order to mitigate the difficulties that separate procedures can cause, a co-ordinated response is required to ensure continuity and consistency.

'Where complaints are about both NHS and Local Authority Services, the new regulation 3A provides that, where the complainant so wishes, the organisations involved must co-operate to deal with the part of the complaint that relates to them and provide a co-ordinated response to the complaint.'

Department of Health. *Supporting staff, improving services – guidance to support implementation of the National Health Service (Complaints) Amendment Regulations (SI 2006 No. 2084).* Department of Health, 2006.

In the UK, reform of government department complaints procedures is recognised as an important component in improving the quality of complaints handling and therefore of public service delivery. This extends to the procedures relating to the public sector Ombudsmen and the aim of any such reform is to provide greater flexibility both to enable cross-departmental complaints to be handled from a single point of entry, and also to extend the range of alternative complaints resolution methods, including mediation or conciliation where these are considered more appropriate than a formal investigation.

'There are a number of methods of resolution that do not require a full investigation that can be applied, including:
→ the provision of an apology or explanation
→ conciliation and mediation
→ a reassessment of the service user's needs
→ practical action specific to the particular complainant
→ an assurance that the local authority will monitor the effectiveness of its remedy; and
→ consideration of the need for a financial payment.'

Department of Health. Learning from complaints: social services complaints procedure for adults. Department of Health, 2006. Paragraph 6.1.4.

The reform of Social Services complaints procedures in England is now enshrined in the *Health and Social Care (Community Health and Standards) Act 2003*, for which there is statutory guidance (Statutory Instrument 2006 No. 1681. *The Local Authority Social Services Complaints (England) Regulations 2006*). The guidance, *Learning from complaints* highlights the value of conciliation and mediation in relation to the resolution of complaints as part of the local resolution procedure, and emphasises some key issues relating to these forms of dispute resolution.

'The key to effective mediation is to:
→ offer it as early as possible before positions become entrenched
→ promote an understanding of the benefits of mediation and conciliation among staff who may find themselves the subject of complaint; and
→ be clear that this is a confidential process.'

Department of Health. Learning from complaints: social services complaints procedure for adults. Department of Health, 2006. Paragraph 6.2.4.

Using conciliation to clarify the issues: the hidden agenda or unacknowledged motive underlying the complaint

Complaints staff are sometimes presented with situations where it is not clear what the complainant is hoping to achieve by making the complaint. This may be because the complainant makes generalised or non-specific references to their treatment or care. In other situations the complainant focuses on what seems to be a straightforward issue but continues to express dissatisfaction despite receiving a comprehensive response. Conciliation can provide a valuable means of enabling healthcare staff to understand the reasons that prompted the complaint when these are not self-evident.

Clinicians will be familiar with those patients who, while expressing concern about a minor physical ailment, do not reveal immediately the underlying reason for their attendance at the surgery or clinic. If there are no clues to the contrary, the patient may be treated for the presenting problem only to return again until it becomes apparent that there is an unspoken issue that is the real cause for their presence.

Sometimes the patient is unaware that there is a connection between their physical symptoms and the fact that they have experienced a life-changing event like losing their job or retiring, or have suffered bereavement or have separated from a partner. At other times they feel they need a concrete, physical symptom as a way of opening the dialogue with their practitioner before explaining what is really troubling them.

Likewise, experienced conciliators become adept in recognising that in some situations the ability to bring about the resolution of a complaint will be linked closely to achieving an understanding and a recognition of the hidden agenda, which may not be apparent to the complainant and may not be linked consciously in their mind as a motivating factor for making the complaint.

Complaints about attitude and manner

Health professionals sometimes underestimate the value of giving honest responses to complainants, whether it be in relation to clinical mistakes or medication errors, the way in which they have carried out a particular procedure, or where their behaviour towards patients has provoked complaints in relation to their attitude and manner.

Patients are much more ready to accept apologies when a practitioner acknowledges that their brusque or offhand manner has caused offence, and admits that they were tired or under pressure that day, or had to deal with a difficult clinical emergency or whatever may have been the perceived cause, once they have had time to reflect on it. Equally, if there is no excuse or mitigating circumstance they need to acknowledge that they regret the lapse, and the distress, anxiety or irritation felt by the patient.

Where complaints relate to the manner or behaviour of the practitioner carrying out a particular procedure or treatment, conciliation may highlight a number of key issues the practitioner has not considered before:

- the procedure may be routine to the practitioner but distressing or uncomfortable for the patient
- the patient's tolerance or experience of the procedure will be influenced by the practitioner's manner both prior to, during and after the procedure
- if the patient feels that the process, including explanations and information about the procedure, has been rushed, it may have a negative effect on their relationship with the practitioner
- a common response from the practitioner to a complaint in such a situation may be '. . . but I didn't do anything differently. That's how I behave with all my patients.'

Through conciliation, the practitioner may appreciate that patients' circumstances and levels of anxiety and vulnerability can differ markedly, and that some may need greater reassurance, empathy and explanation than others.

> 'Patients say that the quality of the patient experience is determined primarily by quality of interpersonal care they receive, with less emphasis on technical aspects of care.'
>
> National Audit Office. *Progress in implementing clinical governance in primary care: lessons for the new primary care trusts.* London: The Stationery Office, 2007.

Using conciliation to rebuild or restore relationships

There are occasions when practitioners request conciliation as a means of preserving a relationship, with either a patient or a carer, which they feel is deteriorating to the point where they will be obliged to withdraw from providing further healthcare themselves to the individuals concerned. Difficulties with the doctor–patient or doctor–carer relationship are more likely to arise when ongoing healthcare is being provided as, for example, in general practice, where there may be frequent contacts between the individuals concerned. Secondary care specialists who provide treatment and care over a long period of time in relation to either physical or mental disorders may also experience similar problems.

'Patients in poor health and those with a disability were consistently more likely to report negative experiences than those in good health and without a disability.'

Healthcare Commission. *Variations in the experiences of patients using the NHS services in England: analysis of the Healthcare Commission's 2004/2005 surveys of patients.* Commission for Healthcare Audit and Inspection, 2006.

Conciliation can be valuable in enabling the parties concerned to identify the reasons for the deterioration in their relationship. Carers, for example, may feel that healthcare staff do not involve them sufficiently in decisions regarding the patient, or value their input. Conversely, they may not appreciate the patient's right to restrict the information that staff are empowered to share. Where a child or person without capacity is concerned, carers may disagree with the treatment proposed and find themselves in direct opposition to healthcare staff.

The primary purpose of conciliation in such circumstances is to restore the relationship by encouraging both parties to recognise that they have a common objective, which is the health of the individual concerned. Each needs to reflect on the situation from the other's perspective, acknowledging misunderstandings where they have occurred and agreeing actions which will address the areas that have the greatest potential for causing concern or future conflict. In situations such as these, the demands of caring cannot be over-emphasised and where a carer has a pivotal role in relation to the patient, their needs require ongoing consideration, whether or not a formal assessment is warranted.

Conciliation can also be used where there has been a deterioration or breakdown of inter-staff relationships. If these are not addressed there can be deleterious consequences for service delivery and, ultimately, clinical care. This particular use of conciliation is discussed more fully in Chapter 5.

'Conciliation is often useful in resolving difficulties arising from a breakdown of a relationship, for example between a clinician and a patient.'

Scottish Executive, Health Department. *Guidance for NHS complaints: hospital and community health services.* Scottish Executive, Health Department, 2005.

Conciliation following termination of the doctor–patient relationship

Conciliators may be involved in relation to complaints that arise in primary care following the formal removal of a patient from a medical or dental practitioner's care. Where a patient has left a practice, either under their own volition or because they have been removed formally from that practice's list, it is unlikely that the restoration of the relationship is regarded by the parties concerned as a likely or desirable outcome for the conciliation process. The patient who has left voluntarily may have complained about an incident or series of incidents that precipitated their decision to leave, and wish for specific responses to the issues they have raised. Where a patient has been formally removed from the practice's list they may wish to complain about the process by which this happened or to dispute the circumstances given to support this action.

> '. . . ending of doctor–patient relationships may . . . be a very negative experience that is profoundly disrupting, producing new problems rather than resolving old ones. For patients, the consequences of the "lock-out" by GPs may be far more serious than the consequences of the "walk-out" by patients.'
>
> Stokes T, Dixon-Woods M, McKinley RK. Ending the doctor–patient relationship in general practice: a proposed model. *Family Practice*. 2004; 21: 507–14.

It should be noted that from 1 March 2004, changes were introduced in relation to the removal of patients from general practitioners' lists as a result of the *NHS (General Medical Services Contracts) Regulations 2004*. Key points relating to this are as follows.

- It must be recorded in writing that the patient has been warned that this might happen.
- The warning must be given in the 12 months preceding the removal.
- A reason for the removal must be given.

The Annual Report of the Parliamentary and Health Service Ombudsman 2005–06 refers to a small number of complaints which were made after the regulations came into force, and shows that the process outlined above was not always followed.

Similar situations can also arise in secondary care where a clinician may feel that they can no longer maintain a therapeutic relationship with a patient and that transferring the patient's ongoing care to another practitioner will be beneficial for all concerned. Despite recognising that their relationship with the clinician has deteriorated, the patient may complain about the manner in which they were informed of the transfer of their care, or dispute the reasons given for this. Conciliation in these cases can further the understanding of both parties with regard to the circumstances that precipitated the action resulting in the termination of the doctor–patient relationship, and can have the effect of providing closure for both the patient and the practitioner.

> 'Given the impact on patients, there is a need to recognize the phenomenon of broken-down relationships in general practice and for them to be dealt

with in ways that are sensitive to the needs of both parties ... There is a need to evaluate the role and effects of mediation-type interventions on fragile relationships in general practice.'

Stokes T, Dixon-Woods M, McKinley RK. Ending the doctor–patient relationship in general practice: a proposed model. *Family Practice*. 2004; 21: 507–14.

'Vexatious' complaints and persistent complainants

It is important to identify any vexatious complaints so that they can be dealt with appropriately, and to recognise that for various reasons some complainants may be described as 'vexatious' or 'persistent'. The unreasonable behaviours commonly defined as 'vexatious' include the following:

- bombarding the complaints department with telephone calls, emails, faxes and reams of written material which may raise other issues apart from those contained in the original complaint (in these circumstances, it is important that genuine issues are not overlooked)
- persistent contact with the complaints department (sometimes continuing when all aspects of the complaints procedure have been exhausted)
- refusal to accept explanations, even when these relate to incontrovertible facts supported by documentary evidence
- verbal abuse or use of aggressive language
- threats of physical violence (or actual violence).

'At all times NHS staff should treat patients, carers and visitors politely and with respect. However, violence, racial, sexual or verbal harassment should not be tolerated. Neither will NHS staff be expected to tolerate language that is of a personal, abusive or threatening nature.'

Department of Health. *Guidance to support implementation of the National Health Service (Complaints) Regulations*. Department of Health, 2004. Paragraph 3.4.

While conciliation can have a place in relation to some seemingly vexatious complaints, careful consideration needs to be given to what can be achieved realistically. The approach may most usefully be focused on trying to discover what is driving the behaviour, and negotiating an agreed way forward in relation to the key issues, rather than attempting to address what may be a huge number of illogical, trivial or apparently frivolous complaints. The risks of suggesting conciliation in such a situation need to be carefully assessed, not least because of the possibility that the process itself may merely generate further complaints, including ones focused on the conciliator's own behaviour. For this reason it may be prudent, with the complainant's consent, to ensure the presence of an independent third party at any conciliation meeting in such circumstances. Clinical advice may also prove extremely valuable when deciding on an appropriate course of action.

> 'If you label a complaint as vexatious from the start then it will never be anything else. This may get in the way of your ability to understand why the complainant is so persistent, and may only prolong the time it takes to reach a conclusion.'
>
> Department of Health. *Handling complaints in the NHS – good practice toolkit for local resolution.* Department of Health, 2005.
> http://www.dh.gov.uk/en/Publicationsandstatistics/Publications/
> PublicationsPolicyAndGuidance/Browsable/DH_5133265

Healthcare organisations will inevitably receive a number of such complaints and should ensure that staff have the necessary training and support to deal with these, as well as access to the appropriate organisational policies, procedures and guidance. Where persistent contact amounts to harassment of staff, appropriate security management measures need be taken to protect them. However, every effort should be made to ensure that genuine issues are not missed among what may be a welter of seemingly inconsequential matter.

> 'Labelling people as persistent, habitual or vexatious complainants should be the weapon of last resort.'
>
> Department of Health. *Handling complaints in the NHS – good practice toolkit for local resolution.* Department of Health, 2005.
> http://www.dh.gov.uk/en/Publicationsandstatistics/Publications/
> PublicationsPolicyAndGuidance/Browsable/DH_5133265

CHAPTER 3

How to set up conciliation

- ➥ Key issues.
- ➥ Appointing a conciliator.
- ➥ Observing confidentiality.
- ➥ Breaching confidentiality.
- ➥ Access to health records and complaints documentation.
- ➥ Consideration of special needs.
- ➥ Clinical advice and expert reports.
- ➥ Telephone contact.
- ➥ Delays and postponements.
- ➥ Location of conciliation meetings.
- ➥ Meetings held in the complainant's home.
- ➥ Meetings held in health service premises or other locations.
- ➥ Support for complainants.
- ➥ Support for staff.
- ➥ Support for conciliators.

Key issues

Once conciliation has been identified as a potential means of resolving the complaint, there are a number of issues which need to be considered. Healthcare organisations will find that the process can be managed more effectively and speedily if staff have access to, and an understanding of, practical guidance relating to the conciliation process. This will need to cover the issues highlighted below ensuring reference is also made where applicable to any relevant national or locally agreed policies or procedures.

▶ Ensure that the parties involved in the complaint are provided with information explaining the conciliation process, and that someone who understands the process is available to answer any questions.

▶ Obtain the parties' written agreement to participate in the process.

▶ Identify an appropriate conciliator, taking into account any preference the complainant might express for someone of their own gender.

▶ Establish that no conflict of interest exists between the conciliator and the parties involved with the complaint.

▶ Identify whether the complainant will require advocacy, interpreting or signing services or other provision as a result of disability, physical or psychological condition.

▶ Identify an appropriate venue.

▶ Ensure the complaints file is comprehensive and includes outcomes of any investigations or reviews where relevant.

▶ If appropriate, gain the complainant's consent for the conciliator to have access to such parts of their health records as relate solely to the complaint.

▶ Provide any additional factual background information which may be helpful to the conciliator, for example, about the service area concerned.

▶ Identify an appropriate clinical adviser or expert if required.

▶ Identify staff support for the person(s) against whom the complaint has been made.

▶ Ensure the availability of the person empowered by the organisation to take part in negotiating any form of redress, or to undertake appropriate action to prevent a recurrence of the issues relating to the complaint.

Information about the conciliation process should be in a format appropriate to the complainant's needs. It is therefore important to make provision for:
▶ enlarged font size for written material
▶ Braille
▶ audio recordings if appropriate
▶ translations into the languages relevant to local populations
▶ access to interpreting and signing services
▶ material suitable for young people or those with a learning difficulty or disability.

Appointing a conciliator

In some areas in the UK, conciliation services are provided by a lead healthcare organisation which maintains the services on behalf of a number of primary and secondary care providers. In England, primary care trusts may, for example, be directly involved or may provide total or partial funding together with partner agencies. It is common practice for NHS organisations, or commissioning bodies acting on their behalf, to appoint conciliators on either a case-by-case or annual basis. Private providers of conciliation services may also be used.

Staff from healthcare organisations with little or no experience of using conciliation, especially those in the secondary care sector, will need to assess the provision available locally and determine how this can best meet their needs. They may also benefit from providing input to any local training or professional development programmes organised for conciliators, since they can use this opportunity to highlight any special requirements relevant to their own services.

> '10.-(1) Every Health Authority shall appoint one or more persons to be known as conciliators for a period, to be agreed between the Authority and any conciliator, of not more than one year (but without prejudice to any re-appointment), to conduct the process of conciliation . . .'
>
> Secretary of State. *Directions to health authorities on dealing with complaints about family health services practitioners and providers of personal medical services National Health Service, England and Wales, in exercise of powers conferred on him by section 17 of the National Health Service Act 1977(a), and sections 9(2) of the National Health Service (Primary Care) Act 1997(b).* Department of Health, 1998.

The 1998 guidance relating to the appointment of conciliators for use in primary care in England also states that health professionals should not undertake this role.

> 'A person who is or has been a registered medical practitioner, a registered dental practitioner, a registered optician, registered pharmacist, member of a supplementary profession or a person who is or has been included in the register maintained by the United Kingdom Central Council for Nursing, Midwifery and Health Visiting under section 7 of the Nurses, Midwives and Health Visitors Act 1997(a) shall not be appointed as a conciliator.'
>
> Department of Health. *Directions to health authorities on dealing with complaints about family health services practitioners and providers of personal medical services.* Department of Health, 1998.

The Community Health Services Complaints Procedure in Scotland specifically excludes 'serving members of Local Health Councils' from posts as lay conciliators to avoid any potential conflicts of interest and also recommends that this role should not be fulfilled by 'those engaged in advocacy'.

In New South Wales, Australia, conciliators used by the Health Conciliation

Registry are drawn from a wide range of professional backgrounds, including healthcare.

> 'There is currently a panel of 37 conciliators with extensive training in dispute resolution, conciliation and conflict resolution. Most of these have a legal background, while others come from the fields of medicine, nursing, social sciences, education and administration.'
>
> Parliament of New South Wales, Committee on the Health Care Complaints Commission. *Discussion paper on the health conciliation registry. Report No. 4.* Committee on the Health Care Complaints Commission, 2004.

Healthcare organisations will need to satisfy themselves that the appropriate recruitment and selection procedures have been followed, including consideration of equality and diversity issues. Depending on the local governance arrangements with the healthcare providers, the conciliators may be appointed on a case-by-case, yearly or other basis. Contracts between the conciliator and the healthcare organisation are essential and should cover terms and conditions of engagement, whether the conciliator is remunerated, or acts in a voluntary capacity. Key issues for consideration will include:

- indemnity cover for conciliators
- confidentiality
- relevant occupational health requirements
- disclosure of criminal offences where relevant
- adherence to the organisation's policies or procedures where applicable
- expenses.

Depending on the issues involved in the complaint, consideration may need to be given not only to the experience of the conciliator but also to their gender and understanding of particular ethnic issues, since the cultural and religious background of the complainant may have significant implications. Knowledge of the individual conciliators who may be appointed with regard to a particular complaint is important, since selecting the right person can be key to engaging the parties and enhancing the likelihood of a successful resolution of the complaint. It is also important to establish whether there is any conflict of interest which could compromise the independence or integrity of the conciliation process; for instance, if the complaint concerns a medical or dental or other practitioner who also treats the conciliator.

Those who are unfamiliar with the competencies or qualities required for conciliation may find it helpful to note that experienced conciliators should have:

- knowledge of the agreed model used locally in relation to healthcare complaints

- good listening skills
- the ability to work with people from widely differing backgrounds
- awareness of ethnic and cultural issues, special needs, and disabilities.

Conciliators should also be able to:
- facilitate neutrally and impartially
- paraphrase and summarise complex issues
- respond appropriately to unexpected events or situations, including interruptions, emotional outbursts and signs of distress.

Observing confidentiality

Conciliators observe the same requirements for absolute confidentiality in relation to patient information as other professionals involved in handling personal data. For example, in England, conciliators will need to comply with the guidance given in *Confidentiality – The NHS Code of Practice* (2003). Contracts and terms of engagement, or appointments which are made on either a case-by-case basis or sometimes (as in the NHS) annually, to individuals providing a conciliation service, should include explicit reference to confidentiality, highlighting the key issues relating to this.

Confidentiality is fundamental to the conciliation process. The conciliator does not divulge the content of the private discussions held with the individual parties without their explicit consent. It is essential that the conciliator should be able to inspire trust so that the participants feel encouraged to talk freely in what can be regarded as a 'protected' environment. This is key to ensuring that the parties gain a mutual understanding of each other's situation, either through the conciliator as intermediary, passing on the agreed information, or where the conciliator acts as facilitator, for example, when the parties involved come together for a joint meeting.

Although all healthcare staff involved in complaints handling must observe the strict code of confidentiality governing patient identifiable information, and must ensure that health records and complaints information are held separately, they are able to share and exchange information with others involved in the investigation or in the preparation of a response to the complainant. All aspects of the investigation, including the interviews with staff and, where appropriate, with the complainant, detailing the questions and answers covered, are recorded and filed.

This is where conciliation differs significantly from other aspects of the complaints procedure. The confidential nature of the process precludes any form of information sharing between the conciliator and complaints handling staff beyond the dates and times of meetings, and the final outcome to confirm whether or not the complaint has been resolved. Resolution of the complaint may have been based on agreement that certain actions will be undertaken and with the consent of the parties concerned such outcomes can be communicated by the conciliator.

At this point it is important to highlight the distinction between what will be communicated to appropriate staff within the healthcare organisation in which the complaint originated (for example, a general practice or provider Trust), and the healthcare organisation (for example, a primary care trust or health authority), which may have responsibility for making conciliation services available. Clearly those staff empowered to take responsibility for negotiating a way forward which may help to resolve the complaint will share the action plan within their own organisation, but neither they nor the conciliator will pass on details about the conciliation process itself to the organisation providing the conciliation services, beyond confirming whether conciliation has or has not resulted in a resolution of the complaint.

Care should be taken when confidential information is passed on to the conciliator by the staff involved in handling the complaint. If referring to a complaint via email, a reference number should be used rather than the name of either party. It is also good practice to avoid committing any detailed information to an email. Difficulties can arise when passing on messages to the parties if they are not available to speak directly by telephone, but confidential information should not be left on answering machines or other voicemail facilities. This highlights the importance of agreeing arrangements for appropriate communication with those involved in the complaint at the earliest opportunity.

It is usual practice for healthcare providers to ensure that conciliators return all relevant documentation relating to the complaint, including any copies of health records, once the conciliation process has been concluded. This requirement can also be included in any form of contract when the conciliator is appointed. It should be noted, however, that this should not normally include any of the conciliator's own notes of the process, correspondence or written material provided direct to the conciliator by either of the parties concerned, or their advocates or interpreters. In England, the importance of preserving confidentiality in relation to the conciliation process is clearly stated in the guidance notes for the NHS Complaints Regulations (2004). Conciliators also have a responsibility themselves to ensure the security or disposal of any identifiable information following the process; for example, by shredding. Some conciliators ensure that initials only are used in any notes they make, and that other details are anonymised.

'Confidentiality must be strictly observed during the conciliation process. Consequently, conciliators should never be required to report to NHS bodies the details of cases in which they are involved.'

Department of Health. *Guidance to support implementation of the National Health Service (Complaints) Regulations.* Department of Health, 2004.

It is important to note that the conciliator's independence extends not only to the parties directly involved in the complaint, but also in relation to those complaints officers with overall responsibility for the handling of complaints. The conciliator will not divulge the content of conciliation meetings to them, or anyone else outside the process itself, without the express consent of the parties concerned.

Breaching confidentiality

In certain rare situations a conciliator may have to breach confidentiality where there is a threat to the physical or mental health of an individual, or if information that could impact on patient safety or clinical care emerges during the course of the conciliation process. Such issues of concern might also relate to children or vulnerable adults. In addition, the document *Confidentiality: the NHS Code of Practice* (2003) points out that actual or potential harm can be a consequence of crimes such as theft or fraud, so evidence of these might also provide grounds for disclosure. In any of these circumstances, the conciliator will need to have contact details of individuals within the healthcare organisation best placed to handle such issues and provide appropriate guidance.

Where the conciliator believes that confidential information must be disclosed, they should attempt, if possible, to obtain the consent of the individual(s) involved. Depending on the circumstances this may be achieved by careful explanation from the conciliator, outlining the reasons for believing that the information needs to be shared. This most commonly applies where considerations relating to an individual's health are concerned.

Access to health records and complaints documentation

In some circumstances the conciliator may need to have access to the health records relating to the person who is the subject of the complaint. Healthcare organisations should have a policy and procedure for accessing records in these circumstances, including the records of deceased persons.

It is essential that the appropriate consent is obtained. Examples are given on the following page.

▶ Where the complainant is also the patient, and is making the complaint on their own behalf, they should sign a form authorising access to all the relevant documentation as well as the parts of their health records relating to their complaint, and should specify to whom this is granted.

▶ Where a complaint is made on behalf of someone else, it is important to ensure that the complainant is acting with the consent of that individual. Where the patient has capacity, they must give written consent themselves for their health records to be made available, and state to whom this applies.

'3.28 It is for the complaints manager, possibly in discussion with the senior person or chief executive, to determine whether the complainant has "sufficient interest" in the deceased or incapable person's welfare to be suitable to act as a representative. The question of whether a complainant is suitable to represent a patient depends, in particular, on the need to respect the confidentiality of the patient. For example, the patient may earlier have made it known that information should not be disclosed to third parties.'

Department of Health. *Guidance to support implementation of the National Health Service (Complaints) Regulations.* Department of Health, 2004. Paragraph 3.28.

In the case of complaints made in relation to deceased persons, or children, or people who are deemed unable to act for themselves by reason of mental or physical incapacity, it is for the complaints manager to determine whether the complainant fulfils the necessary requirements in the complaints procedure (regulation 8), to act as the patient's representative in respect of the complaint.

Consent should also be obtained to ensure that the relevant information, including access to health records, can be made available, where appropriate, to a designated professional acting in an advisory capacity to the conciliator (for example, a medical or dental practitioner); or to an independent clinician who may be asked to provide an expert opinion in the form of a report.

It should be noted that there are circumstances in which access to the record may be denied or restricted by the record holder; for example, if this is considered detrimental to an individual's physical or mental health, or if information confidential to a third party would otherwise be disclosed. However, any such refusal must be able to withstand scrutiny and could further exacerbate the situation relating to the complaint.

While parents or guardians have rights of access to a child's health record, there may be circumstances in which a young person wishes to ensure that confidential information is not divulged. A practitioner needs to consider the possible damage caused by disclosure, and also the child or young person's rights to withhold consent if they are regarded as 'Gillick competent' (*see* Glossary).

Consideration of special needs

Any special circumstances relating to the parties involved in the complaint should be identified by the complaints handling staff and highlighted to the conciliator. This will ensure that appropriate advice, services or facilities are obtained and that information is provided in the correct format.

Specialist advocates may also be involved to represent or support people with learning disabilities or mental health conditions. Similar services may also be provided in some cases for children or young people. The aim is to ensure that the views and input of those who are central to the complaint are considered wherever possible.

Conciliators may also find it helpful to have clinical advice in relation to complainants who have any kind of physical or psychological condition which may impair their ability to concentrate or participate fully in the conciliation process. It is also important that clinical advice is obtained in relation to complaints involving someone with a serious mental health condition to assess their suitability for conciliation, and to ensure that the appropriate risk assessments are undertaken. The fact that the complainant is detained in a mental health facility is not in itself a barrier to using conciliation. Subject to the necessary safeguards, conciliation may also be appropriate in relation to some prison healthcare complaints.

Sometimes family members may offer themselves as interpreters in situations where the complaint has been made by, or on behalf of, a non-English speaking relative. Caution needs to be exercised in such situations, since ideally a professional interpreter should be used, wherever possible, particularly in the context of complaints or conciliation meetings. Similar consideration needs to be given to those who require the use of professional signing services for people with hearing impairment.

It is important that the health service staff have confidence in the interpreter's ability to express their responses accurately and in a culturally appropriate and acceptable way to the complainant. The risks of relying too heavily on the services of a relative, however well intentioned, are twofold:

- this may impede the complainant's ability to speak freely; they should always be given the opportunity to express themselves through an interpreter without a family member being present
- when using an interpreter who is a family member, there is always the danger that the views of the different parties involved in the conciliation will not be expressed adequately or accurately.

Interpreting impartially for someone, in what can be an emotional and highly charged situation, requires special skill and expertise as well as an explicit agreement to observe the confidentiality of the process. For this reason it is advisable to use trained interpreters with experience of working in a healthcare situation. It is also important to ensure that all written information about conciliation, as well as the rest of the complaints procedure, is available in languages that reflect the local population.

Clinical advice and expert reports

It is essential for conciliators to have access to appropriate clinical advice and the means to access expert reports, when required, from relevant professionals. The adviser should be from the same profession as the person who is the subject of the complaint. The extent to which conciliators make use of this facility will vary from case to case. However, it is often helpful to take independent clinical advice prior to discussing the records with either the complainant or the person against whom the complaint has been made, since this may enable the conciliator to note any outstanding clinical issues which require further explanation from the healthcare provider.

In some instances it may be sufficient for a conciliator to have telephone contact with an adviser in order to clarify a particular aspect of medical jargon or to obtain a better understanding of the diagnosis or treatment relating to the complaint. At other times the conciliator may also wish to involve a clinical adviser in a meeting with the complainant. At such a meeting the complainant will be able to put questions directly to the adviser as well as relying on the conciliator to ensure that all areas of concern, which have been identified previously, are addressed.

The clinical adviser may be asked to interpret clinical terminology, and explain about conditions or treatments that may seem unintelligible to the layperson. They may also be asked to state if a particular guideline, procedure or protocol was being followed. They should not be asked to make an *ad hoc* judgement or to comment about the quality of clinical care unless this has been stated clearly as part of their remit.

Sometimes it becomes apparent during the conciliation process that details provided as part of the healthcare organisation's response to the complaint were either not known previously to the complainant, or that discussion of these points causes distress. This might occur, for example, when the complaint relates to a deceased relative and the medical record is being used as a basis for addressing issues raised by the complainant. The person who has died may have had a long-term chronic condition and the general practice notes may show that there have been repeated reminders from the surgery requesting the individual to attend for blood pressure monitoring or dietary advice. There may be issues with drug interactions, especially if these relate to alcohol intake. If the complainant has raised concerns about a lack of care in such circumstances, the clinical adviser will be able to explain the relevance of such information while appreciating the impact this knowledge may have on the complainant.

The value of appropriate involvement from an independent clinician cannot be overstated even when the clinicians and investigating managers concerned in the complaint consider the issues to be straightforward, and addressed comprehensively in their own responses to the complainant. The fact that the clinical adviser is independent of the circumstances relating to the complaint often enables them to present the situation to the complainant in a way that facilitates:

- a better understanding of the organisation's response
- the evidence base, guidelines or best practice for the particular treatment or care provided
- the data on outcomes for the particular condition if this is relevant.

The use of an expert's report may be of particular relevance in complaints involving secondary or specialist care. An expert opinion should be delivered as part of a written report and will usually need to show that the following have been considered.

- Is there a *prima facie* case of negligence? (It would be hoped that indications of this would have been evident at an earlier stage, even prior to a complaint being submitted.)
- Were the healthcare professional's actions in respect of the clinical care based on the responsible exercise of clinical judgement such as could reasonably be expected of his or her peers in similar circumstances?
- Did the healthcare professional respect the rights of the patient (and the relatives or carers with the patient's consent) to influence decisions about his or her care?
- Did the actions of the healthcare professional conform to the codes of practice and regulations of his or her profession?
- Were the necessary information and support or expert professional advice available to the healthcare professional to enable him or her to form a proper judgement and offer appropriate care?
- Did the healthcare professional fail to recognise the limits of his or her professional competence?
- Was care delegated, and if so, was it to someone suitably qualified, supervised, and competent to undertake that care?
- Was there a failure to refer the patient to another healthcare professional?

The expert may need to be asked to bear in mind that the contents of their report will be shared with others apart from the healthcare provider requesting the report; for example, with the complainant, and with the person against whom the complaint has been made. The expert may also be requested to take part in a meeting with one or both parties; for example, with the complainant and the conciliator, to answer any questions about, or to discuss any issues arising from, the content of the report. It is also important that all the parties to the conciliation are kept fully informed by the conciliator about the remit of the clinical adviser or independent expert.

When requesting a report it is important to agree a time frame with the expert in order to maintain the momentum of the conciliation process. This is important whether the complaints file to be considered is substantial or relatively slim. Those representing the healthcare organisation must be ready to respond to the report with appropriate actions, particularly if the report highlights significant shortcomings or areas of practice that could be improved. The extent to which such findings are acknowledged and acted upon will be crucial in determining the outcome of the conciliation process.

An expert report may also be helpful even when a healthcare organisation considers it has demonstrated unequivocally that appropriate action was taken at each stage in relation to a patient's treatment and care. For example, a complainant may be concerned that a patient's death was attributable directly to a delayed or inaccurate diagnosis. The patient may have had a complex medical history with symptoms that could have been consistent with an existing, chronic condition. The presentation of these symptoms may have resulted in a series of investigations with negative findings. It may not have been until the patient's health deteriorated to a point at which hospital admission was indicated that the underlying cause was finally diagnosed. The expert's report may support the healthcare organisation's own response to the complaint by confirming that the earlier symptoms could have had a number of possible causes and did not in themselves suggest the condition which resulted in the patient's death.

However, even when faced with an independent expert's report that exonerates a clinician's actions and states unequivocally that they have acted appropriately, the complainant may not agree automatically that the complaint has been resolved. Feelings of anger, resentment and the need to blame someone can be very strong and will not simply disperse when a person from the same profession, albeit independent of the situation, gives a view that the clinical outcome could not have been avoided. This will apply particularly where there are issues which could have been handled differently, as well as poor communication, misunderstanding or insensitivity.

The complainant may express disbelief about the opinion given in an independent clinician's report, or voice concerns about the process followed, including the quality and relevance of the information on which the opinion is based. This is why it is essential that the complainant is given accurate information about:

- the documentation that was sent to the independent clinician (which should include all the information relating to the complaint, together with the medical record and any other relevant details or clinical findings)
- the precise instructions given, which show clearly the parameters of the advice required and the issues on which comment and opinion is sought
- the clinician's current professional position – ideally, they should be independent from the healthcare provider concerned and it should be made clear that there are no conflicts of interest.

The complainant may need time to reflect on the contents of the expert's report, and the opportunity to refer again to the original issues in the complaint together with the responses from the person against whom the complaint has been made, especially if these have been amplified as a result of the conciliation process. The conciliator needs to lead the complainant through the points reached to date and then refer to the report. The complainant may ask to have a copy (permission should have been sought in advance for this, from the author and from the healthcare organisation) and may also need further time to consider and discuss the issues with other family members, perhaps agreeing to make contact with the conciliator within a specified time. If contact is not made within the agreed time, the conciliator should follow this up.

The Parliamentary and Health Service Ombudsman's Annual Report 2005–06 highlights the value of independent clinical advice and includes the response from a primary care trust following resolution of a complaint which had been achieved through the judicious use of clinical advice, facilitated by the Ombudsman.

'We have noted that your clinical adviser has provided detailed background information about brain tumours. We believe that your adviser's report has shed more light on the clinical decision making process, and the symptoms and incidence of brain tumour, than all previous efforts by the practice at the local resolution stage, or by the IRP [Independent Review Process]. The lesson learned . . . is to encourage and facilitate the use of independent clinical advice where appropriate in dealing with complaints in future. We will amend our Complaints Policy and Procedures to include the option at the local resolution stage for an independent clinical adviser to discuss concerns with a complainant face to face, or to provide a written report.'

Parliamentary and Health Service Ombudsman. *Making a difference: Annual Report 2005–6.* (HC 1363). London: The Stationery Office, 2006. Page 42.

Telephone contact

It is not considered advisable for conciliators to give personal contact details to either party. Depending on the circumstances relating to the complaint, the conciliator may either contact the parties directly by telephone to initiate the meetings, or may decide that it is more appropriate for these arrangements to be made by administrative staff within the healthcare organisation concerned. However, even a brief telephone conversation can be useful since it may enable the conciliator to:

▶ establish a rapport which may help to reassure the complainant or staff member about the process in advance of a meeting
▶ address immediate concerns, allay anxieties and answer any specific questions
▶ facilitate a resolution of the complaint between the parties concerned.

There may be occasions when it is more appropriate to avoid initial telephone contact; for example, where the complaint involves a serious incident or bereavement, so that the first contact between the conciliator and the complainant is made in person. Telephone conversations may, however, be helpful between meetings to clarify points or provide feedback between the parties concerned.

Delays and postponements

Occasionally one of the parties who has agreed to take part in the conciliation process impedes its progress by failing to attend or by postponing the date of the first meeting on more than one occasion. If spurious or implausible reasons are given for this, the conciliator needs to consider carefully if it is appropriate to proceed with the process.

Possible causes for apparently unreasonable delays may relate to:

▶ the venue
▶ the dates or times of meetings
▶ unwillingness to proceed with the complaint
▶ anxiety about the conciliation process.

The venue may be inappropriate because its location presents difficulties in terms of convenience or accessibility, or the complainant may be anxious about returning to healthcare premises because of an association with unpleasant or distressing memories.

It is important to bear in mind that complainants may wish to avoid arranging meetings on certain dates that have a religious or cultural significance for them. Equally, where the complainant has been bereaved they may not wish to attend meetings on, or too close to, the anniversary of the deceased person's death. To ensure that offence is not caused inadvertently, it is advisable to ask the complainant to suggest times that are most suitable for them and also to highlight any dates that they would like to avoid.

Careful consideration may need to be given to the timing of the conciliation meetings. Under normal circumstances meetings take place during the day at times which are acceptable to all parties. Staff must be able to demonstrate a proper commitment to the process, and their attendance at the meetings should be regarded as a priority by the healthcare organisation concerned. If the complainant is unable to attend during the day, some conciliators are prepared to work in the evenings, but this will need to be established at the earliest opportunity.

An unwillingness to proceed with the conciliation meetings can sometimes arise when the complaint has been initiated by the patient's relative or carer. Although the patient may have given their consent at the outset, their feelings or perceptions about the issues may have changed and they may no longer wish to pursue the complaint. The relative or carer may, however, be less willing to allow the matter to rest.

The conciliator will need to ascertain whether the complainant has changed their mind about pursuing the complaint, and wishes to withdraw from the process after reflecting on the issues, or if there is some perceived or actual barrier which is preventing their participation in the conciliation meetings.

If the health professional fails to attend, or cancels conciliation meetings, this may be because they are not taking the complaint sufficiently seriously. They may regard other duties as having higher priority, or they may lack cover to enable them to take the time away from their normal work. Since staff participation is essential, any difficulties of this kind need to be raised with the healthcare organisation as soon as they are identified.

Occasionally delays are caused because members of staff wish to consult with their professional organisations or defence societies, especially if they are concerned about the prospect of litigation as a result of the complaint. Every effort should be taken to minimise such delays since they can impact adversely on the conciliation process, especially if practitioners decline to attend meetings while awaiting a response from their defence society or solicitor. The usual advice in such circumstances is for practitioners to attend conciliation meetings in the hope that the issues can be resolved at an early opportunity.

In advance of the first meeting either party may feel anxious or apprehensive about the conciliation process, regardless of the quality of information that may have been provided. A telephone conversation at this stage, with either of the parties, will enable the conciliator to build a rapport and explore the reasons for the apparent unwillingness to proceed with the process.

Conciliators should not allow significant delays or postponements of meetings without good reason. There may come a point where the conciliator has to withdraw from the process, having provided ample warning that this will be the case, and complaints procedures should provide clear guidance to complaints handling staff about the action they should take in situations of this kind. It is clearly important to ensure that neither party is left wondering indefinitely what is happening.

Location of conciliation meetings

The location used for the conciliation meetings will be influenced by the following considerations:
- the circumstances in which the process is being used; for example,
  - at an early stage in the complaints procedure
  - outwith the complaints procedure, to assist with the process of addressing issues arising in relation to serious incidents or complex clinical situations
  - as a means of restoring clinical relationships
- the health of the complainant.

A neutral venue is normally promoted as the best location for the meetings so that each of the parties is seen to be treated equally. If the meetings do take place within the healthcare organisation concerned, consideration should be given to locating them away from the clinical area involved in the complaint, or in an appropriate meeting place elsewhere. If the complainant is an inpatient this will clearly limit the options available; but, whatever the circumstances, the overriding consideration should be to ensure that the complainant's views and sensitivities are taken into account.

Sometimes the complainant is asked to meet with members of staff during an investigation into the complaint. Care needs to be taken to ensure that the complainant is not outnumbered in what can be an intimidating and overwhelming situation. A negative experience of this kind may be referred to by the complainant at the initial conciliation meeting; and it can impact on their attitude towards the whole complaints handling procedure, including the conciliation process.

Meetings held in the complainant's home

Occasionally the complainant may request that the conciliator visits them in their own home. This may be because either the complainant, or the person on whose behalf the complaint is being made, is unable to attend meetings elsewhere because of health-related or other difficulties. Lack of transport should not be regarded as an insurmountable obstacle, and consideration should be given, where appropriate, to providing a taxi if this would enable the complainant to attend a meeting outside their home.

Sometimes the complainant wishes to ensure that the conciliator has been to their home so that they can demonstrate specific issues relating to the complaint. A carer, for example, may wish to highlight the need for special resources or equipment; or to draw attention to specific difficulties presented by the caring situation itself.

Some conciliators are not prepared to do home visits and it should not be assumed that every conciliator will have the experience or skills necessary to undertake these. If conciliation meetings take place in the complainant's home, the conciliator inevitably has less control over the conduct of the meetings and must be sufficiently flexible to ensure that the issues are covered within whatever constraints arise. It is sometimes possible for an acceptable compromise to be reached, whereby an initial meeting takes place in the complainant's home, but any subsequent meetings are held in a neutral venue.

The positive benefits of acceding to a request for a home visit may be that

- the conciliator gains deeper insight into the key issues and is therefore able to use this knowledge effectively towards the resolution of the complaint; equally
- the complainant may feel more at ease in their home surroundings, particularly if they have a physical or psychological condition, or caring responsibilities, that inhibit their ability to engage positively in the conciliation process.

Depending on the circumstances, the same procedures applying to health service personnel working alone in the community should be used in relation to conciliators, and the risks to personal safety should be assessed carefully. In addition to this the following issues should be considered:

- conciliators who may not wish to visit alone may be prepared to do so if other professionals are to be present; for example, an independent clinician, advocate, or interpreter
- there should always be appropriate risk management measures in relation to security and personal safety
- the conciliator should be prepared to terminate the meeting if there is any verbal abuse or physical threat
- if the complainant has included additional relatives or friends in the meeting, without prior consultation, the conciliator must decide whether their presence will be helpful or detrimental to the process, and must be prepared to act accordingly (*see* Chapter 4).

Meetings held in health service premises or other locations

Where possible, the room chosen should be appropriate to the number of people attending the meeting, since over-large rooms can be intimidating. The purpose of the meeting (for example, whether those present will include all parties to the complaint) also influences the type of room used. Ideally, the room used for the meeting should be within easy reach of toilet facilities and administrative support in case the conciliator needs to have any additional documents or requires further copies for the complainant. In some circumstances it may be advisable to have a telephone in the room. Sometimes people become very distressed when recounting the circumstances relating to a complaint and may appreciate a glass of water and access to a box of tissues. The offer of refreshments at the beginning of the meeting is often appreciated by the complainant and helps to give a welcoming and informal touch to the proceedings.

It is sometimes assumed that low, easy chairs arranged informally, perhaps around a coffee table, create the most acceptable atmosphere. Depending on the purpose of the meeting and any special needs which should be considered, this may be an appropriate arrangement. However, there are several advantages to sitting at an appropriately sized table:

- the parties may feel less vulnerable when discussing contentious or emotionally charged issues
- participants can spread out papers
- it is much easier to refer to the complaints documentation and to make notes when the participants sit around a table rather than trying to balance files on their knees.

In giving consideration to the seating arrangements, the conciliator may wish to avoid a situation where the complainant, and the clinician against whom the complaint has been made, are facing each other across the table. This is achieved more easily if the conciliator conducts the meeting from the side rather than from the head of the table, at the same time inviting the other parties to sit in particular places without appearing too directive. Circular tables are often considered especially appropriate for conciliation or mediation meetings because any sense of hierarchy is avoided.

It is important to ensure that there are no unnecessary interruptions during the meeting. Staff members should therefore be given 'protected time', and should not be expected to be on call. This ensures that all parties treat the meeting as a priority.

Support for complainants

Information relating to the complaints procedure should not only refer to the way in which the complaint may be handled, but should also include details of any complaints advocacy service or similar support that can be made available to the complainant. In England, this role is undertaken by the Independent Complaints Advocacy Service (ICAS), a statutory service which aims to provide appropriate advice and guidance, and in certain circumstances may also provide an advocate to accompany the complainant to conciliation meetings. A similar function is provided in Scotland by Citizens Advice Bureaux; in Wales by the local Community Health Councils, and in Northern Ireland by Health and Social Services Councils.

The complainant may also wish to be accompanied to the conciliation meetings by a friend or relative. Sometimes a number of relatives may wish to attend and complaints staff should confer with the conciliator, who has ultimate responsibility for making such decisions, if this issue arises. Other forms of support have been considered earlier in this chapter in relation to any special needs or requirements; for example, the provision of interpreting or signing services.

Support for staff

It is vital that the person against whom the complaint has been made receives both written information about the complaints procedure and also advice in relation to how the specific complaint may be handled. If conciliation is being considered as an appropriate way forward it is helpful for all concerned if the health professional is well informed about the nature of the process. Participation demonstrates a willingness on the part of the health professional to try to address the complainant's concerns, especially if other attempts have failed. Since conciliation meetings usually take place within the working day, it is important that arrangements are put in place to enable staff to attend the meetings.

While a colleague or staff representative may accompany the person against whom the complaint has been made, it is also essential that someone with sufficient authority or seniority is involved to consider any proposed actions which the healthcare organisation could take to resolve the complaint. This will demonstrate to the complainant that the issues are being taken seriously. Ideally, an undertaking should be given to inform the complainant when the agreed actions have been implemented.

Sources of support for staff within the organisation may come from:

- complaints handling staff
- senior staff in the relevant service area

- colleagues
- occupational health services
- confidential counselling services.

External support for staff may come from:

- professional associations, including local area representatives who may have particular expertise in providing support and guidance in relation to complaints
- family members or close friends outside the workplace
- defence associations, which can provide an important source of support especially if practitioners are concerned about the possibility of litigation.

Support for conciliators

To ensure that conciliators are able to function as effectively as possible, healthcare organisations need to consider how best to provide them with appropriate support. The key issues relating to administrative support have been considered earlier in this chapter.

These are briefly summarised here:

- providing information about the conciliation process to all parties
- arranging appointments and venues, being mindful of accessibility, safety and security issues
- obtaining relevant written consents including authorisation for the conciliator and any independent clinician to access health records where appropriate
- ensuring that documentation regarding the complaint is complete and up-to-date
- responding effectively and without undue delay to requests from the conciliator for further information
- arranging for expert reports as well as input and/or advice from an independent clinician where this is requested by the conciliator.

As well as ensuring that effective administrative procedures are in place to help make the conciliation process run smoothly, healthcare organisations should also consider the possible need for emotional support for the conciliator. The need for this will depend on factors such as the conciliator's own experience and professional networks, but there may be occasions when a conciliator needs to debrief anonymously following involvement in a complaint of a particularly harrowing or distressing nature.

It may, therefore, be useful for conciliators to have access to the same confidential counselling services as other healthcare staff, with the option of either a face-to-face meeting or telephone counselling as appropriate. Where conciliation services are provided by, or on behalf of, a number of healthcare or social care organisations, support may be accessed through peer group networks, mentoring or supervision arrangements. This is especially important for those new to conciliation.

Support may also be necessary for conciliators who become subject to a complaint themselves arising directly from their role in the conciliation process. This is particularly important if the complainant has already shown signs of making vexatious or habitual complaints. In such circumstances, it is a recognised risk that the conciliator will not be immune from this kind of behaviour, and this underlines the importance of both screening complaints and also taking steps to reduce the impact of such a complaint in the circumstances described.

An uncommon but occasional complaint is that the conciliator is favouring one party over another. Where the complaint comes from the healthcare professional concerned it may be that the conciliator appears to be acting as an advocate for the patient and is failing to maintain a sufficiently neutral position. Conversely, the complainant may feel that the conciliator is showing a bias in favour of the views expressed by the person against whom the complaint has been made. Complaints staff need to be aware of the potential for such possibilities and may find it helpful if they have clear guidance for handling complaints against conciliators.

CHAPTER 4

Conduct of the conciliation

- → Telephone contact.
- → Initial meetings between the conciliator and the complainant.
- → Meetings between the conciliator and the staff member(s) against whom the complaint has been made.
- → Psychological aspects of conciliation – feelings as well as facts.
- → Looking at the issues from the other party's point of view.
- → Keeping the parties informed.
- → Numbers of people attending meetings.
- → Taking notes.
- → Length of meetings.
- → Meetings between the conciliator and all parties involved in the complaint.
- → Concluding the conciliation process.
- → Recording the outcome.
- → Letter from the healthcare practitioner to the complainant.
- → Letter from the healthcare organisation to the complainant.

Telephone contact

It was noted in the previous chapter that it is occasionally possible for the conciliator to bring about the resolution of a complaint using telephone contact alone. The following are examples of how this may occur.

▶ It may become apparent to the conciliator during a telephone conversation with the complainant that a key point has been overlooked or misunderstood in the initial response from the healthcare organisation. With the complainant's agreement, the conciliator may be able to highlight and clarify the issue with the healthcare provider so that a further response can be made that addresses fully all aspects of the complaint.

▶ The conciliator can also use telephone contact to facilitate agreement between the parties over issues where a compromise may be negotiated which will prove acceptable to all concerned. Complaints about dental charges, for example, can sometimes be resolved in this way.

More usually, however, if there is telephone contact between the conciliator and the complainant, this will be to make arrangements for an initial meeting. It will also provide an opportunity for the conciliator to begin to build a rapport with the complainant and to allay any anxieties the complainant may express about meeting with the conciliator.

Issues that need to be considered prior to the meeting have been discussed in the previous chapter but a telephone conversation may also raise awareness of:

▶ the most appropriate venue
▶ any specific difficulties or special circumstances that should be taken into account
▶ additional support that may be required.

It can also be helpful if the conciliator has a telephone conversation with the person against whom the complaint has been made, or with the person responsible for representing the healthcare organisation, prior to meeting with the complainant. This enables the conciliator to proceed with any arrangements for a meeting between all the parties concerned, should it be appropriate, and demonstrates to the complainant that those who are involved in the complaint are willing to take part in such a meeting if required.

Initial meetings between the conciliator and the complainant

The purpose of the initial meeting with the complainant is to enable the conciliator to:

▶ build a rapport while remaining unbiased and non-judgmental
▶ give a brief overview of the complaints procedure
▶ explain the principles of conciliation, emphasising the confidential and voluntary nature of the process
▶ discuss the healthcare organisation's written response to the complainant
▶ consider the involvement of an independent, clinical adviser
▶ understand the full range of the complainant's grievances.

It is helpful for the complainant if the conciliator explains the place of conciliation in relation to the overall complaints procedure. By emphasising that it is part of the local resolution stage, the conciliator also acknowledges that the complainant can request an independent review of their complaint from the Healthcare Commission if they are not satisfied with the outcome of the process. This ensures that the complainant knows that participation in conciliation will not prevent them from taking their complaint further should they feel this to be necessary. In addition, they may wish for an explanation of the role of the Health Service Ombudsman. It should also be noted that if a complainant requests an independent review of their complaint, without having had the opportunity to take part in a conciliation process, the complaint may be referred back to the healthcare provider by the Healthcare Commission with recommendations for further action, which could include conciliation.

First stage: Health Service Provider
Local resolution, which may include conciliation.

Second stage: Healthcare Commission

Third stage: Health Service Ombudsman

The complaint can be referred back to the Health Service Provider by the Healthcare Commission for conciliation if deemed appropriate.

FIGURE 4.1 The place of conciliation within the NHS Complaints Procedure

Complainants sometimes find it reassuring to be reminded that the conciliation process is voluntary, and that there is no compulsion on them to meet with the person against whom the complaint has been made if they do not wish to do so. Also, at the outset of the meeting, the conciliator will highlight the fact that confidentiality is an integral part of the conciliation process, which ensures that the complainant is able to share their feelings about the issues in a private and 'protected' environment. The conciliator should explain that any notes they make will be for their own personal use to ensure that they capture the complainant's views accurately, and that no details of the discussion will be disclosed without the complainant's express agreement.

Although uncommon, there are occasions when complainants who are particularly angry may express themselves by being verbally aggressive or abusive about the professional against whom the complaint has been made. In some circumstances, therefore, the conciliator may feel there is a need to reduce the likelihood of this happening by setting clear parameters for the meeting and, while referring to the limits of confidentiality, may need to highlight the obligation to disclose threats of harm should these be made against any individual. If this is included as part of what is clearly an introduction to the conciliation process it need not cause offence. Although conciliators occasionally find themselves defusing situations where emotions are highly charged, threats of violence towards healthcare staff should be taken very seriously, and conciliators working within the NHS should be aware of the organisational procedures in relation to security management.

The initial meeting should also allow the complainant to:

- express their view of the complaints handling to date, including any actions taken as a result of the complaint
- highlight their outstanding concerns
- indicate the desired outcome they hope will be achieved through the conciliation process.

The complainant's expectations of the conciliation process need to be discussed fully. It is important that the conciliator not only states what *can* be achieved by the process, but also what *cannot*. For example, the complainant may demand that immediate disciplinary action be taken against the member of staff involved in the complaint, or that a report be made to their professional body with the expressed intention of preventing them from practising. The complainant may also make a request for damages or compensation. The issue of monetary outcomes or *ex gratia* payments in relation to the complaints procedure has been discussed in Chapter 1. However, what most complainants hope to obtain are:

- an apology, which they sometimes feel should extend to cover the way in which the complaint has been handled up to this point
- an acknowledgement of the distress or inconvenience they have experienced
- explanations regarding issues they have raised
- appropriate redress
- assurance that actions will be taken to prevent any similar occurrence in the future.

Complainants often stress that they are pursuing their complaint in order to prevent other people suffering the same experience.

The conciliator will use the correspondence that has already taken place between the complainant and the healthcare organisation, together with any other supporting documentation, as the basis for the discussion with the complainant. This discussion provides an opportunity for the conciliator to note not only outstanding concerns but also whether the complainant considers that any issues have been addressed appropriately. Where the complainant acknowledges that there has been an acceptable response this needs to be highlighted by the conciliator to emphasise progress that has been made.

The conciliator will need to summarise the issues at appropriate intervals so that the complainant has an opportunity to confirm or correct the conciliator's own understanding of the key points, as well as agreeing those details which may be passed on to the other party involved in the complaint. The conciliator may use advice already obtained from an independent professional in relation to any aspect of the complaint, or they may explore with the complainant the benefits of arranging a meeting with an adviser or requesting an expert report if this course of action is indicated by the circumstances.

Meetings between the conciliator and the staff member(s) against whom the complaint has been made

The conciliator should adopt a common approach to the private meetings held with either the complainant or the person against whom the complaint has been made. This will ensure not only that they maintain an impartial and neutral position, but also that generic information is given at the outset to both parties. The staff member will not necessarily have a greater awareness of the different parts of the complaints procedure or the conciliation process than the complainant. Therefore, the conciliator should ensure that the first meeting with the person against whom the complaint has been made covers:

- the key stages of the complaints procedure and the place of conciliation within the local resolution stage
- the principles of the conciliation process, highlighting the voluntary, impartial and confidential nature of the process
- the role of an independent clinician or other professional, if appropriate.

Prior to the meeting with the staff member, the conciliator should have met with the complainant and will, therefore, be in a position to pass on the outstanding issues and concerns which have emerged, as well as an indication of what the complainant hopes to achieve from the conciliation process. The meeting with the staff member should allow them the opportunity to:

- provide further explanations or comments in relation to the complainant's outstanding concerns
- consider alternative ways of looking at the issues, particularly from the complainant's perspective
- reflect on the original complaint and whether the situation which gave rise to it could have been handled differently

- discuss a way forward which might include an expression of regret at the circumstances which gave rise to the complaint
- consider making an apology if appropriate, especially if mistakes have been made (bearing in mind that an apology is not an admission of liability)
- give further explanations or clarification of issues where misunderstandings have arisen
- request the involvement of an independent clinician or expert if appropriate
- consider possible redress, financial or otherwise
- consider actions to be taken as a direct result of the complaint to prevent a repeat occurrence of the issues in the future.

Where the complaint is made against more than one member of the healthcare organisation concerned, the conciliator will usually expect to meet with each of the individuals separately, prior to passing on the outcomes of the meetings to the complainant. In such circumstances, a person authorised to act on behalf of the organisation to negotiate a satisfactory outcome may also have contributed to the process at this stage.

Psychological aspects of conciliation – feelings as well as facts

The majority of complainants feel hesitant about making a complaint, and where complaints procedures are perceived as lengthy or inaccessible it is only the compelling need to discover exactly what went wrong, or to prevent a similar situation affecting someone else, that motivates them to persist.

Some complainants have experienced extremely distressing events and while the conciliator may wish to express their condolences or sympathy with regard to these circumstances, they must take care to remain unbiased, non-judgemental and impartial in their approach. The conciliation process can be effective only where the conciliator is able to empathise with each of the parties concerned, since it is this ability to empathise which enables the conciliator to view the issues from the standpoint of the parties themselves, and in turn to encourage each to gain an understanding of the other's position.

Where a complaint involving a deteriorating clinical relationship is made on behalf of a relative or person other than the complainant, it is important to establish some common ground. For example, it may be appropriate at the beginning of the conciliation to gain agreement to the principle that all parties regard the best interests of the patient as paramount. This principle can then be used by the conciliator in discussion with both parties so as to facilitate an understanding of each other's positions. This may provide the motivation necessary for the parties to address their concerns through an agreed action plan in order to secure the best possible outcome for the patient.

Sometimes, the complainant may be unsure whether they wish to meet with the other party, and this may be determined as the process progresses. For example, they may wish to hear an apology direct from the person concerned rather than in writing or via the conciliator; or after hearing more detail about the issues they may feel a dialogue with the other party would be helpful. A particular advantage of the conciliation process is that it is adaptable and centred on the complainant's needs, which may themselves change as the process develops. Although most health professionals express a willingness to participate in a joint meeting if this is suggested, in situations where they are no longer responsible for the complainant's healthcare they may also show a degree of relief if the complainant declines to meet with them.

Where the complainant sees no benefit in meeting with the other party, and indeed has sought steps to avoid this in the future, the outstanding issues relating to the complaint can still be resolved as part of the conciliation process. This is where the conciliator's ability to communicate the key issues, as agreed by each party in terms of feelings and perceptions as well as facts, is crucial to the success of the process.

Sometimes, the meeting with the conciliator provides the first opportunity the complainant has been given to express their feelings about the complaint and the way in which it has been handled, in a supportive atmosphere. This may be because the only contact they have had with the healthcare provider has been in writing. In such a situation misunderstandings can arise between both parties and the tone of any letters can also affect the eventual outcome. The situation may be exacerbated further if the complainant feels that their concerns have not been taken seriously, especially if there have been unexplained delays between their contacts with the organisation and any written responses. In other circumstances, there may have been telephone calls as well as an exchange of letters, and the complainant may have found these unsatisfactory for a variety of reasons. A short, brusque or offhand tone, a less-than-helpful response to a request for advice in making the complaint, or a defensive reaction to the issues raised may all compound the original problem.

Alternatively, the complainant may have met with the healthcare staff concerned as part of an investigation into the issues, or at a meeting arranged to discuss the complaint. If the meeting has not had a satisfactory outcome this may have been for any of the following reasons.

- There were misunderstandings on both sides in relation to the complainant's concerns and the explanations of the staff involved.
- Neither party could see the other's point of view.
- Whatever the staff had said, the issues were too emotive at that point for the complainant to accept the explanations given, however accurate.

▶ Where a serious incident or bereavement had occurred, the staff did not acknowledge the complainant's distress sufficiently, or appeared unwilling to accept that mistakes had been made.
▶ The complainant's belief that someone was to blame was too powerful to admit any other explanation.

If the complainant attended the meeting with a number of friends or relatives, the member of staff involved in the complaint may have felt intimidated or outnumbered, especially if the meeting was not chaired effectively and there were constant interruptions with several people trying to talk at once. Equally, if there were several members of staff present the converse could have been the case, with the complainant feeling they had no control over the proceedings and finding it difficult to express their point of view in the presence of a number of people. In addition, the behaviours of the parties may have inflamed an already difficult situation. The meeting may not have been managed effectively, with the result that:

▶ the complainant may have felt they were not given sufficient opportunity or support to state their concerns
▶ the staff may not have been able to offer the explanations or responses required
▶ the complainant may have become physically or verbally threatening or aggressive
▶ the staff may have become increasingly defensive or shown signs of irritation or exasperation.

The interaction between family members may also significantly affect the progress of the conciliation process. It cannot be assumed that there will be general acceptance of the practitioner's explanations from all concerned. Occasionally, it is possible that other family members will be influential in encouraging the complainant to acknowledge that the issues have been addressed. While other relatives may have an important perspective to add to the process, it is the complainant who must feel satisfied with the outcome.

If the complaint follows a death, for example, it may be that the complainant was the patient's carer, and as well as being involved more deeply in the circumstances surrounding the complaint, was also attached more emotionally to the patient than the other relatives. It may be that the successful resolution of the complaint in such circumstances is dependent less on demonstrating to the complainant the accuracy or truth of the practitioner's response, and more on ensuring that the complainant's emotional distress in relation to the situation has been acknowledged, whether or not the patient's death was expected or considered inevitable.

The complainant may, therefore, come to the first conciliation meeting experiencing a range of emotions. They may be apprehensive about the process and unsure of what to expect. They may feel the whole process will be a waste of time but have decided to go along with it as a prelude to moving to the next stage in the complaints procedure. They may also be feeling vulnerable, distressed or angry. Often they will comment to the conciliator that this is the first time anyone has *listened* to them. The importance of this cannot be overemphasised.

Good listening and communication skills are essential, as is the conciliator's ability to empathise appropriately. The complainant needs to be encouraged to focus on the issues of greatest concern but doing so may also trigger strong emotions. This can sometimes have a cathartic or therapeutic effect for the complainant. It may be the first time they have shared their feelings of grief or sense of loss, or felt able to show just how angry they feel towards the person whom they hold accountable.

The way in which a complaint is expressed in writing may give little indication of the extent to which the issues have affected the complainant, or indeed the motivating factors driving the complaint. Part of the purpose of the conciliation meetings is also to explore any hidden agenda, or unacknowledged motive, and the way it impacts on the concerns which have been expressed already in the complaint.

Looking at the issues from the other party's point of view

Sometimes the complainant is convinced that the staff member against whom the complaint has been made has no understanding or appreciation of the distress caused by the circumstances relating to the complaint. This view may have been reinforced further by the initial response the complainant received. Part of the conciliator's role is to ensure that the parties to the complaint not only look at the issues from each other's point of view but also have an understanding of the feelings each has experienced in relation to the situation.

For example, the complainant may be surprised, or even disbelieving, when the conciliator passes on expressions of deep regret from the clinician at the adverse outcome which has initiated the complaint. The clinician may also have felt profoundly distressed by the events, and may wish the conciliator to ensure that the complainant does not believe that they have been unmoved by the incident. Encouraging the parties to acknowledge each other's feelings is an important step in enabling them to understand each other's positions.

During the initial meeting with the complainant the conciliator will also give time for reflection by summarising key issues so that the complainant has confidence that the conciliator has understood what they have been trying to convey. This will encompass their feelings as well as the facts relating to the situation. The conciliator will also reassure the complainant at the outset of the meeting of the confidential nature of the process, emphasising that nothing will be passed on to the person against whom the complaint has been made without the complainant's express agreement.

The written documentation relating to the complaint will provide a starting point for focusing on the issues that have been raised initially, but as the meeting progresses, these may become qualified or amplified as a result of additional detail emerging. The conciliator will need to ensure that the focus of the meeting is maintained, while giving the complainant the opportunity to elaborate on the situation that gave rise to the complaint. It is during this process that it may become clear to the conciliator that there are other issues driving the complaint, apart from those which were at first apparent.

Once the conciliator has demonstrated that they have a clear understanding of the complainant's position, they are often given *carte blanche* to say whatever is needed to the other party. At this stage it is advisable for the conciliator to explain to the complainant exactly how they will pass on the points to the other party, so that there is no confusion about how the issues will be shared. This also applies when the conciliator is relating in a similar way to the person against whom the complaint has been made.

The complaint is more likely to be resolved if the conciliator is able to convey the feelings each party experiences in relation to the facts as accurately as possible. Where the complainant has raised criticism of the attitude or manner of staff members, or the complainant has been perceived as hostile or aggressive to the staff, the conciliator's ability to communicate the background to this will ensure that each party begins to view the other differently as they gain insight into each other's emotions, motivation, or situation at the time. This is an essential part of the process for enabling movement from previously entrenched positions.

Keeping the parties informed

Prior to the conciliation meetings the parties should have been provided with appropriate information about the complaints procedure, as well as details relating to the conciliation process. In between meetings, the conciliator may telephone or communicate otherwise with the parties to report any relevant progress in relation to the complaint, to pass on additional information or to clarify issues.

Although the conciliator will wish to maintain the momentum of the conciliation process, this is not always possible. Delays may occur for a variety of reasons and meetings may, therefore, have to be postponed, occasionally for several weeks at a time. It is most important that the parties are kept informed about any changes to the original timetable for meetings. Sometimes, the complainant's or patient's health is a factor, or the meeting may be deferred because it is close to the anniversary of the incident – particularly if this resulted in a death – which gave rise to the complaint. Healthcare staff should make every effort to avoid delaying the process themselves by failing to give the meeting sufficient priority, since this will be viewed negatively by the complainant.

Numbers of people attending meetings

The complainant may wish to be accompanied to the conciliation meetings by a friend, relative or an advocate. Sometimes a number of relatives may wish to be involved in the process and it will be for the conciliator to decide how this can be managed most appropriately. It is usual for the complainant to act as the spokesperson for the family, although the conciliator should ensure that all family members present have an opportunity to participate if they wish to do so.

Where the complaint involves the death of a patient, a number of immediate family members may wish to attend not only to ensure that they understand what is happening, but also in order to contribute to discussions about outstanding concerns and about any additional issues which may have been overlooked. The exact conduct of the meetings is the responsibility of the conciliator who also has to exercise discretion when deciding on the most appropriate way forward.

Some healthcare staff, like some complainants, may prefer to attend conciliation meetings alone. Others may wish to be accompanied by a supportive colleague, or a senior manager who is empowered to propose or comment on any actions which may help to resolve the complaint. Involvement of a person with appropriate seniority and authority will also ensure that any systems failings or other learning points are captured and addressed.

Taking notes

The meetings between the conciliator and the parties concerned are confidential and any notes made by the conciliator are for their own personal use to ensure key issues are captured accurately. Conciliators may also wish to make fuller notes immediately following the meeting. Note taking should not be a distraction from listening to the complainant and it should be emphasised to all concerned that the notes will not be passed on to the other party, nor used at any further stage in the complaints procedure.

Occasionally notes may also be made by an advocate accompanying the complainant or by a member of staff accompanying the healthcare professional to ensure, for example, that agreed action points are followed up. The exact conduct of the meetings will be for the conciliator to decide in the light of the particular circumstances, but it should be emphasised that the conciliation meetings are held 'without prejudice', and so their content is not considered admissible should any legal proceedings arise at a later date as a result of the complaint.

Length of meetings

In advance of the meetings the conciliator should give an indication of their likely time frame. Circumstances vary and it is unwise to be dogmatic but meetings are normally more effective if there is a clearly focused agenda and they are not too long.

Whether the meetings occur over a day/days as in the commercial mediation model, or with an interval of several days or weeks, each session needs to be carefully time managed. Allotting one-and-a-half to two hours to the meeting allows a degree of flexibility and ensures that the key points can be covered.

Sometimes more than one meeting with the complainant is necessary at the outset to cover all the relevant issues, before involving the person against whom the complaint has been made. This may be dictated by the complexity of the complaint or by the health or other circumstances of the complainant. The conciliator may also need to ensure that the complainant has appropriate breaks during the meetings which will extend the time required.

Meetings between the conciliator and all parties involved in the complaint

It is a common misconception that it is a requirement of conciliation that the parties involved have to meet at some stage in the process. It is helpful if this is made clear in any information, verbal or written, that is given to the parties involved, at the point where conciliation is first being suggested. Concern about the possibility of a meeting with the person against whom they have made the complaint is sometimes given by complainants as a reason for their reluctance to participate in the conciliation process. Others are adamant, at the outset, that they do not wish to meet with the other party in any circumstances. In such cases the conciliator will emphasise the voluntary nature of the conciliation process, and assure the complainant that joint meetings involving all parties are not mandatory and would only ever be arranged with their explicit consent. In situations where complainants require ongoing healthcare they may have made arrangements to ensure that they are treated by a different professional at the earliest opportunity, and sometimes, for example, in relation to general medical or dental care, in a different practice altogether.

Where a joint meeting has been agreed between all the parties it is important that there is advance preparation. This is crucial in order to achieve the best possible outcome. To ensure this, the conciliator will have met with both parties individually, and will have agreed with the complainant the key issues they wish to cover. With the complainant's permission, the conciliator will also have highlighted these issues to the health professional and will, therefore, be aware of the issues that may prove contentious or sensitive.

Where the complaint relates to the circumstances surrounding a death, conciliators may sometimes find that a bereaved complainant will bring a photograph of the deceased person to the meetings. In other circumstances, where the complaint involves a child or vulnerable person, the complainant may wish the conciliator to see or meet with them in advance of the meeting. This is to ensure that the person whose care is at the centre of the complaint is not forgotten, and it may be appropriate at the outset of a meeting with all parties present for the conciliator to refer to this.

In opening the meeting the conciliator will, if appropriate, provide an opportunity for any apologies to be made, having ensured that this has been discussed and agreed in advance. Some complainants prefer the conciliator to put their initial questions to the health professional on their behalf, while others prefer to do this themselves. The conciliator will try to be as flexible as possible, ensuring the key issues are covered while intervening where necessary if the complainant becomes distressed or angry. It has to be recognised that occasionally complainants express themselves very forcefully. While the conciliator will try to avoid interrupting the complainant unnecessarily, it is important to prevent the proceedings from losing focus, or the health professional from being subjected to any kind of verbal abuse. In such circumstances, the conciliator may suggest a short adjournment as a means of defusing tension, and may have to make it clear to the complainant that the meeting cannot proceed unless they undertake to behave appropriately.

The conciliator needs good chairing and active listening skills to ensure that the best use is made of the time and that appropriate progress is maintained. Techniques employed will include summarising key points, highlighting those areas of agreement and disagreement, and listing issues that need to be returned to later. Amplifying or seeking clarification from the parties at different stages in the meeting ensures that each appreciates the other's perspective and that the different areas of the complaint are covered. The conciliator will also need to observe what the participants' body language reveals, and to act responsively to signs of discomfort or distress. The conciliator should also be aware of what their own body language reveals, and ensure that their actions are not open to misinterpretation.

It may not be possible to achieve resolution on all the issues at a single meeting between the parties, and the conciliator will need to consider whether a further meeting will be helpful, or whether to follow up outstanding issues with the parties separately. Even if all the issues are not resolved, the positive aspects of the meeting should be highlighted, emphasising where the complainant agrees that the explanations are acceptable, or approves any actions which the organisation or individual has agreed to take as a result of the conciliation.

Concluding the conciliation process

A point will be reached where the conciliator considers it appropriate to conclude the conciliation process. This may be for any of the following reasons.

- All the issues have been addressed and the complainant has expressed satisfaction with the outcome.
- Some of the issues have been resolved but the complainant remains dissatisfied with the responses or explanations in relation to other aspects of the complaint, and there is no further prospect of achieving resolution regarding these.
- The complainant does not consider that the responses or explanations received have addressed any aspects of the complaint.
- The conciliator considers it inadvisable to continue because of
  — the behaviour or health of one of the parties
  — the emergence of issues which cannot be addressed within the conciliation process, for example:
    — possible criminal activity
    — clinical failings of a serious nature
    — risk of harm to any individual, or the wider public.

The following extract from the New South Wales *Health Care Complaints Act 1993* defines the conclusion of the conciliation process in that jurisdiction in Australia.

'(1) The conciliation process is concluded:
   a. if either party terminates the conciliation process at any time, or
   b. if the parties to the complaint reach agreement concerning the matter the subject of the complaint.

(2) The complainant must notify the Registrar without delay if the parties reach agreement otherwise than during the conciliation process.

(3) The conciliation process is terminated if the conciliator terminates the process after having formed the view:

a. that it is unlikely that the parties will reach agreement, or

b. a significant issue of public health or safety has been raised.'

New South Wales Consolidated Acts. *Health Care Complaints Act 1993.*
Section 52, 'Conclusion of the conciliation process'.

In some cases the conciliation may be concluded in the following situations:

‣ in a final meeting between the parties where apologies are made, explanations given, offers of appropriate redress accepted and possible changes to services or practices proposed as a positive outcome of the complaint;

‣ in a final meeting between the complainant and the conciliator, where the issues relating to the complaint are resolved satisfactorily as a result of the responses provided by the person or the organisation against whom, or which, the complaint was made.

Recording the outcome

In the absence of national guidance in the UK, the exact procedure used by the conciliator following the conclusion of the process will be determined locally. However, it is advisable for the conciliator to write formally to the parties involved so that no misunderstandings occur in relation to the outcome of the process.

Any further details can be included only with the consent of the parties concerned, and it is usually preferable for the organisation or individual against whom the complaint has been made to confirm in writing to the complainant their understanding of the outcome of the conciliation process, together with apologies and explanations where appropriate. Where proposed actions cannot be implemented immediately, there should be reference to the timescale or process that will be followed to ensure that relevant changes or improvements are made, and there should be a follow-up letter to confirm when these have been carried out.

Letter from the healthcare practitioner to the complainant

Where complaints involve individual practitioners who have taken part in the conciliation process, a possible outcome from the conciliation meetings is that the clinician concerned will write personally to the complainant. The complainant may have indicated previously, through the conciliator, the key issues which they expect any such letter to cover, and the conciliator will have passed this on to the clinician. Alternatively, this outcome may have been agreed as a result of a joint meeting between all the parties concerned.

Such a letter might contain some of the following points:

- reference to the conciliation process that had enabled the practitioner to appreciate the complainant's perspective of the key issues
- acknowledgement of the inconvenience, anxiety, distress or discomfort caused by the circumstances that precipitated the complaint
- expressions of regret in relation to any of the issues raised by the complaint
- apologies, which might also include reference to any actions, aspects of behaviour or manner, which, following conciliation, the practitioner realises contributed to the complainant's existing concerns or led directly to the complaint
- additional information which might explain, although not necessarily justify or excuse, any mistake, error of judgement or lapse in behaviour or manner on the part of the practitioner
- the practitioner's own feelings with regard to the situation; for example, if the circumstances surrounding the complaint had been distressing for them, too
- examples of how the practitioner may have altered their own practice as a result of the complaint to avoid a similar situation in the future
- agreed action plans with timescales, where possible, for implementation.

Where the complaints handling process or administrative procedures themselves have further exacerbated the situation this should be acknowledged, and the complainant given assurances that the failings identified will be addressed.

Letter from the healthcare organisation to the complainant

It is a requirement of the NHS complaints procedure that the final letter responding to a complaint is sent by the healthcare organisation concerned. It is, therefore, appropriate that where conciliation has been used as part of the local resolution process the outcomes are recorded in this letter. This provides an opportunity for:

- apologies to be made
- mistakes to be acknowledged
- explanations to be given, together with details of investigations into different aspects of the complaint
- learning points to be highlighted, together with recognition of any training needs
- agreed action plans to be included, together with timescales for implementation where possible.

'The complaints manager must prepare a written response to the complaint which summarises the nature and substance of the complaint, describes the investigation under regulation 12 and summarises its conclusions.'

Statutory Instrument 2004 No. 1768. *The National Health Service (Complaints) Regulations 2004*. London: HMSO, 2004. Section 13 (1).

It is advisable to give the complainant the option of contacting the organisation for further clarification where necessary. The complainant should also be advised of their right to apply to the Healthcare Commission for consideration of their complaint if they are not satisfied with this final letter of response.

'The response must notify the complainant of his right to refer the complaint to the Healthcare Commission in accordance with regulation 14.'

Statutory Instrument 2004 No. 1768. *The National Health Service (Complaints) Regulations 2004*. London: HMSO, 2004. Regulation 13 (4).

It is also important to recognise that the complainant and the person against whom the complaint has been made can have differing views as to the outcome of the conciliation process. The person complained against may feel that they have done everything possible by way of offering apology where appropriate, explanation, evidence of individual or organisational learning, or service improvements. The complainant, however, may feel that nothing short of disciplinary action against the staff member, or financial redress equating to an offer of compensation, will suffice. This attitude may persist even if the conciliator has explicitly discussed with the complainant the possible range of outcomes from an early point in the process.

Since confidentiality is an essential feature of the conciliation process, there must be no expectation from healthcare organisations that any details will be passed on by the conciliator, unless this has been agreed explicitly by the parties involved. Where the process has been facilitated by, for example, an external body such as a primary care trust (PCT) in relation to the health service provider concerned, the outcome recorded for the PCT may be no more than whether the complaint has been 'resolved' or 'not resolved' as a result of conciliation. Any further information would be given only with the express consent of the parties concerned. This might be a record of any apology or explanation, service change or remedial action agreed, and contained in the final letter of response from the healthcare organisation, which the complainant might request to have copied to the PCT.

What is not always recorded by healthcare organisations or individual practitioners is where some, but not all, of the issues have been addressed through

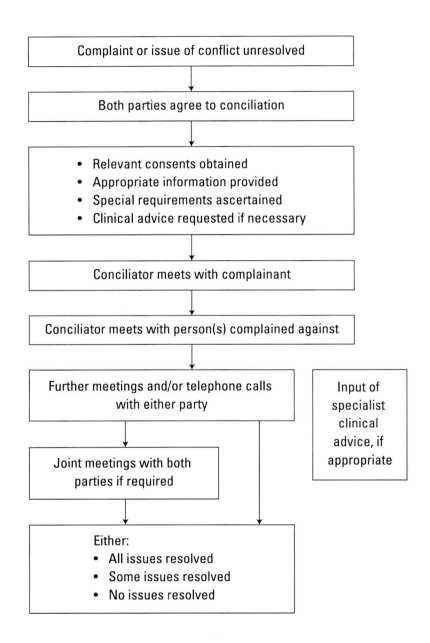

FIGURE 4.2 Typical workflow for the conciliation process

conciliation. In such cases the complainant may be left feeling dissatisfied that outstanding concerns remain, and their overall view of the conciliation process will, therefore, be that the complaint is unresolved. There is a value in considering a third category when recording conciliation outcomes that acknowledges those aspects of the complaint that have been 'partially resolved' through the conciliation process and highlights these to the complainant.

This option is possible only if there is agreement between all the parties for such a record to be made, and in cases where it is possible to identify the distinct facets of the complaint. It also provides acknowledgement that the conciliation process has been of some value and has progressed issues further than might have occurred otherwise. The areas of agreement reached through the conciliation process can thus be captured in the final letter sent to the complainant by the healthcare organisation concerned, even if other issues remain unresolved. Should the complainant wish to refer the outstanding issues to the Healthcare Commission for an independent review of their complaint, this process will be expedited if what has been addressed already through conciliation has been documented clearly.

CHAPTER 5

Conciliation and health service staff

- ➡ The impact of complaints on healthcare staff.
- ➡ Grievances and conflicts within teams.

The impact of complaints on healthcare staff

A feature of the conciliation process is that it provides a supportive and 'protected' environment in which the parties concerned can address issues arising from complaints or situations of conflict or disagreement. Healthcare organisations need to consider the impact complaints can have on individual members of staff and ensure that these are mitigated by appropriate training and complaints handling, including, where appropriate, the use of conciliation. The importance of support for all parties involved in a complaint should not be underestimated. Earlier chapters in this book highlight this point in relation to the complainant, but the staff against whom a complaint has been made may also need support. This will depend not only on the individual's own coping skills in the face of a potentially stressful situation, but also on the extent to which the organisational culture encourages a positive view of complaints. Staff can be greatly supported if those who are experienced in handling complaints provide additional information and advice, beyond that which may be available through the policies and procedures which focus on the process.

'. . . within medicine a major and increasing stressor includes a fear of making mistakes and of litigation and complaints.'

National Clinical Assessment Authority. *Understanding performance difficulties in doctors.* NCAA, London, 2004.

The conciliation process itself can be very supportive for staff. For example, where the complaint involves the death of a patient, particularly if this was unexpected, staff may feel affected personally by their inability to have prevented this outcome. They may have differing attitudes towards the prospect of meeting with the complainant in such circumstances. Some may feel relieved if this is not required, and also reassured to discover that it is still possible for the complaint to be resolved through conciliation without a face-to-face meeting.

Alternatively, a health professional may be particularly anxious to meet with the complainant to try to achieve some kind of reconciliation at the same time as resolving the issues. Where the complainant does not wish for such a meeting, the conciliator will need to explain to the staff member that it may still be possible for the complainant to view the situation differently and to gain an understanding of the health professional's perspective. Sometimes the health professional assumes that the restoration of their relationship with the complainant will be a natural corollary to the resolution of the complaint. This may be expecting too much in a short time frame, especially if the complainant continues to believe that the health professional is responsible for whatever loss or distress they have experienced.

Where conciliation is being considered, practitioners may have a number of concerns about what this involves, and it will be of considerable benefit to the organisation if the complaints handling staff have a good understanding themselves of what conciliation entails. In addition, accurate written information for staff involved in a complaint can help to dispel some of the misconceptions surrounding this process, such as the belief that both parties are always brought together for a joint meeting.

Members of staff against whom a complaint has been made may also need emotional support. It should never be assumed that because someone is a highly skilled and experienced professional they may not feel vulnerable and distressed when a serious complaint is made against them. This may apply as much to a senior member of staff as to a newly appointed practitioner. Neither may have received a complaint before, and depending on the nature of the issues raised, each may, in equal measure, feel angry, bemused, anxious or distressed. They may question their professional ability and competence just as closely and critically as the complainant.

> 'While it is easy to say that complaints should be welcomed as a means of improving services, it is a very human response to feel undermined and personally criticised.'
>
> Department of Health. *Making amends: a consultation paper setting out proposals for reforming the approach to clinical negligence in the NHS. A report by the Chief Medical Officer.* Department of Health, 2003.

The circumstances in which the complaint has been made will inevitably impact on the way the member of staff reacts.

- There may have been a serious incident:
  — they may feel that an adverse outcome could not have been prevented
  — they may be aware that mistakes were made that could have been avoided.
- They may feel that given the particular circumstances, they acted appropriately.
- They may have been subject to verbal or written allegations of incompetence, or negligence.

The complainant may hold the practitioner personally accountable for the situation which led to the complaint, and may believe that the complaints process itself is equivalent to a disciplinary process. It is, therefore, important to clarify this, where necessary, to avoid any misunderstandings and to ensure that the person who has been complained against also clearly understands the distinction. Certainly there is evidence that health professionals occasionally view the complaints process in the same light as disciplinary action. They may also feel that participation in the process is in itself a form of punishment. Some complainants too may state, quite explicitly to the conciliator, that part of their reason for complaining is a desire to punish the health professional. Where this desire to punish the health professional is not expressed explicitly it may, nevertheless, be an underlying issue which prevents or inhibits resolution of the complaint. Equally, where the complainant believes the health professional to be responsible for the situation which led to the complaint, their anger or grief may prevent them from accepting any explanations. It may be difficult for the practitioner to appreciate this if all the issues have been covered as thoroughly as possible, but it is nevertheless a reality in some circumstances.

> 'Although the complaints process is distinct from the disciplinary process, the term "disciplinary complaints process" is widely understood by doctors in New Zealand.'
>
> Cunningham W. The medical complaints and disciplinary process in New Zealand: doctors' suggestions for change. *New Zealand Medical Journal.* 2004; 117(1198). www.nzma.org.nz/journal/117-1198/974/

A speedy and effective complaints process benefits the person against whom the complaint has been made as much as it does the complainant. An unduly protracted process helps neither party nor the organisation itself. Complainants sometimes comment that 'life has been put on hold', and this can apply to the health professional too. When researching the effects of complaints on general practitioners, Jain and Ogden noted in 1999 that there was a negative outcome for some participants in their study, including practising defensively, and even leaving general practice. Few at that time described the complaint as a learning experience.

➡ 'Patients' complaints against general practitioners are increasing.

➡ Negative experiences of a complaint were shock, being out of control, depression, suicide, doubts about clinical competence, conflicts with family and colleagues, defensive practice, and a decision to leave general practice.

➡ A minority of participants expressed immunity towards complaints and a small minority saw complaints as a learning experience.'

Key messages from: Jain A, Ogden J. General practitioners' experiences of patients' complaints: qualitative study. *BMJ.* 1999; 318: 1596–9.

The stressful effects of the experience may also be evident when staff take sick leave on receipt of a complaint. Some organisations hold the view that the complaint cannot be pursued until the member of staff has returned to work. However, an offer of support may be appropriate, together with an opportunity for the staff member to receive advice and guidance about the complaints process. Periodic training relating to complaints handling, and an awareness of the relevant procedures, may also enable staff to cope more effectively should a situation arise where a complaint is made against them.

'A complaints system is of no value unless those who are intended to use it (customers, clients, patients, etc.) know of its existence and unless staff within the organisation are trained to operate it effectively.'

Smith J. *Shipman Inquiry. Six reports, published between 2002 and 2005.* (Command Papers: Cm 5853, 5854, 6249, 6349) (The fifth Shipman report, 2004, Chapter 12, 'Clinical Governance', paragraph 12.8)

Ideally, all new staff should receive training in complaints handling as part of their induction, while even experienced staff should receive it as part of their ongoing professional development, and specific training needs should be identified through regular appraisal.

'Training for staff at all levels will help overcome the defensive reaction which most claimants and complainants feel is the current automatic response to their concerns.'

Department of Health. *Making amends: a consultation paper setting out proposals for reforming the approach to clinical negligence in the NHS. A report by the Chief Medical Officer.* Department of Health, 2003.

The nature of the support provided to staff may also help to ensure that any negative effects on a health professional's clinical practice are minimised. It is not uncommon for a practitioner's confidence to be shaken severely, resulting in either defensive practice or heightened anxiety generated by similar circumstances to those in which the complaint arose. Conversely, where practitioners are encouraged to view complaints positively as a learning experience, there is potential for clinical practice to be enhanced. The effects of complaints on health professionals' clinical practices, as well as the psychological impacts, have been observed in a number of studies across the world and highlight an area in which further research could prove beneficial.

'It is possible, however, that the delivery of patient care may be impaired if the complaints process has a negative impact on the self of the doctor and on the doctor–patient relationship.'

Cunningham W. The medical complaints and disciplinary process in New Zealand: doctors' suggestions for change. *New Zealand Medical Journal.* 2004; 117(1198). www.nzma.org.nz/journal/117-1198/974/

The private meetings held during the conciliation process between the conciliator and the health professional can provide an opportunity for the expression of the strong emotions which are sometimes experienced in relation to a complaint. A sense of loss of control is not uncommon in relation to either party, although practitioners may express bewilderment at this particular effect of the complaint on themselves. Occasionally, they may refer to the impact the complaint is having on their home or work life and express a willingness to do whatever is necessary to resolve the situation. In some cases they may also show deep distress and comment on general feelings of worthlessness.

A key feature of the conciliation process is that the parties concerned should find it a supportive experience, and that the conciliator is able to generate an atmosphere of trust through the separate meetings with the participants. This is as important in relation to the person against whom the complaint has been made as it is for the complainant, and provides an opportunity for the expression of those emotions described earlier.

The conciliator aims to make both parties active participants in the conciliation process, thereby ensuring ownership of any agreed outcomes. An experienced conciliator can help the practitioner to regain a sense of perspective about the situation and, most importantly, enable them to become an active participant in the resolution process. One of the reasons that practitioners sometimes feel powerless to resolve the complaint is because they feel it is trivial or unimportant, and represents an unreasonable response from a patient whom they may regard as difficult and demanding. In such situations the conciliation process aims to enable the practitioner to view the complaint through the eyes of the patient, and to understand the context in which the complaint arose.

Another positive outcome from conciliation is that some of the deleterious effects of the complaint can be minimised for both parties. In relation to the professional concerned this can have far-reaching consequences.

> 'This study indicates that receiving a medical complaint has a significant impact on the doctor, and on important components of the doctor–patient relationship. It suggests that in the first few days and weeks after receiving a complaint, a doctor may need emotional and practising support.'
>
> Cunningham W. The immediate and long-term impact on New Zealand doctors who receive patient complaints. *New Zealand Medical Journal.* 2004; 117(1198). www.nzma.org.nz/journal/117-1198/972/

Encouraging a positive attitude towards complaints is important not just from an organisational point of view. Staff who feel properly supported are more likely to regain their confidence and enjoyment in their work more quickly. They are also less likely to experience an inability to relate effectively to other patients, which can be a damaging consequence of receiving a complaint.

> 'In the long-term, the impact of a complaint softened – but feelings of persisting anger, reduction in trust of patients, and of reduced feelings of goodwill toward patients was reported.'
>
> Cunningham W. The immediate and long-term impact on New Zealand doctors who receive patient complaints. *New Zealand Medical Journal.* 2004; 117(1198). www.nzma.org.nz/journal/117-1198/972/

As well as providing appropriate support for staff in such circumstances, there are explicit training requirements. These should include encouraging a positive attitude towards complaints so that they are seen as providing a valid means of feedback which can lead to improvements in both practice and clinical services. It should also be acknowledged that clinical relationships may be damaged as a result of a complaint, and there will be some practitioners who feel that their ability to continue in a therapeutic relationship with the complainant has been compromised. This highlights the importance of ensuring that staff are aware of the value of conciliation, not only as a means of resolving complaints, but also as a process for restoring clinical relationships where this is essential for a patient's ongoing healthcare needs.

'[Conciliation] can be particularly useful where there are multiple issues involved or where the doctor–patient relationship has already broken down significantly.'

Royal College of General Practitioners. *Complaining and commenting in general practice.* (Information sheet). RCGP, 2006.

Grievances and conflicts within teams

Conciliation may sometimes be used as a means of resolving situations where issues of concern or conflict arise between individual members of staff. Unless such issues are addressed effectively, staff may feel that they have no alternative but to make formal complaints through the organisation's grievance procedure. When considering the use of conciliation in such circumstances, the same degree of thoroughness needs to be applied to the process as is observed in relation to patient or client complaints.

A careful and thorough review of the situation should be undertaken to consider not only the preferred outcome of any resolution but also the most effective means of achieving it. This will depend on the specific circumstances and may be influenced by:

- the number of individuals involved
- the length of time the difficulties have been apparent
- the catalyst that triggered the need for action.

For example, a situation may have developed to a point where a team is no longer functioning properly and it may be deemed more appropriate to make radical changes in personnel so that certain individuals no longer work together. This type of action may be necessary where a culture has developed which is found to be having detrimental effects on the individuals within the team, or is affecting the quality of services provided by the organisation. Conversely, a review may reveal that considerable benefits may be achieved if working relationships can be restored through the conciliation process.

Conflicts in the workplace can also involve imbalances of power between the individuals involved; for example, someone with an aggressive management style may be unaware of the distress their behaviour is causing to a more junior colleague. The conciliation process can provide a non-confrontational means of enabling the parties concerned to consider the situation from each other's point of view.

Situations where conciliation may prove helpful in resolving issues in the workplace may be identified as a result of:

- one or more incidents observed by staff who raise concerns

- one or more incidents reported by the individual affected by the circumstances involved
- an appraisal highlighting problems with inter-personal relationships.

Sometimes the difficulties which an individual is experiencing become apparent only following investigation of other issues of concern which may be identified by:

- frequent episodes of sickness or absence
- mistakes, which may include clinical errors
- patient complaints
- reduced interest in and enthusiasm for work.

Where any of the above issues are linked to inter-personal difficulties, conciliation may provide an effective means of addressing them.

Issues to consider in setting up the conciliation process are discussed in Chapters 2 and 3, but key points are reiterated here.

- The choice of conciliator is important and any specific issues relating to the individual parties concerned, or the specific circumstances involved, may need to be taken into account so that the most appropriate person is identified.
- The parties concerned must be fully informed about what the conciliation process entails and must be willing to take part.
- The confidential nature of the conciliation meetings should be explained clearly.
- It should be emphasised that transcripts will not be made of the meetings.
- Notes made by the conciliator will be used exclusively in relation to the conciliation process.
- The conciliator will require access to all documentation relevant to the issues.
- The venue should be acceptable to all parties and if necessary should be a neutral location chosen away from the workplace.
- The parties should be offered appropriate support and the opportunity to invite a friend or colleague to accompany them to the meetings.
- Proposed timescales for the conciliation process should be agreed with those concerned. Undue delays between meetings should be avoided wherever possible. This will ensure that the momentum of the process is maintained, and also help to minimise any anxiety felt by the participants about taking part.
- The organisation should ensure that a senior individual with appropriate authority can participate in the conciliation process if required, especially at the point where consideration is given to any possible action which may need to be taken in order to resolve the issues.

The desired outcomes of the conciliation process, both from an individual and from an organisational point of view, will need to be explored. Actual outcomes may include:

- apologies
- identification of training needs
- changes in working practices
- acknowledgement that external relationship difficulties, health or family concerns have contributed adversely to the current situation.

Where resolution of the issues requires the implementation of agreed actions, these should be documented and accompanied by appropriate timescales.

The conciliator will need to terminate the process if it becomes apparent that conciliation is not an appropriate means for dealing with the issues; for example, if allegations of a serious nature are made which suggest that an individual is at risk or has suffered physical or psychological harm. Further details regarding the conduct of the conciliation meetings, together with reasons for concluding or terminating the process, are discussed in Chapter 4.

CHAPTER 6

Conciliation in relation to clinical and corporate governance

➥ Quality and accountability.

➥ Compliance with statutory timescales.

➥ Conciliation in relation to complaints policies and procedures.

➥ Organisational learning.

Quality and accountability

The approach to healthcare conciliation in the UK is to encourage organisations to develop arrangements which will best suit their own requirements, while ensuring these are consistent with the principles set out in the relevant complaints procedures. Some general guidance can be found in government publications, including the complaints regulations and its accompanying guidance; and information relating to conciliation can be found on the Department of Health website under the title *Handling complaints in the NHS – good practice toolkit for local resolution.*

Quality is most effectively assured if there is a robust recruitment, selection and training process for conciliators, whether this is undertaken by local healthcare organisations or by private providers. Complainants and those complained against should have confidence that the conciliator has:

▸ appropriate training

▸ experience relevant for handling the complaint

▸ understanding and awareness of:

— the codes of confidentiality

— the regulations governing the access to health records

— the current legislation in relation to equality, disability and human rights

— issues of consent.

These and any other specific requirements can be included in a contract between the individual conciliator and the healthcare organisation concerned.

Organisations that recruit to, and manage, a conciliation service, should be responsible for ensuring that conciliators are able to undertake appropriate continuing professional education and development. Opportunities need to be provided for conciliators to learn from one another, reflect on their own experiences and practice, and take part in evaluation and quality assurance. It is particularly important to ensure that people with the appropriate skills are recruited for conciliation, so the job description, the person specification and the interview process should all reflect this, regardless of whether the person will be acting in a voluntary capacity, as in some parts of the UK, or will be remunerated.

The Report of the Committee on the Health Care Complaints Commission in New South Wales, Australia, *Seeking closure: improving conciliation of health care complaints in New South Wales* (2002), highlights the key areas of concern that were identified in a survey of the conciliation process used by the Health Conciliation Registry in relation to complaints which had not been resolved at local level. These included concerns about:

- the process of referral for conciliation
- perceived unfairness on the part of the conciliator
- concerns about pressure to achieve an outcome, or that written outcomes failed to reflect the parties' own understanding of the outcomes.

The report made a number of recommendations focusing on specific areas for improvement. Those that are of general relevance in any country are:

- consideration of the recruitment and training of conciliators
- ensuring appropriate scrutiny of the process itself to identify and address specific problems; for example, unacceptable delays caused by a lengthy referral process
- obtaining relevant and appropriate feedback about the process from all parties involved, ideally using an external agency.

Care should be taken with regard to the type of information requested, for monitoring or evaluation purposes, from the individual parties following a conciliation. The range of questions which can be asked by the healthcare organisation involved directly in the complaint will necessarily be limited, and may be part of an evaluation procedure relating to the complaints handling process as a whole. For this reason, more detailed feedback should be obtained by an independent third party rather than the healthcare organisation concerned. This should attempt to capture not only quantitative information about the process, but also qualitative information about the experiences of the complainants and health professionals involved.

Providing the parties concerned with the opportunity to give feedback about their experiences of the process would ensure that good practice is highlighted, and would allow for the identification of areas that require improvement. If this information is then analysed in relation to the overall complaints handling process, valuable data might be provided not only for the individual organisations concerned but also for comparable bodies to use for benchmarking purposes. Independent surveys covering responses from a large number of complainants would also allow for a greater range of issues to be covered, while ensuring that anonymity and confidentiality could be preserved.

Where external conciliation services are provided, either by a primary care trust (as in England) or through a healthcare complaints commission (as in Australia), the provider of such services can monitor the use of the service, raise its profile and note the generic issues arising from the complaints, as well as the actions taken to address any failings. These issues should be communicated routinely to provider organisations; for example, through the use of annual reports, to ensure further opportunities for organisational learning.

A provider of conciliation services may find it particularly useful to evaluate the conciliation process alone. However, any evaluation of conciliation by individual healthcare organisations should, ideally, be considered as part of an evaluation of the whole of the complaints handling process. This will allow for appropriate review of the context in which conciliation has been used.

As described in Chapter 4, the complainant's experiences in relation to the complaints handling process itself, prior to the first conciliation meeting, can affect the progress of the conciliation and, if this has been negative, the issues can impact adversely on the matters to be resolved. Delays in acknowledging the complaint, or in passing on the results of relevant investigations or enquiries, are among the issues which can have additional implications. Some important points to ascertain in relation to the conciliation process are listed below.

- Did the parties feel they were provided with sufficient information about the conciliation process in advance of the meetings?
- Did the parties receive information or advice about any support available to them?
- Was the venue chosen acceptable to all parties?
- Did the complainant feel the organisation was trying to learn from the complaint?
- Did the health professional, against whom the complaint had been made, feel that the conciliation process enabled them to gain a better understanding of the complainant's concerns?

▶ Did the complainant feel that the conciliation process enabled them to achieve the desired outcome from the process, in terms of apologies, explanations, remedial actions or appropriate redress?

As well as evaluating the experiences of those directly involved in the complaints process as a means of improving quality of services, other sources of information relating more generally to patients' experiences are also invaluable. Local and national studies or surveys can highlight predisposing factors which may lead to dissatisfaction as well as to the possibility of generating complaints. For example, the Healthcare Commission in England published a report in November 2006 which focused on the way in which patients' attitudes differed in relation to the healthcare services they experienced. The questionnaire study included over 312,000 patients, and among its conclusions the report noted that those people with the most complex and disabling conditions were the most likely to respond negatively to the questions about their experiences. Understanding some of the reasons behind the expressions of dissatisfaction may enable healthcare providers to identify potential areas for improvement.

'. . . patients with a disability or poor health are more likely to have a negative experience of healthcare services.'

Healthcare Commission. *Variations in the experiences of patients using the NHS services in England: analysis of the Healthcare Commission's 2004/2005 surveys of patients.* Commission for Healthcare Audit and Inspection, 2006.

Some primary care trusts in England, especially those providing conciliation services for both the primary and secondary healthcare sectors, include information about the conciliation process in their annual reports for the year under review. These may cover, as a minimum:
▶ the number of complaints referred for conciliation
▶ outcomes, recorded as 'resolved' or 'not resolved'.

'An indication of how beneficial conciliation is in resolving complaints at local resolution, is that of the 26 cases referred to conciliation, only two cases have not been resolved following conciliation.'

Camden Primary Care Trust. *Annual complaints report, 2004–2005.* Lodged in online document store at: www.documentstore.candinet.nhs.uk/

The Health Care Complaints Commission *Annual Report 2005–6*, New South Wales, Australia, includes the following details relating to complaints referred to the Conciliation Registry:

- the number of complaints where the parties agreed to participate in the conciliation process and the outcomes
- the number of complaints resolved as a result of the Registry's involvement where conciliation meetings were not required
- the number of complaints where the parties did not consent to take part in the conciliation process.

If the use of conciliation in relation to healthcare complaints becomes more widespread in England, as a result of regulation 12(2) of the 2004 complaints procedures ('. . . the NHS body must ensure that appropriate conciliation or mediation services are available'), there will be a greater incentive for organisations to include more detailed information about the complaints in which conciliation has been used in their quarterly and annual complaints reports. For convenience, this could most easily be added to the categories already used for recording complaints information, and would therefore capture not only the numerical and basic outcomes data, but also a greater level of detail regarding the use of conciliation; for example:

- the categories of complaints concerned
- the service areas involved
- the professions of the healthcare staff involved
- more detailed outcomes which might include additional categories; for example, apology, service improvement or other form of redress
- generic feedback from participants, ideally captured by an independent third party.

It is important to ensure that where data relating to conciliation is included in complaints reports this is anonymised appropriately, and does not include any references that could identify the individuals involved or compromise the integrity of the process.

Compliance with statutory timescales

Timescales have the potential to ensure that the momentum is maintained in addressing the issues relating to the complaint, and the organisation's performance may be monitored externally in relation to its compliance with the timescales. It is clearly advantageous for all parties concerned if resolution is achieved speedily rather than being part of a long and protracted process. However, there are occasions when a rigid approach to timescales may be detrimental. For example, a degree of flexibility may be important in relation to achieving a successful outcome through the conciliation process. This issue is recognised in the 2006 amendments to the 2004 Complaints Regulations in England, and healthcare organisations can extend the 25-working-day limit for a final response with the agreement of the complainant.

> '. . . the response must be sent to the complainant within 25 working days beginning on the date on which the complaint was made, unless the complainant agrees to a longer period in which case the response may be sent within that longer period.'
>
> Statutory Instrument 2006 No. 2084. *The National Health Service (Complaints) Amendment Regulations 2006.* London: HMSO, 2006.

Situations where conciliation is deemed appropriate may require an extension of the statutory time limit. The complexity of the issues, the health of the complainant and the speed with which an investigation can be completed or expert reports obtained, can all impact on the time needed. Where revised timescales are proposed to the complainant they should be realistic, and achieve a balance between allowing sufficient time to resolve the issues and merely creating an unreasonable delay in providing a response to the complaint.

Evaluation of the complaints handling process should include consideration of the timescales applied, not only to monitor compliance, but also with a view to determining the extent to which these may have assisted or hindered the quality of the process. Where delays have occurred, the organisation should assess whether these could have been avoided and, where appropriate, implement improvements for the future.

Conciliation in relation to complaints policies and procedures

Healthcare organisations should ensure that their complaints handling policies include appropriate references to conciliation as a means of complaints resolution. Key issues should be highlighted with cross-referencing to other relevant policies and procedures. Specific note should be made, for example, to those relating to access to health records as well as issues of consent and confidentiality.

In addition, staff need to have access to practical guidance that encompasses all aspects of the process. This is discussed fully in Chapter 3. Staff should be familiar with the range of services available to support the process, and should know how to access them when necessary. Local information should include, for example, contact details for advocacy and interpreting services as well as other forms of support for the parties involved in the complaint, and the means to access appropriate clinical or other professional advice as necessary.

There should be clear guidance relating to the appointment of the conciliator, who may also require general information about the organisation, including, for example, details of the service area concerned or the role of the health professional involved in the complaint.

Each organisation will need to produce guidance best suited to their own requirements but consideration should be given to the issues listed below.

- Have the parties involved in the complaint been given information about the conciliation process in a form appropriate to their needs?
- Have the parties agreed in writing to take part in the process?
- Has the conciliator been appointed in accordance with the relevant procedures?
- Has appropriate information been made available to the conciliator?
- Has the complainant given written authorisation for documentation relating to the complaint (including health records where relevant) to be made available to the conciliator or clinical adviser/expert, as required?
- Has a clinical adviser/expert been identified, if required?
- Have the parties been offered appropriate support; for example, from advocacy services or professional bodies?
- Does the complainant wish to be accompanied by a relative or friend?
- Does the member of staff wish to be accompanied?
- Has consideration been given to the most appropriate person to take part in negotiating any form of redress or action to resolve the complaint, or intended to prevent a recurrence of the issues relating to the complaint?

As well as providing a useful checklist to staff involved in the administration of the conciliation process, appropriate procedures can also provide a valuable means of tracking adherence to the key requirements for administering the conciliation process. This will also ensure that routine audit and evaluation of the complaints handling procedures include the way in which the conciliation process is being managed within the organisation. Any procedural failings or areas requiring improvement can then be identified and addressed.

Organisational learning

The complaints handling procedures in a number of countries require organisational learning as an outcome from complaints. This is evident especially in the UK, Australia and New Zealand, where improvements to healthcare may be generated directly by issues arising from complaints.

Healthcare organisations need to identify any common themes and trends from complaints that can be benchmarked against those identified by similar organisations, as well as evidence of timely and appropriate responses. Where mistakes or serious incidents have occurred, failures should be acknowledged to the complainant and the issues investigated at a level commensurate with the circumstances. It is the responsibility of the healthcare organisations themselves to ensure that the lessons learnt in one particular service area are shared throughout the whole organisation. In England, the ability to demonstrate organisational learning from complaints is a component of the *Standards for better health* against which healthcare organisations are assessed by the Healthcare Commission.

'Healthcare organisations have systems in place to ensure that patients, their relatives and carers . . . are assured that organisations act appropriately on any concerns and, where appropriate, make changes to ensure improvements in service delivery.'

Department of Health. Standards for better health. Department of Health,
July 2004, updated April 2006. Core standard C14.

Quarterly and annual complaints reports can be used to demonstrate an organisation's ability to identify trends and areas requiring more in-depth work, as well as tracking progress and improvements arising from any learning points. With wider use of conciliation, these reports could include key themes from complaints where conciliation had been used, and further analysis might highlight other situations in which the conciliation process could have been applied. The extent to which conciliation is used, together with the outcomes of the process, could be benchmarked against the data from other comparable organisations and would have the potential to become an integral part of performance monitoring in relation to complaints.

'(1) For the purpose of monitoring the arrangements under these Regulations each NHS body must prepare a report for each quarter of the year for consideration by its Board.

(2) The reports mentioned in paragraph (1) must –
   a. specify the numbers of complaints received;
   b. identify the subject matter of those complaints;
   c. summarise how they were handled including the outcome of the investigation; and
   d. identify any complaints where the recommendations of the Healthcare Commission were not acted upon, giving the reasons why not.'

Statutory Instrument 2004 No. 1768. The National Health Service (Complaints)
Regulations 2004. London: HMSO, 2004. Regulation 21.

In some countries there is a statutory requirement for certain healthcare providers to submit annual complaints reports to their regulatory bodies. In England, NHS Trusts are required to submit these to the Healthcare Commission. The value of such reports lies in the extent to which the data they contain is analysed and made accessible to all healthcare organisations. This emphasis on organisational learning is also apparent in relation to those complaints which have not been resolved at a local level and have been sent to the Healthcare Commission for review.

'The Healthcare Commission is in a unique position to offer a broad view of complaints about the NHS . . . We are therefore committed to sharing our learning to allow NHS organisations to respond better to complaints.'

> Healthcare Commission. *Spotlight on complaints: a report on second-stage complaints about the NHS in England 2007.* Commission for Healthcare Audit and Inspection, 2007.

Rigorous evaluation of the complaints procedures, including the use of conciliation, is consistent with the principles of integrated governance with which NHS organisations are required to comply.

'Integrated governance arrangements representing best practice are in place in all health care organisations and across all health communities and clinical networks.'

> Department of Health. *Standards for better health.* Department of Health, July 2004, updated April 2006. Developmental standard D3.

One of the aims of integrated governance is to prevent the development of silos which exist independently of each other, thus preventing the lessons learnt in one part of an organisation from being applied to another.

'Integrated Governance is defined as: "Systems, processes and behaviours by which trusts lead, direct and control their functions in order to achieve organisational objectives, safety and quality of service and in which they relate to patients and carers, the wider community and partner organisations".'

> Department of Health. *Integrated Governance Handbook. A handbook for executives and non-executives in healthcare organisations. Department of Health,* 2006.

Conciliation can prove valuable not only as a means of resolving situations where conflict has arisen, but also in identifying the conditions which gave rise to the issues in the first place. An integrated approach, therefore, is essential and may highlight areas requiring special consideration. For example, there may be a correlation, in a specific service area, between patient complaints and significant staffing issues (which may be reflected in high sickness levels, staff grievances, and the use of temporary or agency staff). It may be noted within the organisation that the figures recorded for staff sickness, grievances or the use of temporary staff, as well as patient complaints, are higher than average, but the exact nature of the problems giving rise to this may not be apparent without an awareness that these figures may have their origin in a common source and signal a need for careful investigation. Equally, patient complaints may focus on certain aspects of care but deeper analysis may be required in order to reveal the extent of the underlying causes involved. This is sometimes achieved through the conciliation process and may therefore be an unexpected but highly desirable outcome from a patient complaint.

The benefits of subjecting complaints to rigorous analysis is recognised in a number of different countries. For example, the use of root cause analysis techniques, which are applied to adverse incidents in the UK, can also be used in the context of complaints, and a similar approach is promoted in parts of Australia.

'The techniques of root cause analysis, for which training is being developed by the NPSA in the context of adverse events, are equally applicable to complaints.'

Department of Health. *Making amends: a consultation paper setting out proposals for reforming the approach to clinical negligence in the NHS. A report by the Chief Medical Officer.* Department of Health, 2003.

The Health and Community Services Complaints Commission Annual Report 2004–05, Northern Territories, Australia, highlights the value of applying risk management techniques to issues raised as part of the conciliation process. This enables service providers to ensure that the risks which are identified by the complainant are quantified, analysed, and minimised, as a result of actions taken, so as to reduce the likelihood of a similar situation arising in the future.

'It is the risk management exercise that has been conducted by service providers in response to the conciliations that is heartening to the Commission and demonstrates the value of the Commission's work in enhancing and improving the performance of service providers for the benefit of the citizens of the Northern Territory.'

Northern Territories Health and Community Services Complaints Commission. *Seventh Annual Report, 2004–2005.* http://www.hcscc.nt.gov.au

Importantly, organisational learning can arise out of the negotiations and discussions with the complainant. The person against whom the complaint has been made will sometimes be in a position themselves not only to address the issues which apply specifically to their own clinical practice or behaviour, but also to identify procedural or other system improvements. However, additional members of staff may also be necessary to assist in this process. For example, where complaints relate to individual medical or dental practices in primary care, practice managers sometimes contribute significantly to the conciliation process where complaints handling itself, or the manner of reception staff, has been a component of the complaint, by proposing actions to address administrative or systems failings, as well as identifying training needs for clerical and secretarial staff. Where larger organisations are concerned, the specific circumstances and service area affected will determine which members of staff are most appropriately placed to respond to the complainant's concerns, participate in the conciliation process, and to facilitate the implementation of any agreed actions.

> 'Perhaps as important as changes in process are changes in outlook: the NHS must come to value complaints as a vital learning resource.'
>
> Chief Medical Officer. *Good doctors, safer patients: proposals to strengthen the system to assure and improve the performance of doctors and to protect the safety of patients*. Chief Medical Officer, 2006.

There may also be other issues of an urgent nature that emerge from a conciliation and become apparent to those empowered to propose actions to address the complaint. For instance, it is imperative to ensure that any health and safety issues which may impact on patients, staff or members of the public are addressed as soon as possible, and remedial action taken where appropriate.

> 'We also accept that some complaints may raise issues which go beyond the needs of the individual complainant and point to some more general issue of patient safety.'
>
> HM Government. *Safeguarding patients: the Government's response to the recommendations of the Shipman Inquiry's fifth report and to the recommendations of the Ayling, Neale and Kerr/Haslam Inquiries.* (Command Paper: Cm 7015). London: The Stationery Office, 2007.

The conciliation process may also highlight training or support issues that need to be managed through an individual staff member's ongoing professional supervision. For example, an important concern that patients express is a fear that if they complain they will receive a lower standard of treatment or be discriminated against in the future. In England, the *Standards for better health*, which are monitored by the Healthcare Commission, require that 'systems are in place' to prevent this happening. However, complainants sometimes give the conciliator examples of situations in which they feel they have been discriminated against as a result of making a complaint. This can occur even when the issues relating to the complaint have been addressed by the organisation or individual concerned.

'Health care organisations have systems in place to ensure that patients, their relatives and carers . . .
. . . b) are not discriminated against when complaints are made;'

Department of Health. *Standards for better health.* Department of Health, July 2004, updated April 2006. Core standard C14.

It is sometimes difficult for complainants in such situations to articulate clearly how they have been treated differently, but they may refer to changes in a health professional's attitude and manner towards them. When a further incident occurs which generates a complaint they may attribute this to the fact that their relationship with their practitioner never recovered fully after their initial complaint. This emphasises that it is sometimes necessary for practitioners to be supported in their subsequent contacts with complainants for a period of time following a complaint, and highlights the value of rebuilding relationships, wherever possible, through the conciliation process.

Some organisational changes are relatively easy to bring about, others are more difficult. Cultural changes are among the most challenging to make, yet these are often necessary, and it is sometimes through complaints that the need for cultural changes achieves recognition by senior management. It should also be recognised that the procedures or processes which are put in place will be effective only if those who are expected to implement or use them are trained appropriately to do so. The extent to which an organisation can gain assurance that this is the case will depend on the quality of routine audit and evaluation.

Early in 2007 the Healthcare Commission published *Spotlight on complaints: a report on second-stage complaints in England.* The report is based on some 16,000 complaints, received by the Commission between July 2004 and July 2006, which had not been resolved at local level.

'The top 10 issues raised in complaints reviewed by the Healthcare Commission were:
1. Safety of clinical practices (22%)
2. Poor communication by providers and not enough information for patients (16%)

3. Ineffective clinical practices and administrative procedures (5%)
4. Poor handling of complaints (5%)
5. Discharge and coordination of care (4%)
6. A lack of dignity and respect (4%)
7. Poor attitudes of staff (4%)
8. Failure to follow agreed procedures relating to consent (4%)
9. Poor environments for patients, including unhygienic premises (3%)
10. A lack of access to personal clinical records and disputes about personal clinical records (3%)'

> Healthcare Commission. *Spotlight on complaints: a report on second-stage complaints about the NHS in England 2007*. Commission for Healthcare Audit and Inspection, 2007.

Poor complaints handling is among the issues highlighted by the report which also states that of the complaints received by the Commission during the period under review, approximately one-third were returned to the healthcare organisations concerned for further action. Behind these figures are costs which are not easily quantified. Unnecessary delays can have significant consequences from both an individual and an organisational perspective. Frustrated complainants may resort to litigation as a means of achieving the explanations they had hoped for from the complaints process, and early opportunities for identifying systems failings or other weaknesses may be lost, thereby exposing the organisation to unnecessary risks.

There may also be emotional costs for the individuals involved in the complaint in terms of additional stress and damaged relationships as a result of a protracted and ineffectual process. In addition to raising standards in relation to all aspects of the procedure, improved complaints handling should also include greater awareness of the possibilities for resolution offered by conciliation.

This book has sought to raise the profile of conciliation as an effective means of resolving complaints and other situations of conflict. The practical implications of implementing this process have been considered in the context of the guidance available both within and beyond the UK. Conciliation has value not only for the individual parties concerned, but also as an important resource in supporting the ongoing improvement of healthcare services through clinical and organisational governance.

Glossary

access to health records
In the UK, access to the records of living persons is covered by the *Data Protection Act* (1998), with guidance from the Department of Health, and model consent forms, that can be found at www.dh.gov.uk/PolicyAndGuidance/ by following the links. For deceased persons, the relevant legislation is the Access to Health Records Act (1990).

adjudication
'Adjudication involves an impartial, independent third party hearing the claims of both sides and issuing a decision to resolve the dispute. The outcome is determined by the adjudicator, not by the parties. Determinations are usually made on the basis of fairness, and the process used and means of decision-making are not bound by law. It can involve a hearing or be based on documents only'. (Secretary of State for Constitutional Affairs and Lord Chancellor. *Transforming public services: complaints, redress and tribunals.* (Command Paper: Cm 6243) London: HMSO, 2004)

Advisory, Conciliation and Arbitration Service (ACAS)
ACAS is a publicly funded body operating in England, Scotland and Wales. Its stated aim is 'to improve organisations and working life through better employment relations'.

alternative dispute resolution (ADR)
This term is used to refer to those dispute resolution processes which can be used as an alternative to court proceedings.

arbitration
'Arbitration involves an impartial, independent third party hearing the claims of both sides and issuing a binding decision to resolve the dispute. The outcome is

determined by the arbitrator, is final and legally binding, with limited grounds for appeal. It requires both parties' willing and informed consent to participate. It can involve a hearing or be based on documents only.' (Secretary of State for Constitutional Affairs and Lord Chancellor. *Transforming public services: complaints, redress and tribunals.* (Command Paper: Cm 6243) London: HMSO, 2004)

Bristol Royal Infirmary Inquiry
This enquiry focused on the management and care of children receiving complex heart surgery at the Bristol Royal Infirmary. The terms of reference were 'to make recommendations which could help to secure high quality care across the NHS' and its recommendations influenced the complaints procedures introduced in England in 2004. (Bristol Royal Infirmary Inquiry. *Learning from Bristol: the report of the public inquiry into children's heart surgery at the Bristol Royal Infirmary 1984–1995: final report.* (Command Paper: Cm 5207). Bristol Royal Infirmary Inquiry, July 2001)

bullying
'Offensive, intimidating, malicious or insulting behaviour, and abuse or misuse of power through means intended to undermine, humiliate, denigrate or injure the recipient.' (Advisory, Conciliation and Arbitration Service (ACAS))

capacity
The Mental Capacity Act (2005) states that a person lacks capacity 'if . . . he is unable to make a decision for himself in relation to the matter because of an impairment of, or a disturbance in the functioning of, the mind or brain.' The test is 'if he is unable a) to understand the information relevant to the decision, b) to retain that information, c) to use or weigh that information as part of the process of making the decision, or d) to communicate his decision . . .'

claim
Claims are defined by the National Health Service Litigation Authority (NHSLA) as 'allegations of clinical negligence and/or a demand for compensation made following an adverse clinical incident resulting in personal injury, or any clinical incident which carries significant litigation risk for the Trust'.

clinical adviser
This term is used to refer to any health professional whose expertise enables them to provide advice relating to the clinical aspects of a complaint.

clinical governance

'A framework through which NHS organisations are accountable for continuously improving the quality of their services and safeguarding high standards of care by creating an environment in which excellence in clinical care will flourish.' (Scally G, Donaldson LJ. The NHS's 50th anniversary: clinical governance and the drive for quality improvement in the new NHS in England. *BMJ*. 1998; **317**: 61–5)

complaint

The NHS Complaints Toolkit gives the succinct definition of a complaint used by The Citizen's Charter complaints task force (*The Citizen's Charter Complaints Task Force. Information note: accessible complaints policies*, 2003) quoting the Cabinet Office (1997) as 'any expression of dissatisfaction that needs a response.'

conciliation

'Conciliation is essentially a process of facilitating agreement between the complainant and complained against, whether it be an organisation or person' (*National Health Service (Complaints) Regulations 2004*). 'NHS Conciliation is a method of facilitating a dialogue to resolve an issue. It is an intervention whereby a third party helps the parties to reach a common understanding. It gives space to resolve issues, preserve on-going relationships and time to defuse or calm heightened situations' (Department of Health. *Handling complaints in the NHS – good practice toolkit for local resolution*, 2005. www.publications.doh. gov.uk/complaints/toolkit/conciliation.htm).

confidentiality

'A duty of confidence arises when one person discloses information to another (e.g. patient to clinician) in circumstances where it is reasonable to expect that the information will be held in confidence. It –
a. is a legal obligation that is derived from case law;
b. is a requirement established within professional codes of conduct; and
c. must be included within NHS employment contracts as a specific requirement linked to disciplinary procedures.'
(*Confidentiality – The NHS Code of Practice* (2003))

consent

'For consent to be valid, it must be given voluntarily by an appropriately informed person (the patient or where relevant someone with parental responsibility for a patient under the age of 18) who has the capacity to consent to the intervention

in question. Acquiescence where the person does not know what the intervention entails is not "consent".' (Department of Health. *Reference guide to consent
for examination or treatment*, 2001)

coroner

Coroners are independent judicial officers appointed and paid for by the relevant
local authorities who are responsible for investigating violent, unnatural deaths
or sudden deaths of unknown cause and deaths in custody that are reported to
them' (Ministry of Justice).

Criminal Records Bureau (CRB)

This organisation's stated aim is 'to help organisations in the public, private
and voluntary sectors by identifying candidates who may be unsuitable to
work with children or other vulnerable members of society.' (http://www.crb.
gov.uk)

Disability Conciliation Service

'Through conciliation, the DCS offers disabled people a uniquely accessible and
empowering alternative to court or tribunal action, as a way of exercising their
civil rights under the Disability Discrimination Act 1995.' (Disability Conciliation
Service (www.dcs-gb.com/))

ex gratia payments

These are discretionary payments which may be made in relation to claims or
complaints where financial redress is considered appropriate but is not based on
legal liability.

general practitioners

'General practitioners (GPs) are best defined by the unique nature of the
doctor–patient relationship. GPs are personal doctors, primarily responsible
for the provision of comprehensive and continuing medical care to patients
irrespective of age, sex and illness. In negotiating management plans with
patients they take account of physical, psychological, social, and cultural factors,
using the knowledge and trust engendered by a familiarity with past care. They
also recognise a professional responsibility to their community.' (Royal College
of General Practitioners (http://www.rcgp.org.uk/))

'Gillick competence'

The ruling of the House of Lords in the case *Gillick* v. *West Norfolk and Wisbech
Area Health Authority* [1985] 3 All ER 402 (HL) states that 'As a matter of

law the parental right to determine whether or not their minor child below the age of 16 will have medical treatment terminates if and when the child achieves sufficient understanding and intelligence to enable him to understand fully what is proposed.' A doctor has to judge whether a child aged under 16 is 'Gillick competent'. 'Gillick competence' is also referred to as 'Fraser competence' after Lord Fraser who ruled on the case.

harassment
'Unwanted conduct affecting the dignity of men and women in the workplace. It may be related to age, sex, race, disability, religion, nationality or any personal characteristic of the individual, and may be persistent or an isolated incident. The key is that the actions or comments are viewed as demeaning or unacceptable to the recipient.' (Advisory, Conciliation and Arbitration Service (ACAS))

Healthcare Commission
This is the title commonly used for The Commission for Healthcare Inspection and Audit, which is the independent regulatory and inspection body for the NHS in England (www.healthcarecommission.org.uk). It was created on 1 April 2004 under the *Health and Social Care (Community Health and Standards) Act 2003*. It took over responsibility for the second stage of the NHS complaints procedure on 31 July 2004, which involves considering requests for independent review of complaints which have not been resolved through local resolution. This function is performed in Wales by the Healthcare Inspectorate Wales; in Scotland by NHS Quality Improvement Scotland; and in Northern Ireland by the Health and Personal Social Services Regulation and Improvement Authority. Similar bodies exist in other jurisdictions, particularly Australia and New Zealand.

Health Care Complaints Commission, New South Wales, Australia
'The New South Wales Health Care Complaints Commission (HCCC) acts in the public interest by receiving, reviewing and investigating complaints about health care in NSW.' (http://www.hccc.nsw.gov.au/)

Health Quality and Complaints Commission, Queensland, Australia
'The Health Quality and Complaints Commission (HQCC) is an independent body dedicated to improving the quality and safety of health services in Queensland.' (http://www.hrc.qld.gov.au/)

Health Service Ombudsman
see Parliamentary and Health Service Ombudsman

healthcare provider

This term may be used to refer to professionals who are qualified to give healthcare in any setting, and it is also used to refer to the organisations providing healthcare.

indemnity

'Under National Health Service indemnity, NHS bodies take direct responsibility for costs and damages arising from clinical negligence where they (as employers) are vicariously liable for the acts and omissions of their healthcare professional staff.' (Department of Health. *Health Service Guideline HSG (96)48*. www. dh.gov.uk/PublicationsAndStatistics)

Independent Complaints Advocacy Service (ICAS)

In England, section 12 of the *Health and Social Care Act 2001* places a duty on the Secretary of State for Health to make arrangements to provide independent advocacy services to assist individuals making complaints in relation to NHS treatment or care. The service started on 1 September 2003. In Scotland this role is undertaken by Citizens Advice Bureaux; in Wales by local Community Health Councils, and in Northern Ireland by Health and Social Services Councils. More details can be found at: www.dh.gov.uk/en/PolicyAndGuidance/ OrganisationPolicy/ComplaintsPolicy/NHSComplaintsProcedure/.

inquest

This is an inquiry, held in public by a coroner, to find out who has died, and how, when and where they died. The coroner's duty is to establish the cause of death, where it is not known, and to enquire into the cause of a death if it seems to be unnatural (for instance, accidents, poisoning, and medical mishaps).

integrated governance

Integrated governance is defined as: 'Systems, processes and behaviours by which trusts lead, direct and control their functions in order to achieve organisational objectives, safety and quality of service and in which they relate to patients and carers, the wider community and partner organisations.' (Department of Health. *Integrated Governance Handbook. A handbook for executives and non-executives in healthcare organisations*. Department of Health, 2006)

investigating officer

This term may be used to refer to the complaints manager or '. . . any other suitable person appointed by the NHS body' who undertakes the investigation of the complaint. (Department of Health. *Guidance to support implementation of the National Health Service (Complaints) Regulations*, 2004. Paragraph 3.45)

Local Government Ombudsman

The Local Government Ombudsmen investigate complaints about councils and certain other bodies. They investigate complaints about most council matters including housing, planning, education and social services. (http://www.lgo.org.uk)

local resolution

'The purpose of local resolution is to provide an opportunity for the complainant and the organisation (or individual) subject to the complaint, to attempt a rapid and fair resolution of the problem. The process should be open, fair, flexible and conciliatory, and should facilitate communication on all sides.' (Department of Health. *Handling complaints in the NHS – good practice toolkit for local resolution*, 2005)

mediation

'Mediation is an intervention whereby a third party helps the parties to reach a new, common understanding. It gives space to resolve issues, preserve on-going relationships and time to defuse or calm heightened situations.' (Department of Health. *Learning from complaints: social services complaints procedure for adults*, 2006.) 'Mediation is a private, voluntary, non-binding process in which a neutral third party – the mediator – assists the parties to a dispute to find a mutually satisfactory outcome.' (National Health Service Litigation Authority. *The Clinical Disputes Forum's guide to mediating clinical negligence claims. Guide to mediation*, 2001) A full discussion of mediation can be found in Chapter 1.

Mental Health Act Commission

The mission statement for the Mental Health Act Commission is 'safeguarding the interests of all people detained under the *Mental Health Act*'. It provides advice on complaints made by persons detained under the *Mental Health Act* (1983, amended 2007) in England and Wales.

National Audit Office

The National Audit Office is a UK institution that is independent of government. Its purpose is to scrutinise public spending on behalf of Parliament. An important recent publication with relevance to complaints management was *Citizen redress: what citizens can do if things go wrong with public services. Report by the comptroller and auditor general.* (HC 21 Session 2004–2005). London: The Stationery Office.

National Clinical Assessment Authority (NCAA)

This UK organisation has become the National Clinical Assessment Service (NCAS), and is now part of the National Patient Safety Agency (q.v.). Its purpose is that it 'promotes patient safety by providing confidential advice and support to the NHS in situations where the performance of doctors and dentists is giving cause for concern.' (www.ncas.npsa.nhs.uk) Relevant publications from this body include *Understanding performance difficulties in doctors* (2004) which highlights the stressful nature of complaints on doctors and dentists.

National Health Service (NHS)

This is the public healthcare system in the UK which was established in 1948.

National Health Service Foundation Trusts

'*The Health and Social Care (Community Health and Standards) Act 2003* establishes NHS Foundation Trusts as independent public benefit corporations modelled on co-operative and mutual traditions.' (Department of Health website, Policy and Guidance) 'The regulatory requirements on local resolution do not apply to NHS Foundation Trusts. NHS Foundation Trusts are able to develop their own local systems for handling complaints' (2.11). '. . . However, where a complainant is unhappy with the outcome of any investigation of their complaint by an NHS Foundation Trust, or the NHS Foundation Trust has no local complaints procedure in place, the complainant can ask the Healthcare Commission for an independent review of their complaint' (2.12). (Department of Health. *Guidance to support implementation of the National Health Service (Complaints) Regulations*, 2004)

National Health Service Litigation Authority (NHSLA)

'The NHSLA is a Special Health Authority (part of the NHS), responsible for handling negligence claims made against NHS bodies in England. In addition to dealing with claims when they arise, we have an active risk management programme to help raise standards of care in the NHS and hence reduce the number of incidents leading to claims.' (http://www.nhsla.com)

National Patient Safety Agency (NPSA)

'The NPSA is a Special Health Authority created in July 2001 to improve the safety of NHS patients.' *Putting patient safety first: The National Patient Safety Agency Annual Report and Accounts 2006–07.* London: The Stationery Office,

2007. (www.npsa.nhs.uk/) The NPSA has no specific role in the complaints process, but in its publications (such as Safer Practice Notice 10, *Being open: communicating patient safety incidents with patients and their carers*) it has emphasised the importance of transparency with patients and families when mistakes and medical accidents occur.

negligence

This word is used medically, legally and colloquially, but it has no statutory definition in English law. In case law, 'Negligence is the omission to do something which a reasonable man, guided upon those considerations which ordinarily regulate the conduct of human affairs, would do, or doing something which a prudent and reasonable man would not do.' Per Alderson B., *Blyth* v. *Birmingham Waterworks Co.* (1856). For professionals (especially doctors) the 'Bolam' test for negligence is used: the 'Bolam' principle is that a doctor is *not* negligent if he or she practises in a manner accepted at the time as proper by a responsible body of medical opinion. *Bolam* v. *Friern Barnet Hospital* (1957). For the purposes of NHS indemnity in England, negligence is defined as 'A breach of duty of care by members of the health care professions employed by NHS bodies or by others consequent on decisions or judgements made by members of those professions acting in their professional capacity in the course of their employment, and which are admitted as negligent by the employer or are determined as such through the legal process.' (National Health Service Executive. *NHS indemnity: arrangements for clinical negligence claims in the NHS*. Department of Health, 1996)

NHS Redress Act 2006

This Act allows for the introduction in England and Wales of 'a scheme for the purpose of enabling redress to be provided without recourse to civil proceedings'. (*NHS Redress Act, 2006*. London: HMSO, 2006)

Northern Territories Health and Community Service Complaints Commission

'The Health and Community Services Complaints Commission is an independent statutory body, co-located within the Office of the Ombudsman for the Northern Territory.' (http://www.nt.gov.au/omb_hcscc/hcscc/)

ombudsman

see Parliamentary and Health Service Ombudsman or Local Government Ombudsman

Parliamentary and Health Service Ombudsman

The Parliamentary and Health Service Ombudsman in the UK states: 'We carry out independent investigations into complaints about UK government departments and their agencies, and the NHS in England – and help improve public services as a result.' (www.ombudsman.org.uk/). Similar roles exist for Ombudsmen in other jurisdictions.

Guidance to support implementation of the National Health Service (Complaints) Regulations 2004 states:

'6.1 The Health Service Ombudsman considers complaints made by or on behalf of people who have suffered an injustice or hardship because of unsatisfactory treatment or service by the NHS or by private health providers who have provided NHS funded treatment to the individual.

6.2 The Ombudsman is independent of the NHS and of government and derives her powers from the Health Service Commissioners Act 1993 (the 1993 Act), as subsequently amended.

6.8 Anyone wishing to complain to the Ombudsman must normally have put their complaint first to the NHS organisation or practitioner concerned. However, the Ombudsman has the power to consider complaints that have not been put to the relevant NHS body and/or where the first two stages of the complaints procedure have not been exhausted where she considers that, in the circumstances of the particular case, it is not reasonable to expect this.'

Patient Advice and Liaison Service (PALS)

'The core functions of PALS are to:
- be identifiable and accessible to patients, their carers, friends and families
- provide on the spot help in every Trust with the power to negotiate immediate solutions or speedy resolution of problems
- act as a gateway to appropriate independent advice and advocacy support from local and national sources
- provide accurate information to patients, carers and families, about the Trust's services, and about other health related issues
- act as a catalyst for change and improvement by providing the Trust with information and feedback on problems arising and gaps in services
- operate within a local network with other PALS in their area and work across organisational boundaries
- support staff at all levels within the Trust to develop a responsive culture.'

(Department of Health/PALS National Development Group. *PALS Core National Standards and Evaluation Framework: Assessing performance against National Core Standards for PALS.* Department of Health, 2003)

practitioner
This term is used synonymously with 'clinician' and can be taken to refer to any health professional. The context in which it is used will make it clear if this relates specifically to a medical, dental, nursing or other practitioner.

primary care
'The frontline of the NHS is officially called primary care. The initial contact for many people when they develop a health problem is with a member of the primary care team, usually their GP. Many other health professionals work as part of this frontline team – nurses, health visitors, dentists, opticians, pharmacists and a range of specialist therapists. NHS Direct and NHS walk-in centres are also primary care services.' (Public Health Electronic Library: http://www.phel.gov.uk/)

primary care trusts
'Primary care trusts (PCTs) are responsible for planning and commissioning health services for their local population. For example, PCTs must make sure there are enough GPs to serve the community and that they are accessible to patients. PCTs must also guarantee the provision of other health services including hospitals, dentists, mental health care, walk-in centres, NHS Direct, patient transport (including accident and emergency), population screening, pharmacies and opticians. In addition, they are responsible for integrating health and social care so the two systems work together for patients.' (Public Health Electronic Library: http://www.phel.gov.uk/)

'rights based conciliation'
This term is sometimes used to refer to the particular conciliation process that is adopted when the individual or organisation against which the complaint is being made has specific obligations toward the complainant.

Royal College of General Practitioners
'The Royal College of General Practitioners (RCGP) is the academic organisation in the UK for general practitioners. Its aim is to encourage and maintain the highest standards of general medical practice and act as the "voice" of general practitioners on education, training and standards issues.' The RCGP gives constructive advice for General Practitioners on how to deal with complaints. For further information go to: www.rcgp.org.uk.

secondary care
'Specialised medical services and commonplace hospital care (outpatient and inpatient services). Access is often via referral from primary health care services.'

(Wanless D. *Securing good health for the whole population: final report*. London: HM Treasury, 2004)

Shipman inquiry

This Independent Public Inquiry was instituted following the conviction, in 2000, of Harold Frederick Shipman for the murder of 15 of his patients while he was a general practitioner. Six reports were published between 2002 and 2005 and a number of comments and recommendations were made in relation to the NHS complaints procedures. (http://www.the-shipman-inquiry.org.uk)

Standards for better health

'The standards describe the level of quality that health care organisations, including NHS Foundation Trusts, and private and voluntary providers of NHS care, will be expected to meet in terms of safety; clinical and cost effectiveness; governance; patient focus; accessible and responsive care; care environment and amenities; and public health.' (Department of Health. *Standards for better health*, 2006)

vexatious complainants

'These are sometimes described as habitual, persistent, or prolific complainants, and are identified by the types of behaviours listed below:
- complains about every part of the health system regardless of the issue
- seeks attention by contacting several agencies and individuals
- always repeats full complaint
- automatically responds to any letter from the trust
- insists that they have not received an adequate response
- focuses on a trivial matter
- is abusive or aggressive.'

(Department of Health. *Handling complaints in the NHS – good practice toolkit for local resolution*, 2005)

'without prejudice'

This is a legal term and is defined under the guidance to the *Civil Procedure Rules* (http://www.justice.gov.uk) as 'Negotiations with a view to a settlement are usually conducted "without prejudice" which means that the circumstances in which the content of those negotiations may be revealed in the Court are very restricted'. The processes by which conciliation and mediation are conducted are referred to as being 'without prejudice'.

Bibliography

Access to Health Records Act 1990. London: HMSO, 1990.

Allsop J, Mulcahy L. Maintaining professional identity: doctors' responses to complaints. *Sociology of Health & Illness*. 1998; **20**: 802.

Australian Council for Safety and Quality in Health Care. *Complaints management handbook for health care services*. Commonwealth of Australia, 2005.

Australian Council for Safety and Quality in Health Care. *Open Disclosure Standard: a national standard for open communication in public and private hospitals, following an adverse event in health care*. Commonwealth of Australia, 2003.

Bendall-Lyon D, Powers TL. The role of complaint management in the service recovery process. *The Joint Commission journal on quality improvement*. 2001; **27**: 278–86.

Bismark MM, Brennan TA, Paterson RJ, *et al*. Relationship between complaints and quality of care in New Zealand: a descriptive analysis of complainants and non-complainants following adverse events. *Quality and Safety in Health Care*. 2006; **15**: 17–22.

Bristol Royal Infirmary Inquiry. *Learning from Bristol: the report of the public inquiry into children's heart surgery at the Bristol Royal Infirmary 1984–1995: final report*. (Command Paper: Cm 5207). Bristol Royal Infirmary Inquiry, July 2001.

British Standards Institute. *British Standard on Complaints Management Systems* (BS 8600: 1999).

British Standards Institute Quality Management. *Customer satisfaction: guidelines for complaints handling in organizations*. (BS ISO 10002: 2004).

BSI – *see* British Standards Institute.

Burstin HR, Conn A, Setnick G, *et al*. Benchmarking and quality improvement: the Harvard Emergency Department Quality Study. *The American Journal of the Medical Sciences*. 1999; **107**: 437–49.

Cabinet Office, Citizen's Charter Complaints Task Force. *Effective complaints systems, principles and checklist*. London: HMSO, 1995.

Cabinet Office, Citizen's Charter Complaints Task Force. *Good practice guide*. London: HMSO, 1995.

Cabinet Office. *How to deal with complaints*. London: Cabinet Office, 1997. Archived at: http://archive.cabinetoffice.gov.uk/servicefirst/1998/complaint/bk5top10.htm

Camden Primary Care Trust. *Annual complaints report, 2004–2005*. Lodged in online document store at: www.documentstore.candinet.nhs.uk/

Chief Medical Officer. *Good doctors, safer patients: proposals to strengthen the system to assure and improve the performance of doctors and to protect the safety of patients.* Chief Medical Officer, 2006.

Citizen's Charter. *The Citizen's Charter Complaints Task Force. Information note: accessible complaints policies.* Citizen's Charter, 2003.

Citizens Advice Bureau. *Independent Complaints Advocacy Service annual report September 2004 – September 2005.* Citizens Advice Bureau, 2005.

Cunningham W. New Zealand doctors' attitudes towards the complaints and disciplinary process. *New Zealand Medical Journal.* 2004; **117**(1198). www.nzma.org.nz/journal/117-1198/973/

Cunningham W. The immediate and long-term impact on New Zealand doctors who receive patient complaints. *New Zealand Medical Journal.* 2004; **117**(1198). www.nzma.org.nz/journal/117-1198/972/

Cunningham W. The medical complaints and disciplinary process in New Zealand: doctors' suggestions for change. *New Zealand Medical Journal.* 2004; **117**(1198). www.nzma.org.nz/journal/117-1198/974/

Cunningham W, Crump R, Tomlin A. The characteristics of doctors receiving medical complaints: a cross-sectional survey of doctors in New Zealand. *New Zealand Medical Journal.* 2004; **117**(1198). www.nzma.org.nz/journal/116-1183/625/

Daniel AE, Burn RJ, Horarik S. Patients' complaints about medical practice. *Medical Journal of Australia.* 1999; **170**: 598–602.

Data Protection Act 1998. London: HMSO, 1998.

Department for Education and Skills. *Getting the best from complaints: social care complaints and representations for children, young people and others.* Department for Education and Skills, 2006. www.everychildmatters.gov.uk/resources-and-practice/IG00152/

Department of Health. *Confidentiality: NHS code of practice.* Department of Health, 2003.

Department of Health. *Creating a patient-led NHS: delivering the NHS Improvement Plan.* Department of Health, 2005.

Department of Health. *Directions to health authorities on dealing with complaints about family health services practitioners and providers of personal medical services.* Department of Health, 1998.

Department of Health. *Directions to NHS Trusts, health authorities and special health authorities for special hospitals on hospital complaints procedures.* Department of Health, 1998.

Department of Health. *Guidance to support implementation of the National Health Service (Complaints) Regulations.* Department of Health, 2004.

Department of Health. *Handling complaints in the NHS – good practice toolkit for local resolution.* Department of Health, 2005. Accessible at: www.dh.gov.uk, Home > Publications and statistics > Publications > Publications policy and guidance.

Department of Health. *Health Service Guideline HSG (96)48.* Department of Health, 1996.

Department of Health. *Integrated Governance Handbook. A handbook for executives and non-executives in healthcare organisations.* Department of Health, 2006.

Department of Health. *Learning from complaints: social services complaints procedure for adults.* Department of Health, 2006.

Department of Health. *Making amends: a consultation paper setting out proposals for reforming the approach to clinical negligence in the NHS. A report by the Chief Medical Officer.* Department of Health, 2003.

Department of Health. *Making things better? A report on the reform of the NHS complaints procedure in England.* (HC 413). London: The Stationery Office, 2005.

Department of Health. *NHS Complaints Procedure National Evaluation. System Three Social Research and the York Health Economics Consortium.* Department of Health, 2001.

Department of Health. *NHS redress: improving the response to patients.* Department of Health, 2005.

Department of Health. *Reference guide to consent for examination or treatment.* Department of Health, 2001.

Department of Health. *Standards for better health.* Department of Health, July 2004, updated April 2006.

Department of Health. *Supporting staff, improving services – guidance to support implementation of the National Health Service (Complaints) Amendment Regulations (SI 2006 No. 2084).* Department of Health, 2006.

Department of Health and King's Fund. *Improving the patient experience – celebrating achievement: enhancing the healing environment programme. Best practice guidance.* Department of Health, 2006.

Department of Health/PALS National Development Group. *PALS evaluation framework: Assessing performance against National Core Standards for PALS.* Department of Health, 2003.

Doig G. Responding to formal complaints about the emergency department: lessons from the service marketing literature. *Emergency Medicine Australasia.* 2004; **16**: 353.

Furniss R, Ormond-Walshe S. An alternative to the clinical negligence system. *BMJ.* 2007; **334**: 400–401.

General Medical Council. *Good medical practice.* General Medical Council, 2006.

GMC – *see* General Medical Council.

Gunn C. *A practical guide to complaints handling in the context of clinical governance.* London: Churchill Livingstone, 2001.

Health and Social Care Act 2001. London: HMSO, 2001.

Health and Social Care (Community Health and Standards) Act 2003. London: HMSO, 2003.

Healthcare Commission. *Complaints* (leaflet). Commission for Healthcare Audit and Inspection, 2007. www.healthcarecommission.org.uk/ Homepage > contact us > complaints > complaints about the NHS.

Healthcare Commission. *Effective responses to complaints about health services – a protocol.* http://www.healthcarecommission.org.uk/ (accessed September 2007).

Healthcare Commission. *Putting patients first: a better experience of health and healthcare. Annual report 2005/2006.* Commission for Healthcare Audit and Inspection, 2006.

Healthcare Commission. *Spotlight on complaints: a report on second-stage complaints about the NHS in England 2007.* Commission for Healthcare Audit and Inspection, 2007

Healthcare Commission. *Variations in the experiences of patients using the NHS services in England: analysis of the Healthcare Commission's 2004/2005 surveys of patients.* Commission for Healthcare Audit and Inspection, 2006.

Health Care Complaints Commission. *Annual Report 2005–6.* New South Wales: HCCC, 2006.

Health Rights Commission, Queensland. *Annual Report 2005–6.* Queensland: HRCQ, 2006.

Health Service Ombudsman for England. *Annual Report 2003–4.* London: The Stationery Office, 2004.

HM Government. *Safeguarding patients: the Government's response to the recommendations of the Shipman Inquiry's fifth report and to the recommendations of the Ayling, Neale and Kerr/Haslam Inquiries.* (Command Paper: Cm 7015). London: The Stationery Office, 2007.

HM Prison Service. *Handling complaints about prison health.* (Prison Service Instruction 14/2005). London: HMSO, 2005.

ICAS – *see* Independent Complaints Advocacy Service.

Independent Complaints Advocacy Service. *The First Year of ICAS: 1 September 2003 to 31 August 2004.* Department of Health, 2004.

Information Commissioner. *Use and disclosure of health data. Guidance on the application of the Data Protection Act 1998.* Information Commissioner, May 2002.

International Organization for Standardization. *ISO 10002: 2004* (Note: supersedes BS 8600: 1999). Geneva: ISO, 2004.

ISO – *see* International Organization for Standardization.

Jain A, Ogden J. General practitioners' experiences of patients' complaints: qualitative study. *BMJ.* 1999; **318**: 1596–9.

Javetz R, Stern Z. Patients' complaints as a management tool for continuous quality improvement. *Journal of Management in Medicine.* 1996; **10**: 39–48.

Kraman SS, Hamm G. Risk management: extreme honesty may be the best policy. *Annals of Internal Medicine.* 1999; **131**: 963–7.

Lamb RM, Studdert DM, Bohmer RMJ, *et al.* Hospital disclosure practices: results of a national survey. *Health Affairs.* 2003; **22**: 73–83.

Mazor KM, Reed GW, Yood RA, *et al.* Disclosure of medical errors: what factors influence how patients respond? *Journal of General and Internal Medicine.* 2006; **21**: 704–10.

Medical Council of New Zealand. *Disclosure of harm: 'Good medical practice'.* Medical Council of New Zealand, 2004.

Mental Capacity Act 2005. London: HMSO, 2005.

Mental Health Act 1983: Elizabeth II, 1983. London: HMSO, 1983.

Mental Health Act 2007. London: HMSO, 2007.

Mental Welfare Commission for Scotland. *Memorandum of agreement between the Scottish Public Services Ombudsman and the Mental Welfare Commission for Scotland – September 2002.* http://www.mwcscot.org.uk/web/FILES/mwc-spso-moa.pdf.

Minister of Health. *Improving quality (IQ): a systems approach for the New Zealand health and disability sector.* Wellington: Ministry of Health, 2003.

National Audit Office. *Citizen redress: what citizens can do if things go wrong with public services. Report by the comptroller and auditor general.* (HC 21 Session 2004–2005). London: The Stationery Office, 2005.

National Audit Office. *Progress in implementing clinical governance in primary care: lessons for the new primary care trusts.* London: The Stationery Office, 2007.

National Clinical Assessment Authority. *Understanding performance difficulties in doctors.* NCAA, London, 2004.

National Health Service Executive. *NHS indemnity: arrangements for clinical negligence claims in the NHS.* Department of Health, 1996.

National Health Service Health and Social Care Information Centre. *Workforce publication and dissemination: dataset KO41a.* NHS Health and Social Care Information Centre, 2005.

National Health Service Litigation Authority. *The Clinical Disputes Forum's guide to mediating clinical negligence claims. Guide to mediation.* NHSLA, 2001.

National Health Service (Scotland) Act 1978: Directions to Health Boards, Special Health Boards and the Agency on Complaints Procedures. London: HMSO, 2005.

National Patient Safety Agency. *Being open: communicating patient safety incidents with patients and their carers.* (Safer Practice Notice 10). NPSA, 2005. Available at: www.npsa. nhs.uk/ Public > Alerts and advice > Being open when patients are harmed > safer practice notice – full version.

National Patient Safety Agency. *Putting patient safety first: The National Patient Safety Agency Annual Report and Accounts 2006–07.* London: The Stationery Office, 2007.

NCAA – *see* National Clinical Assessment Authority.

New South Wales Consolidated Acts. *Health Care Complaints Act 1993.* www.austlii.edu.au/ au/legis/nsw/consol_act/hcca1993204/

NHS Redress Act, 2006. London: HMSO, 2006.

NHS – *see* National Health Service.

NHSLA – *see* National Health Service Litigation Authority.

Northern Territories Health and Community Services Complaints Commission. *Seventh Annual Report, 2004–2005.* http://www.hcscc.nt.gov.au

NPSA – *see* National Patient Safety Agency.

Office of National Statistics. *Data on written complaints in the NHS 2004–05.* www.ic.nhs. uk/pubs/wcomplaints

Parliament of New South Wales, Committee on the Health Care Complaints Commission. *Discussion paper on the health conciliation registry. Report No. 4.* Committee on the Health Care Complaints Commission, 2004.

Parliament of New South Wales, Committee on the Health Care Complaints Commission. *Seeking closure: improving conciliation of health care complaints in New South Wales: report.* Committee on the Health Care Complaints Commission, 2002. http://nla.gov.au/nla. arc-55604

Parliamentary and Health Service Ombudsman. *A year of progress: Annual Report 2004–5.* (HC 348). London: The Stationery Office, 2005.

Parliamentary and Health Service Ombudsman. *Making a difference: Annual Report 2005–6.* (HC 1363). London: The Stationery Office, 2006.

Phelps E, Williams A. *The pain of complaining: CAB ICAS evidence of the NHS complaints procedure.* Citizens Advice Bureau, 2005. www.citizensadvice.org.uk/

Pichert JW, Federspiel CF, Hickson GB, *et al.* Identifying medical center units with disproportionate shares of patient complaints. *The Joint Commission journal on quality improvement.* 1999; **25**: 288–99.

Pichert JW, Miller CS, Hollo AH, *et al.* What health professionals can do to identify and resolve patient dissatisfaction. *The Joint Commission journal on quality improvement.* 1998; **24**: 303–12.

RCGP – *see* Royal College of General Practitioners.

Royal College of General Practitioners. *Complaining and commenting in general practice.* (Information sheet). RCGP, 2006.

Scally G, Donaldson LJ. The NHS's 50th anniversary: clinical governance and the drive for quality improvement in the new NHS in England. *BMJ.* 1998; **317**: 61–5.

Schwartz LR, Overton DT. The management of patient complaints and dissatisfaction. *Emerg Med Clin North Am.* 1992; **10**: 557–72.

Scott DJ. Understanding and coping with complaints: a clinician's view. *Current Paediatrics*. 2003; **13**: 376–81

Scottish Executive, Health Department. *Guidance for NHS complaints: hospital and community health services*. Scottish Executive, Health Department, 2005.

Secretary of State. *Directions to health authorities on dealing with complaints about family health services practitioners and providers of personal medical services national health service, England and Wales, in exercise of powers conferred on him by section 17 of the National Health Service Act 1977(a), and sections 9(2) of the National Health Service (Primary Care) Act 1997(b)*. Department of Health, 1998.

Secretary of State for Constitutional Affairs and Lord Chancellor. *Transforming public services: complaints, redress and tribunals*. (Command Paper: Cm 6243). London: HMSO, 2004.

Sibbald B, Enzer I, Cooper C, *et al*. GP job satisfaction in 1987, 1990 and 1998: lessons for the future? *Family Practice*. 2000; **17**: 364–71.

Smith J. *Shipman Inquiry. Six reports, published between 2002 and 2005*. (Command Papers: Cm 5853, 5854, 6249, 6349). http://www.the-shipman-inquiry.org.uk

Statutory Instrument 1996. *The National Health Service (Functions of Health Authorities) (Complaints) Regulations 1996*. London: HMSO, 1996.

Statutory Instrument 2004 No. 291. *The National Health Service (General Medical Services Contracts) Regulations 2004*. London: HMSO, 2004.

Statutory Instrument 2004 No. 1768. *The National Health Service (Complaints) Regulations 2004*. London: HMSO, 2004.

Statutory Instrument 2006 No. 1681. *The Local Authority Social Services Complaints (England) Regulations 2006*. London: HMSO, 2006.

Statutory Instrument 2006 No. 2084. *The National Health Service (Complaints) Amendment Regulations 2006*. London: HMSO, 2006.

Stokes T, Dixon-Woods M, McKinley RK. Ending the doctor–patient relationship in general practice: a proposed model. *Family Practice*. 2004; **21**: 507–14.

Strasser F, Randolph P. *Mediation: a psychological insight into conflict resolution*. London: Continuum, 2004.

Tapper R, Malcolm L, Frizell F. Surgeons' experiences of complaints to the Health and Disability Commissioner. *New Zealand Medical Journal*. 2004; **117**: 1198. www.nzma. org.nz/journal/117-1198/975/

Taylor DM, Wolfe RS, Cameron PA. Analysis of complaints lodged by patients attending Victorian hospitals, 1997–2001. *Medical Journal of Australia*. 2004; **181**: 31–5.

Tena-Tamayo C, Sotelo J. Malpractice in Mexico: arbitration not litigation. *BMJ*. 2005; **231**: 448–51.

Treasury Board of Canada Secretariat. *Quality service – effective complaint management* (Guide XI). Treasury Board of Canada Secretariat.

Wanless D. *Securing good health for the whole population: final report*. London: HM Treasury, 2004.

Ward Platt M, Ward Platt A. Conflicts of care. *Archives of Disease in Childhood*. 2005; **90**: 331.

Useful weblinks

Advisory, Conciliation and Arbitration Service (ACAS) http://www.acas.org.uk/
Bristol Royal Infirmary Inquiry http://www.bristol-inquiry.org.uk/
Cabinet Office http://www.cabinetoffice.gov.uk/
Department for Constitutional Affairs http://www.dca.gov.uk/
Department of Health http://www.dh.gov.uk/
General Dental Council http://www.gdc-uk.org/
General Medical Council http://www.gmc-uk.org/
General Optical Council (UK) http://www.optical.org/
Health Care Complaints Commissioner Tasmania
  http://www.healthcomplaints.tas.gov.au/
Health Professions Council http://www.hpc-uk.org/
Healthcare Commission http://www.healthcarecommission.org.uk/
Healthcare Complaints Commission (New South Wales) http://www.hccc.nsw.gov.au/
Healthcare Inspectorate Wales http://www.hiw.org.uk/
Information Commissioner http://www.ico.gov.uk/
Local Government Ombudsman http://www.lgo.org.uk
Medical Council of New Zealand http://www.mcnz.org.nz/
Ministry of Justice http://www.justice.gov.uk/
National Audit Office http://www.nao.org.uk/
National Clinical Assessment Service http://www.ncas.npsa.nhs.uk/
National Patient Safety Agency http://www.npsa.nhs.uk
NHS Quality Improvement Scotland http://www.nhshealthquality.org/
Northern Ireland Health and Personal Social Services Regulation and Improvement
  Authority http://www.rqia.org.uk/
Northern Territories Health and Community Services Complaints Commission
  http://www.hcscc.nt.gov.au
Nursing and Midwifery Council http://www.nmc-uk.org/
Parliamentary and Health Service Ombudsman http://www.ombudsman.org.uk/
Pharmaceutical Society of Northern Ireland http://www.psni.org.uk/
Royal College of General Practitioners http://www.rcgp.org.uk
Royal Pharmaceutical Society of Great Britain http://www.rpsgb.org/
Scottish Executive Health Department http://www.sehd.scot.nhs.uk/
Scottish Public Services Ombudsman http://www.scottishombudsman.org.uk
The Shipman Inquiry http://www.the-shipman-inquiry.org.uk/

South Australia Health & Community Services Complaints Commissioner
http://www.hcscc.sa.gov.au/
The Health Quality and Complaints Commission (HQCC) Queensland
http://www.hrc.qld.gov.au/
Welsh Assembly health http://new.wales.gov.uk/topics/health/

Index

Engaging and
contestd orks
underpi kills
and stite ld, it
locatecr stice
and lim are
encorag ocial
worlr th

Thbook nt of
soal wo and
cntext o nent
critical

efinition hout
he text, itten
y a dive stim-
ulating, peri-
enced so

Christine shine
Coast.

Selma M oria).

Phillip Abl

Engaging with Social Work

A critical introduction

Christine Morley

Selma Macfarlane

Phillip Ablett

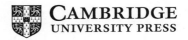 CAMBRIDGE
UNIVERSITY PRESS

CAMBRIDGE
UNIVERSITY PRESS

477 Williamstown Road, Port Melbourne, VIC 3207, Australia

Cambridge University Press is part of the University of Cambridge.

It furthers the University's mission by disseminating knowledge in the pursuit of
education, learning and research at the highest international levels of excellence.

www.cambridge.org
Information on this title: www.cambridge.org/9781107622395

First published 2014

Cover designed by Sardine Designs
Typeset by Integra Software Services Pvt Ltd
Printed in Singapore by C.O.S Printers Pte Ltd

A catalogue record for this publication is available from the British Library

A Cataloguing-in-Publication entry is available from the catalogue
of the National Library of Australia at www.nla.gov.au

ISBN 978-1-107-62239-5 Paperback

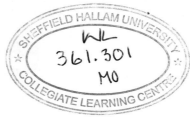

This book is dedicated to critical social workers,
both past and present, whose struggles have contributed
to transforming the conditions that create social inequality
and impede human freedom, and to mitigating
the impacts of these conditions on individuals' lives.

Foreword

In one of the best known quotes from liberation theology, Dom Helder Camara states: 'When I feed the poor, they call me a saint, but when I ask why the poor are hungry, they call me a communist.' This important quote summarises the central point of this book on social work practice. Critical social work is about asking not just 'how can I help?', but also asking *why*. It is only by asking *why* that we can hope to 'help' people in ways that will be more than simply 'band-aid' social work, and that will seek to address the underlying causes of their problems. But asking *why* can be challenging; Dom Helder Camara was called a communist for asking *why*, and social workers have also been called derogatory names for daring to ask *why* the people they work with are suffering names such as do-gooders, interfering busybodies, dangerous radicals, naive, unrealistic and unreasonable. Indeed, if social workers were not called such names it would be a sign that they were not doing their job; being 'unreasonable' from time to time is important for a social worker. And asking *why* is essential; it enables us not only to seek the causes of people's problems, but also to understand that these causes are usually well beyond the control of the person, family or community concerned. Critical social work practice, therefore, seeks to understand and address the causes of disadvantage as well as the lived experiences of people, and this means making the connection, as the sociologist C. Wright Mills argued back in 1970, between private troubles and public issues, or, to use the term made famous by feminist writers, recognising that 'the personal is political'.

This critical approach to social work, as outlined in this book, is not new. C Wright Mills and the feminist writers were not writing yesterday, and social workers have for a long time accepted these ideas as important, and sought to use them as a basis for practice. The history of social work includes many writers who have taken a critical perspective. Pioneers include Jane Addams and Bertha Reynolds in the United States, who worked between the 1920s and 1950s; The 'radical social work' movement of the 1970s was led largely by British writers such as Paul Corrigan, Peter Leonard, Roy Bailey, Mike Brake and many others, mostly influenced by a Marxist analysis. They were followed in the 1980s by feminist writers, such as Helen Marchant and Betsy Wearing; postmodernist writers, such as Peter Leonard; supporters of 'structural social work', such as Bob Mulally; and the anti-oppressive social work writers, such as Lena

Dominelli. Australia has had a strong tradition of critical social work writers, including Jan Fook, Bob Pease, Linda Briskman, John Tomlinson, Stuart Rees, Harold Throssell, Karen Healy, Jude Irwin and Carolyn Noble. Their perspectives vary; many of these authors would disagree with each other, and they have different theoretical lenses, but they all seek to ask *why*, and to understand people's problems within their political, cultural, social, racial, gendered and organisational contexts, seeking ways that social workers can initiate action to address the structures and discourses of oppression and disadvantage.

This book belongs in this critical tradition. But unlike much of the work of the above-mentioned writers, this book is aimed at the beginner student. There has been an unspoken agreement, in many social work schools, that the critical approach belongs later in the course, that students first need to be acquainted with 'conventional' or mainstream social work thinking before being introduced to critical alternatives. Thus, critical social work can become an add-on, an afterthought, an interesting sideline that may be accepted or ignored, but never really seen as central to the task of social work and the institutions of the social work profession. This can marginalise the critical perspective. The refreshing aspect of this book is that it starts with the critical perspective from the first day; critical social work becomes the norm, and more mainstream approaches can be introduced later for comparison. It is an approach to social work that has never been more important or necessary in these troubled times; the context for social work is characterised by runaway growth regardless of social and environmental cost; harsh neoliberal economics, global capitalism 'on steroids' and pervading managerialism; increasing inequality, individualism, consumerism, greed and intolerance of difference; and a blatantly unsustainable social, economic and political order supported by powerful media and corporate interests. Critical social work seeks to contribute to solutions that will address these problems, rather than simply accepting this world as the normal context for living and for professional practice.

One common criticism of critical social work has been that it is fine in theory, is strong on analysis and sounds good in university seminars, but it does little to help the social worker in the 'real world'. It should be noted that the rhetoric of the 'real world' is not just atheoretical but anti-theoretical; it assumes that somehow discussion of ideas takes place in some unreal space, and that ideas can be dispensed with when the 'real' work has to be undertaken. Critical social work must resist this 'real world' narrative; the world of ideas is very real. It is intimately related to the day-to-day work of social workers, and the problems of the people with whom they work. Indeed, the world of the modern university is all too 'real', and the same structures and discourses that are described in the book (neoliberalism, managerialism, outcome focus, 'evidence-based practice', structural inequality, and so on) also impact on the experiences of both students and academics, generally not for the better. There must, therefore, be a clear link between critical social work practice and critical pedagogy; the classroom, the social agency, the welfare bureaucracy and the community group must be seen as connected, and critical analysis and practice must address them all.

This book achieves that end by constantly relating everyday social work practice to critical ideas and analysis. The book's approach cannot be dismissed as irrelevant to the 'real world', however artificial such a construction may be.

Social work is not a value-neutral profession, or a simple set of technical tasks. It has always been premised on ideas and ideals, which have been variously described in terms such as social justice, human rights, values of humanity, interdependence, caring society, public good, liberation and emancipation. These idea(l)s are challenging in the neoliberal managerial world in which social workers have to practise; their values are often out of step with the dominant values portrayed by conservative media, or enacted by managers and political leaders. Hence, social work is a constant challenge: how to help people, families and communities while at the same time addressing those structures and discourses. Some social workers seek to deal with this challenge by working 'below the radar' in their day-to-day work, seeking to artic-ulate and enact the values of humanity and social justice while deliberately not con-fronting powerful interests overtly. Often this can be the most effective way to work, remembering the importance of the 'little things' that can affect people's lives and have a cumulative effect in bringing about change. However, social workers also need to address issues of disadvantage more strongly than this, through either individual or collective action; often a worker has little capacity to address underlying causes of disadvantage as an individual working in an organisation, but by linking with others and working collectively much more is possible. Social workers can readily become affected by the dominant individualism and forget the power of collective understand-ing and collective action.

This book will be, for many readers, the start of a journey: an exciting, challenging journey, which will not be easy, but which can be immensely rewarding. It is a very important journey, even though those who take it will never 'arrive' at their ideal world; critical social work will always be a work in progress, and there is always much more to learn on the journey. It is about involving social workers, and the practice of social work, in the wider project of building a better, fairer, more sustainable world, where the values of humanity underlie all institutions, structures, processes and practices. This book is just a first step on that journey, but it is a really good place to start.

Jim Ife
Melbourne, December 2013

Contents

Acknowledgements

We would not have considered writing this book without the encouragement and support of Professor Jim Ife. Thank you, Jim, for suggesting this book might be possible, connecting us with Cambridge and writing such a thought-provoking foreword.

A number of social work students at the University of the Sunshine Coast (USC) have undertaken library research to assist us with this project, including Lyndall Hall, Tiffany English and Kirsty Roberts. Thank you to each of you for your generous contributions and interest in our work. Other USC social work students, namely Scott Mitchell, Judi Moir and David O'Connor, provided valuable student feedback on a number of chapters, which has been most helpful. We would also like to acknowledge the SWAANs (Social Work Action Advocacy Network of Students) at USC, particularly Liz Duce, Emma Persich, Rachel Dowling, Jennie Briese and Adam Thomas for their positivity and creativity in producing the equality/equity images. A number of friends – Kitty and David Geldard, Julie Matthews, John O'Malley and Trin Davies – have dutifully shared our enthusiasm for the book and given us feedback and encouragement.

Joanne Dunstan, Karen Marshall and Carey Shaw, our much valued research assistants, deserve a special mention for the contributions they have made. Thank you, Jo, for sharing your feedback on the chapters and undertaking the in-depth research, often within very pressured timelines, to help us source definitions and citations for some of the key terms. Thank you, Karen, for assisting us with the compilation of the references section, and for the tireless searches you have undertaken to locate copyright holders across the globe to secure permission for the reproduction of many of the images in this text. We also wish to acknowledge the copyright holders who have kindly granted permission for us to reproduce their material. And thank you Carey for preparing such a comprehensive index.

We wish to acknowledge the Faculty of Arts and Business publication grants scheme at USC, which assisted us to employ the research assistants (named above) who contributed to this book. We also wish to acknowledge the Open Learning and Teaching Grants Program, sponsored by the Centre for Support and Advancement of Leaning and Teaching (C-SALT) at USC, for funding a number of projects that enabled some of the research presented in this book to be undertaken.

We also wish to thank Isabella Mead and Tara Peck from Cambridge University Press for their guidance and support in the composition of our manuscript. We would also like to thank the peer reviewers for their insightful comments and feedback, much of which we have gratefully accepted, and which has helped improve this resource.

Thank you Mike Buky and Angela Damis for your thoughtful comments about our writing and for copyediting the text.

There are too many other people to whom we are indebted to name specifically – they have engaged in the conversations and fuelled the ideas that have contributed to this book. We are grateful to you all, including our students and colleagues who continue to challenge us, and from whom we continue to learn.

■ Publisher's acknowledgements

The publisher would like to thank the following individuals and organisations for contributing to the artwork of this book: Shutterstock.com/Balqis Amran; Michael D Brown; amenic181; panco971; arindambanerjee; Cafebeanz Company; rnl; wrangler; master_art; Dooder; Hollygraphic; ChameleonsEye; Zurainy Zain; Raywoo; gdvcom; cobalt88; Nicku; Sadik Gulec; Adam Gregor; Sergey Baykov; wavebreakmedia; tommaso79; Monkey Business Images; VLADGRIN; Ocskay Bence; Howard Klaaste; Alexey Mhoyan; kwest; Amir Ridhwan; Twin Design; Dirk Ercken; alexmillos; Juliya_strekoza; Harvepino; amasterphotographer; nmedia.

List of abbreviations/acronyms

Australian Association of Social Workers (AASW)

Australian Community Workers' Association (ACWA)

Australian Council for Social Services (ACOSS)

Australian Institute of Health and Welfare (AIHW)

Australian Law Reform Commission (ALRC)

Australian Securities and Investments Commission (ASIC)

Centres Against Sexual Assault (CASAs)

Charitable Organisation Society (COS)

Diagnostic and Statistical Manual of Mental Disorders (DSM)

Human Rights and Equal Opportunity Commission (HREOC)

International Federation of Social Workers (IFSW)

lesbian, gay, bisexual, transgender and intersex (LGBTI)

National Council of Women (NCW)

National Registration and Accreditation Scheme (NRAS)

non-government organisation (NGO)

Organisation of Economic Co-operation and Development (OECD)

Programme for International Student Assessment (PISA)

Psycotherapy and Counselling Federation of Australia (PACFA)

Radical Women's Group (RWG)

Social and Community Services (SACS) (part of the Australian Services Union)

United Nations Development Programme (UNDP)

Workplace Gender Equality Agency (WGEA)

1

The critical potential of social work

■ Introduction

THIS BOOK IS about the potential of social work, and in particular the potential of **critical social work**. It is about what social work is, what social work can be and, from a critical perspective, what social work should be. We use the word 'potential' quite deliberately, as it implies that there are elements of uncertainty in endeavouring to make social work critical that are yet to be fully realised and are never guaranteed. Furthermore, this book will show that to be critical is not to adopt a negative or pessimistic outlook on the world and its problems. Rather, it

> **Critical social work** is a progressive view of social work that questions and challenges the harmful divisions, unequal power relations, injustices and social disadvantages that characterise our society.

is anchored in a spirit of discerning hope. Critical, or educated, hope is not about developing a blind, idealistic sense of optimism, but a hope that is grounded in an analysis of society, and the challenges created by contemporary contexts for anyone seeking to change it for the better (Amsler 2011; Canaan 2005; Giroux 2004, 2001; Webb 2013).

In treating the writing of this book as a conversation, not just among ourselves, but also with you, we have grappled with where to begin the discussion. From the outset, we ask that you keep an open mind, and strive to be humble and courageous, as it is only with these qualities that you can be willing to genuinely consider the potentially challenging and confronting concepts that may lead you to think quite differently, and to practise critically. We invite you to interrogate the ideas presented here and the application of them beyond these pages in a critical way. We also want to invite you to be a little transgressive; to avoid simple conformity with what most people think social work is, or should be, and instead to think critically about what sort of social worker you are or aspire to be.[1]

---

[1] We should note from the beginning that in referring to social workers we are using this term very broadly to include any practitioner (be they a social worker, human services worker, community-based activist, counsellor, welfare worker, social scientist or sociologist) who uses social work knowledge and practices to work in ways that enhance a more socially just, equitable and democratic world. We sometimes also refer to these people as practitioners or simply 'workers'.

In deciding where to begin, we have asked ourselves a number of questions. Should we start by defining what we mean by critical social work, and discussing how this form of social work is different from uncritical (establishment) social work? Should we explain what we mean by **establishment social work** so that we can offer information about the orientation of this book and how it may differ from some of the others you have read? We should say from the beginning that we understand social work as a highly contested enterprise, in that it means different things to different people, encompasses a diverse range of visions and takes numerous forms.

Should we introduce ourselves so that you know where we are coming from? After all, an important part of critical social work is **critical reflection**, and how can we ask you to critically reflect on your own values, assumptions and position in the world if we do not share something of our own reflections about these things? Perhaps we should define critical reflection and discuss the vital importance this holds for critical social work, or talk about why critical social work is particularly important in the current political and practice context. Perhaps we should provide some background information about what the nature of the contemporary context is, and why this matters to social work. Of course we need to cover all of these things as part of this introductory chapter, and we will now work through them one by one.

■ Critical social work

Critical social work has a longstanding and vibrant history (e.g. Allan, Briskman & Pease 2009; Ferguson 2008; Fook 1993, 2012; Healy 2000; Hick, Fook & Pozzuto 2005; Ife 1996; Moreau 1979; Mullaly 2007; Rossiter 1996). This book is about continuing this history and extending its ideas and practices into the future. The word 'critical' is used a lot in social work texts, sometimes with different meanings, and its interpretation depends on the context and the views of the authors. So, it is important to understand how the term is being used here. The word 'critical' comes from the Ancient Greek word *kritikos* (κριτικός), which literally means given to judging, or bringing into question (Liddell & Scott 1940). In Western thought, the word 'critical' has two main meanings. The first has to do with the questioning of ideas and arguments, which most academic disciplines claim to do. The second use of the word has to do with questioning our current society – its harmful divisions, unequal power relations,

---

Establishment social work is a conservative understanding of social work dominant in most welfare systems today, which uncritically accepts existing social inequalities and helps people cope with the impact of injustices instead of challenging them. It is also strongly associated with objective scientific methods for managing the marginalised in the most cost-effective and least disruptive manner possible.

A first step in a **critical reflection** process involves understanding the ways our own values, beliefs and assumptions influence and shape our view of the world. The next part of a critically reflective process is to question how closely aligned our values are with a social justice perspective, and to challenge them when we see a gap between them and our social justice commitments (Fook 2012).

Social or socioeconomic disadvantage refers to those who are low-income earners, temporarily unemployed, or permanently excluded from the labour market (Mullaly 2010).

injustices and disadvantages – with a view to overcoming these. In this latter understanding, adopting a critical position can be a challenging position to take because it means defying the power of those who may benefit from existing divisions, and resist attempts for change (Agger 2013). Being critical may also mean having to seriously question ourselves, where we stand and what role we play in either promoting or attempting to combat the social problems that critical social work seeks to address. We refer to this self-questioning as **critical reflection**. Critical reflection is a core part of critical social work and one that we will ask you to spend significant time engaging in as we work through the chapters.

In simple terms, by favouring a critical approach to social work, we are putting forward a form of social work that is aligned with the people we claim to work with – those who experience **social disadvantage**, those who are **marginalised** and those who experience **oppression**.

> **Marginalisation** is a process of decentring and / or pushing someone or something else to the margins of society (Thompson 1998).

> **Oppression** can be defined as the domination by powerful groups of less powerful groups in ways that restrict their rights, opportunities and access to resources (Mullaly 2010).

REFLECTIVE EXERCISE 1.1

What differences, subtle though they may be, are there between the terms 'disadvantaged' and 'oppressed'? (You might also like to think about any differences in meaning between the terms 'needy' and 'people with unmet needs'.)

Obviously, the world is more complex than understanding it in terms of two sides (later, when we look at theory, **poststructuralism** certainly highlights the limitations of seeing just two sides and alerts us to much more complex possibilities). However, if we simplify our analysis for the moment in order to begin the discussion somewhere, critical social work is about positioning ourselves alongside the people we are working with, rather than trying to protect and maintain the current systemic inequalities and power divisions. It is about being on the side of **social change**, arguing for human betterment rather than keeping the system (with its associated injustices and inequalities) as it is. This is because critical social work is critical of the existing **social structures** that cause some groups (those with power) to be advantaged, and others (those with less access to formal power structures) to be marginalised (Fook 1993). Critical social work is critical of social arrangements that are socially unjust, inequitable and undemocratic, but it is not about simply taking a negative or pessimistic stance; nor does being critical mean

> **Poststructuralism** rejects a singular view of the world to instead encourage multiple understandings based on differing cultural, institutional and individual standpoints and contexts (Seidman 2013).

> **Social change** refers to transformations of societal structures and cultural patterns; not simply of individuals' lives (Van Krieken et al. 2012).

Social structures are enduring social patterns, power divisions, institutions and inequalities that make up a society. Political, economic, gendered, historical and so on, they exist independently of the action of any one individual.

Social justice is an ethical norm holding that society is responsible for, and obliged to prevent, poverty and other extreme forms of inequality. Most definitions of social justice agree that it involves access, equity, rights and participation.

Human rights concern the basic entitlements of every human being.

Self-determination may be defined as 'the belief that the individual or the group has the right to make decisions that affect her/himself or the group' (Berg-Weger 2013, Glossary 1–10).

denouncing everything that the majority of the population values. Critical social work is about acknowledging the limitations of our current society and the systems that characterise it, and exposing oppressive conditions that impede human freedom and **social justice** (Mullaly 2010) in order to think about how things might be different. For example, imagine if we saw the social issue of poverty as being the result of social, political and economic systems that have failed, rather than the fault of the people who are impoverished. How would our analysis of this situation and therefore our response be different if we privileged a social, rather than an individualist, analysis (that ignores the structural context) (Fook 1993)?

While recognising that the problems with our current systems can feel overwhelming at times, being critical involves a constant questioning of unjust and harmful practices based on the hope that they might be otherwise. It prompts us to consider how we might be able to work towards a society that is more socially just – where people have access to the resources and services they need, resources are more equitably (rather than equally) distributed, **human rights** are protected and everyone has the opportunity to meaningfully participate in **self-determination**.

An important distinction to make here is between *equity* and *equality* in the context of social work. Equality means to distribute resources equally. This may sound fair; however, consider the left-hand picture opposite, where the shortest person is given the same amount of help as the tallest person, who can already easily access something. The result only sustains the inequality. Looking at the picture on the right-hand side, we see the shortest person is given a larger (*equitable*) amount of help. That person has an opportunity to participate (access something), resulting in a more socially just outcome.

Similarly, consider a scenario in which one family has a combined income of more than $100 000 per year and another family is trying to survive on less than $17 000 per year. If we gave the same amount of resources to each family, then our intervention would be equal, but only serve to reproduce existing inequalities. If, however, our resourcing of these families was equitable instead of equal, we would give more resources to the poorer family whose need is greater, and reduce the amount given to the wealthy family, which does not need them. This involves distributing the resources unequally, but more fairly, according to need. Hence, *equitable* distribution may appear unequal in allocation, but ultimately results in greater *equality* of outcomes for everyone.

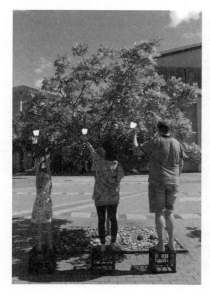
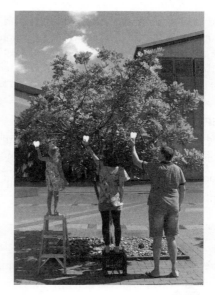

Figure 1.1a   **Figure 1.1b**
[Images reproduced with kind permission of the SWAANS, USC.]

This is not to suggest, however, that all unequal distribution is fair or equitable. Consider the federal Coalition's 2013 policy on paid maternity leave, which if made law will result in women earning very high incomes being far more advantaged than women earning lower or no incomes. This is an example of a **social policy** that causes greater social injustice. For a social policy to be just it must take into account the pre-existing inequalities and differing needs of differently advantaged groups.

> **Social policy** 'is a process of authoritative allocation of material and human resources ... for the purpose of achieving certain social, economic, cultural and political outcomes in society' (Jamrozik 2009, p. 49).

Many authors have written about social justice. For Barker (1995, p. 94), social justice is the 'conditions in which all members of society have the same basic rights, protections, opportunities, obligations, and social benefits'. For former Aboriginal and Torres Strait Islander Social Justice Commissioner Mick Dodson (1993–98):

> Social justice is what faces you in the morning. It is awakening in a house with adequate water supply, cooking facilities and sanitation. It is the ability to nourish your children and send them to school where their education not only equips them for employment but reinforces their knowledge and understanding of their cultural inheritance. It is the prospect of genuine employment and good health: a life of choices and opportunity, free from discrimination (Human Rights and Equal Opportunity Commission (HREOC) 1993).

The current president of the Australian Association of Social Workers (AASW), Professor Karen Healy, suggests that to work towards social justice is 'not a matter of overcoming oppression once and for all, but an ongoing negotiation of power in the current practice context' (Healy 1999, p. 13).

The AASW is the professional body for social workers in Australia; see http://www.aasw.asn.au.

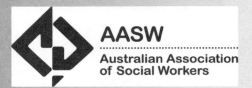

Figure 1.2

In summarising how we understand a critical approach to social work, a number of important elements emerge:

- an emphasis on questioning taken-for-granted assumptions and developing an openness to a range of different sources of knowledge and alternative perspectives (e.g. Fook 2012)
- an emphasis on possibilities for *social change*, and concern with how our everyday actions contribute to social change and *social justice* (or maintaining social arrangements that cause injustices) (e.g. Allan, Briskman & Pease 2009; Ife 2012, 2013; Mullaly 2010)
- awareness that our own and others' personal experiences are shaped by broad inequalities and social structures (e.g. Allan, Briskman & Pease 2009; Fook 1993; Mullaly 2007).
- acknowledgement of how the words that we use to label our experiences create (inter)actions and power relations (e.g. Fook 2012; Healy 2000; Leonard 1997; Parton & O'Byrne 2000)

- openness to being reflexive (locating ourselves in the picture) and engaging in *critical reflection* about our own beliefs, theory and practice (e.g. Fook 2012; Rossiter 2005)
- an emphasis on the importance of understanding others' realities and promotion of respectful relationships (e.g. Allan, Briskman & Pease 2009).

If you have come here to help me, you are wasting our time. But if you have come because your liberation is bound up with mine, then let us work together (Aboriginal activists group, Queensland, 1970s).[2]

REFLECTIVE EXERCISE 1.2
- How comfortable do you feel with the critical ideas that have been presented here?
- Do they sit comfortably with your own values, or are there aspects that you feel challenged by?
- Can you start to make a list of the values that you hold that are affirmed or unsettled by the key tenets of critical social work?

■ Why critical social work?

Some of you may be questioning why we are choosing to focus on critical social work, over and above other approaches to social work. Our answer to this is very simple: for us, critical social work is social work. Although we are favouring a critical approach because this is our preference, it does not have to be yours. We do, however, hope to make a compelling case for choosing a critical perspective, and ask only that you attempt to understand it before making your own decision to embrace it or not. Our reasons for choosing a critical approach relate to our philosophical and ethical positions; in the spirit of critical reflection and a desire to make our **biases** transparent, we share our

Bias is a partial and subjective view that is often seen as negative or undesirable. However, from a critical perspective, all information (including scientific evidence) is connected with values, assumptions and constructions, and is therefore biased (Morley 2013).

---

[2] This quote has served as a motto for many activist groups in Australia and elsewhere, including United Students Against Sweatshops. A possible origin for the quote is a speech given by Lilla Watson at the 1985 United Nations Decade for Women Conference in Nairobi. Watson has said of this quote that she was 'not comfortable being credited for something that had been born of a collective process' and prefers that it be credited to 'Aboriginal activists group, Queensland, 1970s': see http://unnecessaryevils.blogspot.com.au/2008/11/attributing-words.html.

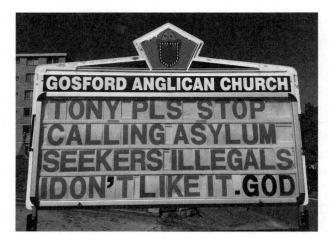

Figure 1.3
Image reproduced with kind permission of Father Rod Bower, Anglican Parish of Gosford.

> Our **biography** is our social, economic, political, cultural, gendered and historical positioning and experiences which shape our interpretive lens of the world (Fook 1999).

> Our **worldview** is the overall beliefs and assumptions that inform our interpretation of life and the world.

> **Critical theories** are 'concerned with possibilities for liberatory, social transformation' (Healy 2000, p. 13).

> **Secular humanism** is the belief that human beings can direct their own *progress* towards greater freedom and equality, without religion.

reflections on our social **biographies** and experiences and how these have shaped our **worldviews** later in this chapter. **Critical theory** is an approach we embrace that shares a vision of every human having equal dignity and worth. With this starting point, any social arrangement that impedes the realisation of human dignity and worth must be challenged. As Karl Marx ([1843] 1977, p. 220), writing almost two centuries ago, put it, the purpose of critical theory is 'To overthrow all conditions under which humankind is oppressed, enslaved, destitute and a despised being'.

This value base, for us, captures the essence of what social work should be, and as we will explore in subsequent chapters, holds particular implications for practice. It is a vision strongly associated with **secular** (non-religious) **humanism** but such ideas can also be found in all the world's major religious traditions and philosophies. See, for example, the photograph above – a message to the Prime Minister of Australia, Tony Abbott, about his lack of care and injustice towards asylum seekers. Without humanist views, the oppression and exploitation of others can be justified.

■ What is the approach taken in this book?

We want to assure you at this point that we are aware that you may be reacting to some of the language we are using. Many of the technical terms we have used so far need to be unpacked, which we intend to do along the way. Over the years our students have told us that we use too many big words. Such words can be considered jargon and our aim in this book is to use the simplest language possible to explain some of the quite complex and sophisticated concepts that we will be covering. Despite this, we remain aware that learning the language of a discipline is part of becoming a professional in that discipline, and each discipline has its own language. For example, you cannot become a lawyer without knowing about torts and contracts. You cannot become a chemical scientist without knowing about molecular structures. And you cannot do social work without knowing about *social structures*, *dominant discourses*, *ideologies*, *hegemony*, *globalisation*, *neoliberalism*, *managerialism*, *capitalism*, and so on. Indeed, you will need to know the language of social work in order to talk to other social workers, to do your job and even to apply for a social work–related position. Understanding such terms will also be invaluable in developing a critical approach to practice. Hence, part of your experience of engaging with this book will be to learn about some of the language of our discipline. You will find key terms bolded and defined in a margin box. These definitions appear again in the glossary at the end of the text, often in extended form. We define many other important terms in the commentary – these do not appear in a margin box but their meanings are included in the glossary as well.

We are also aware that people will be reading this book at different stages of their development as social work practitioners. Some of you will be embarking on your Bachelor of Social Work, Human Services, Community Work, Social Science, or Counselling degrees and hence much of the language that we use to talk about social work knowledge and practice may be new for you. Others will be studying Masters of Social Work (Qualifying) courses, which means some students will bring a strong knowledge base from other disciplines and/or professions, while still others will have been working in the human services sector for a long time. There are also those who may be experienced practitioners who simply want to immerse themselves in the theory and practice of critical social work. Whatever your background, our goal is to introduce you to the world of social work using a critical approach as our lens in a way that is accessible and meaningful.

■ Critical reflection

Consistent with our focus on a critical approach to social work, we will also be adopting a critical approach to education in the writing of this book. You will have already noticed that a key feature of this will be using critically reflective exercises throughout this text. These are to assist you in beginning to think about your own values, assumptions and experiences that are often taken for granted, and about how these may

Transformative learning is deep learning that potentially challenges and changes how one sees the world (Ramsdem 1998).

Socialisation is 'the process by which an individual learns the culture of a society and internalises its norms, values and perspectives in order to know how to behave and communicate' (Germov & Poole 2011, p. 522).

influence your practice as a social worker. The aim of the critical reflection exercises is to confront, disturb and unsettle in ways that promote **transformative learning**.

This learning is not simply about reinforcing what you already know, but assisting you to consider alternative perspectives and to open your mind to ways of thinking that you may not have previously contemplated. Our research indicates that students often describe this process as fun, exhilarating and exciting (Morley & Ablett unpub1; Morley & Ablett, unpub2). Many students, however, also find this process really challenging, particularly at first, as all of us have been influenced by dominant messages that we receive through **socialisation**, our peers, the media, and so on. It can also be angering, unsettling and sometimes painful to question the 'truths' that we (often unquestionably) have held dear.

'Donate to stop the Murdoch media' provides a good example of questioning the ways in which dominant ideas can shape our own views of reality: https://secure.avaaz.org/en/murdoch_fr_nd/?bbnQGab&v=28692.

As DiAngelo (1997, p. 6) states: 'Ultimately undoing oppression means that a privileged individual must come to the realization that everything they have seen as "normal", the true, fair, logical and thus, *cherished*, is actually false illogical, and brutally unfair.' Learning, like social work practice, is not simply a technical exercise; nor is it purely intellectual, but also contains practical, moral, ethical and emotional components. As such, we ask you to sit with the many potential moments of discomfort; keep reading, thinking and reflecting, persist in asking questions, and talk with your peers and tutors. Taking a critical approach requires us to become aware of our own values and assumptions and locate ourselves in our learning about social work theory and practice. Our role is to assist you to challenge not only dominant ways of thinking that are created by society, but also personally held values, biases and assumptions that may create limitations or barriers to critical social work practice.

The basic principle of our approach is that effective social work practitioners are formed through engaging in critical analysis of society and critical reflection on self, rather than the passive reception of information or techniques. Both critical analysis and critical reflection are essential for lifelong, self-directed learning and a vital

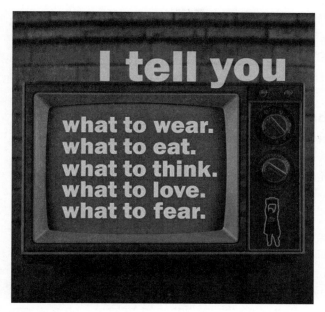

Figure 1.4
Image reproduced with kind permission of Anonymous Art of Revolution.

precondition for any **sustainable** social change (Brookfield 1995; Giroux 2011). Given that contemporary practice contexts may result in students and practitioners feeling unable to make a difference (Ferguson 2008), our research indicates that critical reflection is an important vehicle for assisting students to think critically and independently in terms of how they respond to some of the most complex and challenging dilemmas that currently face the social work discipline (Bay & Macfarlane 2011; Morley & Ablett, unpub2; Morley & Macfarlane, unpub). In this book we will be sharing our

> **Sustainability** means that systems must be able to be maintained in the long term (therefore, resources should only be used at the rate at which they can be replenished) and that outputs to the environment should be limited to the level at which they can adequately be absorbed (Ife 2013, p. 51).

REFLECTIVE EXERCISE 1.3
- What are the main reasons that have led you to study social work?
- What qualities or personal characteristics do you have that will contribute to you being a good social worker?
- What assumptions have you made about what qualities constitute a good practitioner?
- Can you identify some ways that dominant social messages may have influenced your perception?

own and others' practice experiences and research, linking theory to practice (often through using case studies), and assisting you to critically reflect on your own values, assumptions and experiences in relation to social justice in all learning exercises along the way.

■ Our reflections on social work

In the critical reflection exercise we asked you to do, you were asked to identify the main reasons that have led you to study social work. For some, this may have been a fairly straightforward and rational activity; but for others it may have evoked strong emotions in relation to individual or family tragedies, or painful experiences that can remain with us over long periods of time. As part of our professional development as social workers we will sometimes need to make decisions about how much of our own personal experiences to share with others, or, depending on the context and our level of vulnerability, whether such **self-disclosure** is necessary and for what purpose. In writing this section, and reflecting on our own motivations for going into social work, we are making these choices now; deciding how to present our stories and what parts to share.

> **Self-disclosure** is a contentious practice that can be defined as 'The sharing of personal information with a client system' (Berg-Weger 2013, Glossary 1–10).

Christine's story

I grew up in a working-class family and attended public schools. A number of friends had parents with mental health and/or substance abuse issues, or had found themselves as teen parents, and within our school community we experienced a number of deaths owing to car and motorcycle accidents, illness and suicide. I became aware at a young age that there was more complexity and hardship to life than Louis Armstrong's optimistic view of a 'wonderful world'! In fact, far from simply being wonderful, I learnt the world can be a potentially dark, unjust, depressing and dangerous place for many people.

Like many social work students I've subsequently spoken with, I went into social work with a vague notion of wanting to 'help people', not really understanding what social work was. I remember wondering when I started my undergraduate degree: how could they possibly fill four years of study with learning about how to help people? Fortunately, I quickly learnt there was so much more to social work than simply helping people. It became obvious social workers could not help people without a critical analysis of society. Once I realised what this meant, I could not imagine how they could fit everything that we needed to know into just four years – an anxiety

I continue to experience for different reasons now as the head of an academic social work program.

Early on in my social work studies, I became very interested in critical perspectives, particularly in relation to **medical dominance**. I developed a personal and intellectual passion as I read everything I could lay my hands on that questioned psychiatry as the only legitimate way to understand mental health and illness. This became the focus of my Honours degree as I completed my final social work placement in a sexual assault setting. Most of the women with whom I worked in that setting had been prescribed antidepressants, or had some involvement with a mental health service that usually resulted in a diagnosis of mental illness and medication. Yet on very few occasions did the mental health clinician who assessed these women ever enquire about their sexual assault history or take account of the impact of a history of violence on their mental health. Perplexed by this stunning omission, my task then became to find a way to work with each woman and the experiences she presented with, rather than focusing on her diagnosis. I was fortunate to work in a number of Centres Against Sexual Assault (CASAs) over the next few years. The role of being a counsellor/advocate with CASAs gave me the opportunity to offer therapeutic **counselling**, predominantly with women who had been assaulted as children or experienced a recent sexual assault. I enjoyed this work immensely because of the relationships I developed with the women. I admired the tremendous courage these women displayed as they worked to come to terms with the impact of sexual assault on their lives, and still feel incredibly privileged and humbled to have been part of their journey as they moved from being a victim to a survivor.

> **Medical dominance** refers to social arrangements and discourses that legitimate and sanction medical control over the definitions, management and treatment of health and illness.

> From a critical perspective, **counselling** seeks to be both supportive and educational by working in partnership with individuals to explore the ways in which they are disadvantaged by social and political structures and working with them to find ways of resisting injustices in the system (Fook & Morley 2005; Morley 2014).

For about an 18-month period during my seven years of working in CASAs, I was also afforded an opportunity to work with young people who were particularly marginalised, using an outreach model of service delivery. This role was vastly different from working with the adult women and began with an understanding that the traditional, adult-focused style of sitting opposite each other in order to conduct counselling could be completely inappropriate for young people, who may engage more if you go to them. So I would go to them: to cafes, the beach, pinball parlours, the streets, the young person's home or school or wherever they felt most comfortable, to 'hang out' and talk about the things that were of concern to them.

Working as a counsellor/advocate in CASAs also gave me the opportunities to be involved in **advocacy** roles with the police, forensic doctors and other professionals potentially involved in victims'/survivors' lives. These roles enabled me to be involved in **policy development** and **analysis**, **community development** and education projects and **social activism** to raise the public's awareness about the incidence and prevalence of sexual assault in our communities.

My experiences confirmed my belief in the power of education to be a positive force for change. The desire to increase the educative potential of social work practice, coupled with my concern with the inadequate response of the legal system in relation to sexual assault, led me to take on my first teaching and research role, and this has continued in various forms throughout my working life, including my current responsibility of leading the social work program at the University of the Sunshine Coast. I see my teaching and research practices as a form of social activism to maintain the space for critical thought. They are a means of resisting dominant power relations and structures, including **neoliberal** forces, by facilitating transformative student learning through an exploration of the ethical, social and political dimensions of social work theory and practice, and by allowing me to undertake research that contributes to a critical social work agenda. The universities in which I have worked have been based in regional areas where many students are from lower socioeconomic backgrounds and are the first in their families to attend university. These universities service communities where unemployment and homelessness are high, and in the Sunshine Coast in particular, the destructive impacts of rapid urban development on the local environment and community are manifest. Within this context, my teaching and research aim to stimulate students' consciousness about the structural dimensions of social disadvantage, and to connect people with a personal sense of **agency** to facilitate social change for a more socially just, democratic and sustainable world. I have been very fortunate to have been mentored and inspired by the work of Australian social work leaders such as Jan Fook, Linda Briskman, Jim Ife and Fiona Gardner, who have been formative in my journey as a critical social worker.

Social work is a very diverse career path and, alongside working as an academic, I have had opportunities to establish a grief-counselling service within a community centre, working particularly with people who were bereft at losing a companion animal. I have worked as an after-hours worker to respond to people who have been recently raped. My work has enabled me to travel to parts of the world that I never imagined I would visit. This includes Lombok, Indonesia, where I talked to local service providers about undertaking research with them to support their work with the victims of **human trafficking**. I have met with critical practitioners in Finland to talk about globalisation and how social work might make a unique contribution to addressing human-induced **climate change**. I have presented papers about critical social work practice at international conferences in places across Europe. I continue to work with a range of local government and community organisations in a supervisory capacity to assist practitioners to bring a more critically reflective stance to their practice, and have travelled to remote communities in the Northern Territory to meet with workers, community members, Aboriginal elders and town clerks about the key issues they face. After being immersed in social work for almost 20 years, I still feel passionate about its possibilities, humbled by its diversity and inspired to explore how social work can maintain its political core and at the same time make an increased contribution to holistic health and wellbeing.

Agency is the ability of people, individually and collectively, to influence their own lives and the society in which we live (Germov & Poole 2011).

Human trafficking is the recruitment and transfer of people by means of threat, force, abduction, deception, abuse of power or vulnerability, or payments of benefits for the purpose of sexual exploitation, forced labour, slavery or the removal of organs (UNODC 2013).

Selma's story

I came to study social work as a mature age student; 25 years ago my two young daughters had started school and it was time to do something for me and, I hoped, for the world. This may already sound familiar to some of you! In describing my social location I would have categorised myself as a migrant (having moved to Australia in my early twenties from the United States); married; a mother of two children; in my early thirties; of a working-class background (my mother was an office worker and my father a logger); of a low-income status (my husband was an enrolled nurse and I stayed home with the children); a renter; and identified with the peace movement and hippy culture that had characterised northern California – my home-place – in my teens and early twenties. At that time I probably would not have identified myself as white, as that aspect of my status was largely invisible to me; it has only been through some years of developing an understanding of

Climate change 'is the by-product of industrialization models ... [that exploit] natural resources to produce goods that make a profit, while discharging greenhouse gases and other pollutants into the atmosphere and water ... These activities subsequently caused air temperatures to rise to levels that threaten all forms of life on Earth' (Dominelli 2012, p. 12).

Colonialism 'involves the act of colonising, invading, conquering, moving in and then taking over another people's land, resources, wealth, culture and identity' (Ife 2013, p. 198).

Dispossession refers to the denial of citizenship of Aboriginal people by colonising Europeans, resulting in their dispossession from land, physical ill-treatment, social disruption, population decline, economic exploitation, discrimination and cultural devastation (Gardiner-Garden 1999).

Institutionalised racism is the discriminatory behaviours embedded within organisations towards people because of their colour, culture or ethnic origin (Hollinsworth 2006).

Welfare dependence is a derogatory term perpetuated by proponents of neoliberalism to blame and stigmatise people who are receiving government entitlements.

the ongoing impact of **colonialism** and **dispossession** in Australia and the deeply embedded nature of **institutionalised racism** that I have come to a critical awareness of *white privilege* (see Chapter 8).

I had been interested in both psychology and social change for some time and was an avid reader of philosophical, disarmament and self-help literature, alongside my peace movement activities, volunteer work at a local counselling centre, and involvement with various religious and philosophical movements, ranging from the Quakers to the metaphysics of Gurdjieff and Tibetan Buddhism. Lest you think I was particularly fastidious in following these belief systems, I also indulged in various vices, such as smoking and drinking, and lived at times in neighbourhoods that were high in crime and violence, in Sydney and in Melbourne.

It took me nine years to complete my Bachelor of Social Work degree, taking time out for parenting, having another child, experiencing financial difficulties and **welfare dependence**, moving from one place to another and, eventually, taking on single parenting, after separating from my husband. Increasingly, I realised that social work allowed me to encompass my political activist beliefs, my love of learning, my interest in psychological processes and my awareness of oppression and inequality in society, as well as the potential to enter a career in which I could better provide for myself and my children and make a positive contribution to society. After completing my Bachelor degree, I took another eight or nine years to achieve a PhD.

During this time I experienced my own mental health problems, as did a number of members of my family, causing great upheaval and pain. On graduating with my Bachelor of Social Work I was drawn to practising in community mental health where I worked for a number of years in residential, outreach and day programs. It was involvement in this work, along with the experiences of my family and myself, which generated my PhD topic: support and recovery in a therapeutic community. I interviewed many people – service users, former service users and staff – to explore people's experiences and present their narratives. I was particularly drawn to literature about mental health and illness written in the 1970s and 1980s that could be classified as part of an 'anti-psychiatry' movement; while not totally rejecting psychiatry as a whole these writers drew on various forms of knowledge outside the **biomedical model** (Macfarlane 2006) to seek understandings of psychological upheaval. At the same time, I started working as a lecturer in social work within the university system and was heavily influenced by writers and colleagues such as Jan Fook who were developing critical social work approaches that both fitted with and greatly expanded my thinking about social change and the multiplicity of truths around human experience.

Over the past 15 years I have had the opportunity to work with a diverse range of students, colleagues and practitioners from many cultures and backgrounds, and to travel to communities across Australia to see how social workers and others are responding to individual, family and community needs. This involvement has broadened my understanding of ways in which power and knowledge affect our identity and place in the world and I am currently very interested in the **epistemological racism** that pervades Western university and research cultures and how it might be challenged.

> The **biomedical model** refers to the current, dominant approach to health and illness that is based on the biological sciences (Healy 2005).

> **Epistemological racism** is the view that only the wisdom and knowledge of a dominant group (often white and Western) is valid. It serves to delegitimise or invisibilise other forms of knowledge, and is a view so deeply embedded as to become almost invisible and overwhelmingly accepted as the 'norm' (Scheurich & Young 1997).

Phillip's story

I have contributed to this book with feelings of trepidation and enthusiasm. The trepidation stems from the fact that I am not a social worker but a sociologist who supports the vision of critical social work. Consequently, when invited to co-author a book on the core elements of another discipline I had misgivings as to whether I had anything to offer – what did I know as an outsider? However, my social work co-authors have insisted otherwise. They reminded me that sociology and social work share a common ancestry and interest in understanding society. In particular, both examine how social processes produce the major problems we face in the world today – problems such as poverty, inequality, environmental degradation and violence. My co-authors also reminded me that to address these problems effectively requires not only analysing *how society is* but also imagining ways to *change it for the better*. This is the source of my enthusiasm because, like my co-authors, I want to use our understanding of society to work with and advance the interests of those who suffer from its current divisions and injustices. So, I see critical social work as a challenging but profoundly hopeful endeavour, and how I came to support it has been part of a lifelong journey of learning.

I was born into a working-class family in inner Melbourne in 1961, towards the end of the postwar economic boom. The prosperity of those times was spread equally

Discrimination refers to the way marginalised groups are excluded, harassed, ridiculed, intimidated and sometimes attacked by dominant groups because of their physical, behavioural or cultural differences (McDonald et al. 2011).

Conservative refers to a political stance that preserves the existing social order (including its inequities and injustices) (Mullaly 2007).

Marxism is a body of theory associated with the work of Karl Marx that seeks to criticise, and liberate people from, economic oppression.

Feminists are women who advocate the rights of women to overcome patriarchal (male-dominated) inequality and oppression (Dominelli 2012).

Radicalism is the act of advocating for institutional change using the practice of high-risk activity to exert positive or negative influence on mainstream organisations (Cross 2012; Haines 1988).

enough for people like my parents (dad was a gas meter maker, and mum a full-time parent) to pursue the middle-class 'Australian Dream' of home ownership and a better life. So, we joined the migration of 'brick-veneer poor' to the then outer-eastern suburb of Ringwood. Growing up there was lean but relatively comfortable. I was only vaguely aware of the major social changes that were underway in the 1960s and 70s, overturning the cultural and political conservatism of the previous decade. These changes were occurring in communications (television), fashion, music, sexual relations, national identity and Australia's relations with the rest of the world. The Vietnam War was reported on television but I had no awareness of the massive protests it generated.

My only recollections of these wider changes at the time were my parents dressing in black wigs to attend a Beatles party and their impatience for a change of government to Labor after 23 years of Liberal rule. The election of Gough Whitlam's Labor Government in 1972 inspired hopes for radical change and a wave of overdue reforms in every field followed, including the final removal of Australian troops from Vietnam; the outlawing of racial **discrimination**; official recognition of the government of Communist China (Australia had refused to acknowledge China's existence during 1949–72); 'no fault' divorce; a national health insurance scheme; free university education; and the first Aboriginal land rights, human rights and environmental legislation. Regrettably, entrenched **conservative** forces opposed the government's reforms, which eventually culminated in Whitlam's controversial dismissal by the then Governor-General.

Although young, I learnt from these developments that fundamental change to promote people's rights and social justice was possible. It had happened before and could happen again. However, change would also involve formidable opposition, reversals and struggle. Another legacy of this period was that working-class kids could enter university if they had the grades. So, in the early 1980s I enrolled in social sciences at La Trobe University. It opened up new vistas both inside and outside the classroom. Inside, I discovered sociology and its critical questioning of the power structures of society, particularly in the writings of **Marxists** and **feminists**. Outside the classroom, student **radicalism** had peaked and I tried to practise some of these critical theories of change by joining various groups on campus. I became an **activist** in the 'radical Left' of the student movement that contained a broad spectrum of socialists, peace activists, communists, anarchists, progressive Christians, radical feminists and gay and lesbian activists. One of our concerns involved supporting the aspirations of student movements for democracy, justice and self-determination in other parts of the world. In many countries these struggles were a matter of life and death. There was, for instance, the militant struggle of the African National Congress against apartheid in South Africa, and in South Korea and the Philippines mass movements confronted dictatorship and repression.

> An **activist** is someone who engages in social activism.

In 1985 I visited the Philippines and witnessed first-hand the struggles of students, peasants and workers in opposing the Marcos dictatorship. The stark divisions between rich and poor, the abject poverty of millions, the military atrocities and the abuse of power by the elite shocked me. I could see this disparity of power was not going to shift while the dictatorship lasted and I came to support the revolutionary opposition. I was also inspired by the courage and capacity of people from all walks of life to organise and resist these oppressive conditions though trade unions, student unions, women's groups, cooperatives, community organisations and **social movements**. Most intriguing was the role of the Christian churches, which traditionally supported the **status quo**, but there were also priests and nuns who sided with the revolution. Still an activist, I undertook research into the participation of Christians in the Marxist-led revolution, which became my doctorate in sociology. A revolution did occur in 1986 with the ouster of Marcos by a popular uprising but it was co-opted by wealthy elites and did not go according to the plans of the revolutionary left. Once again, there were lessons to be learnt from this experience about change for social justice. These included lessons about the role of professionals (such as clergy, community developers, health providers and social workers) in working with the impoverished and marginalised. I learnt that one could accompany and support the marginalised in their struggles for self-determination, one could dialogue and learn with them, but one should never dictate solutions or predict with certainty the outcome of a struggle. Moreover, I learnt about the grounding of theories in the experience of the poor rather than our own projections of how they should behave.

> **Social movements** are a large collectivity of people who aim to either maintain or challenge the existing social order (Giddens & Sutton 2013).

> **Status quo** refers to maintaining the existing order.

As a university lecturer, I now teach critical social theories about social change for a more just, democratic and sustainable society in a manner that runs counter to the dominant forms of sociology and social work. Many sociologists spend a lot of time studying these goals in academic settings but seldom have time to do anything about them. Many social workers by contrast are so immersed in the daily institutional work of meeting the needs of disadvantaged or marginalised people that they think they have little time for critical theory or reflection. However, having taught in a critical social work program, understood broadly as facilitating justice and freedom in everyday life, I believe it has a vital role to play in transforming our world.

■ Social work: diverse possibilities for justice

Often there is a perception in society that social work only concerns doing paperwork in an office or being the 'softer' police of government to work with the 'bottom rung' of society. Thankfully our experiences of social work indicate that it is far more diverse than that. Our experiences collectively indicate that as a professional career path, social work is incredibly broad, challenging, dynamic and exciting. We cannot imagine wanting to do anything else, as being offered this kind of variety we are able to engage in creative endeavours that are limited only by imagination and always feel like we are making important contributions to a better world. Social work provides opportunities to be part of amazing efforts that genuinely make a difference to the quality of communities and people's lives, but social work does require being creative, courageous and critical – and this, we believe, will be a key challenge for future graduates and practitioners.

Identity refers to who we are as people. From a poststructural perspective identity is fluid and contextual, whereas previously our sense of 'self' was thought of as static or the result of fixed attributes.

While the stories we have written are 'true' they are also limited and partial. In foregrounding some elements of our stories, we have left out others. We have put our stories 'out there', freezing them in textual time, but if we were to write them again tomorrow or next year, would we emphasise and omit the same things? Or how might our accounts be different? Such fluid and complex accounts of **identity** and narrative are arguably part of the poststructural condition: our constructions of our selves, the profession of social work and the way we look at the world are dynamic and always incomplete. Even in the act of **constructing** workers and clients we make the world in particular ways; as critical practitioners we take on the challenge of attempting to understand how our 'making' of ourselves and others creates opportunities for empowerment or oppression.

A **construction** is a product of human organisation or creation (Parton & O'Byrne 2000).

Whatever one's reasons, the point here is to acknowledge the reasoning beneath the way we tell stories of ourselves and others, and acknowledge the partial and dynamic nature of our narratives (stories). This applies to the stories we will tell ourselves about the people and communities that we work with, and the stories that they will tell us about ourselves. This also has implications for how we undertake social work assessments, a practice that is discussed further in Chapter 7.

■ Challenges to critical social work and the increased need for this work

Most social workers would agree in principle with the sentiments of critical social work presented in this chapter. Despite this, much of social work – what we refer to as 'establishment social work', the dominant or mainstream understanding of (uncritical) social work – may engage in practices that, when analysed, reflect more of a commitment to being on the side of the system (that creates the injustices) than to supporting the people who are disenfranchised by these systems.

This is not new; however, the current social and political context arguably exacerbates these problematic practices by affirming establishment social work and discouraging critical social work. The current context has endemic problems: widespread poverty and developing world debt; increasingly powerful transnational corporations and international banks; widening inequalities between powerful groups and socially disadvantaged ones; and a global redistribution of political and economic power and resources resulting in the West's monopoly of technological, financial and communication resources and weapons (see, for example, Ife 2013). Some of the consequences of this include widespread violence in the form of war, ongoing acts of terrorism, and atrocities based on ethnic and religious differences. Rampant consumerism and other excesses of our Western lifestyle have resulted in severe environmental degradation and exploitation, leading to serious changes in climatic conditions and vast increases in the severity and incidence of natural disasters (see, for example, Dominelli 2012; Ife 2013). The potentially catastrophic environmental consequences of these changes place far more than our economies at risk; it also threatens the very survival of the human race and our planet. (The current contexts of social work practice will be explored further in Chapter 2.)

This has created an incredibly broad range of complex social problems and, in some quarters, a sense of moral panic, which leads governments to make conservative policy decisions with the aim of 'treating' and 'managing' the people who are most affected by the adverse conditions, rather than seeking to change the system that creates the adversity. At the same time, we have seen the ascendancy of science and medicine to diagnose, medicate and treat; the promise of evidence-based practices to improve our effectiveness; and the increased reliance on **risk assessment** procedures to try to promote **objectivity** and certainty. All of these approaches are seen to have superior capability to combat the uncertainty and complexity that now characterise the nature of social problems in our world, and yet all of them are severely lacking in the sophistication required to deal with increased uncertainty and complexity. Indeed, by trying to reduce social problems to simplifiable, manageable components that we can study objectively and treat with the right techniques, we hinder our ability to respond to uncertainty and complexity.

We are also continuing to experience a reduction in resourcing the Western welfare states, whereby governments in the Western countries have increasingly cut spending in real terms in the health, welfare and education sectors since the 1970s (Jamrozik 2009; McDonald et al. 2011). We have also seen the introduction of business (**economic rationalist**) principles of competition, such as survival of the fittest, user pays, or services offered at the most cost-effective price and in the most efficient way (despite a reduction in the type and quality of services offered), which results in fewer opportunities for social workers to practise in ways that promote social justice, citizenship and human rights (Baines 2006). Such rapid contextual changes have also left the social work discipline asking questions about its own survival as we grapple with concerns to remain relevant within the contemporary context. This, of course,

Risk assessment is an organisational procedure designed to manage risk for both workers and service users in the name of accountability. However, the dangers in this approach are that workers can become so fixated on assessing, managing and ensuring against risk that they potentially lose sight of what is important and effective in their work with service users. (Gardner 2006).

Objectivity is the idea that one can stand outside of reality and observe it without any subjective interpretations or prejudices.

Economic rationalism (often used interchangeably with 'neoliberalism') is a narrow view of economics that refers to the idea that 'free' markets will provide the best outcomes in all spheres of society. It consistently places economic issues over social concerns (Jamrozik 2009).

raises questions about who social workers aim to be relevant for. While most social workers at times feel some pressure to conform to the system, establishment social work particularly seeks to fit within this and take on the practices that are determined as appropriate by the powerful groups. These practices preserve the existing system rather than challenge it.

Since the birth of social work, we have seen examples of social workers being involved in punishing and disciplining the poor through the practices of conducting home visits (see Chapter 4, specifically on the Charitable Organisation Societies, for more information about this) and being actively implicated in the eugenics movements in the early 1900s, 'in which tens of thousands of mostly poor Americans were subject to involuntary sterilisation in the name of "national regeneration"' (LaPan & Platt 2005, pp. 139–64). In Australia, social workers have been involved in the implementation of forced removal of Aboriginal and Torres Strait Islander children from their family networks (the Stolen Generations) and continue to engage in practices that uncritically subscribe to colonialist views (see, for example, Briskman 2014; Menzies & Gilbert 2013). Social workers have also been complicit in similar acts of injustice and oppression whereby First Nations people in North America and the Maori of Aotearoa/New Zealand have suffered, with a host of ramifications that have carried through to the present day (Alia & Bull 2005; McKendrick 2001). In short, social work has a long history of being implicated in supporting social conditions that have been oppressive for socially disadvantaged groups whose interests we claim to serve (Healy 2000; Morley & Macfarlane 2008; Rojek, Peakcock & Collins 1988). Disturbingly, this history is not a distant memory, but continues in current-day practice and has the capacity to shape the future of social work. The extremely conservative social and political context that is currently prevailing means there is pressure for social workers to become enforcers of oppressive social systems rather than agents of social change (Holscher & Sewpaul 2006).

One of the ways that social workers have tried to retain **professional integrity** is to gain increased professional status, but this comes at a cost. Misguided attempts to gain professional credibility, by aligning with and carrying out practices that promote the interests of the most powerful groups in society, have had disastrous consequences for social work's human rights and social justice commitments (Morley & Macfarlane 2008). While social workers may not always feel powerful in relation to the systems in which they work, they are often in roles that are afforded a large amount of power to make important decisions that impact on the lives of vulnerable people. One of the first steps in being a critical social worker is to recognise the divisions of power in society and to acknowledge that working in

> **Professional integrity** is our capacity to work in a manner consistent with our values as critically reflective practitioners.

the role of a social worker is a potentially powerful role that is not only capable of providing opportunities to create positive change, but also of causing great harm (Fook 2012; Rossiter 1996). One of the ways we can cause harm is by accepting the commonly held beliefs, values and assumptions that benefit and contribute to maintaining the current system (see, for example, Mullaly 2010). We refer to these as *dominant ideologies* or myths, which promote the best interests of the most powerful groups in society. Unlike the myths that may be told to a child as bedtime stories of heroes and monsters, the myths we are referring to here can have profound negative consequences. An example may be that there is a 'queue' that people seeking asylum in Australia are 'jumping'. This has the effect of painting refugees, who constitute some of the most vulnerable populations in the world, as undeserving, and as troublemakers or villains, rather than victims, who have been potentially subjected to a range of social oppressions and are simply exercising their human right to seek asylum under the United Nations Convention Relating to the Status of Refugees (1951), of which Australia has been a signatory since 1954 (for further information see Briskman, Latham & Goddard 2008).

In August 2012 the Australian Government announced that it would increase the total number of refugees it would accept per year across the two components of the Humanitarian Program, from 13 750 to 20 000. Australia is the only country in the world to numerically link its system for granting asylum onshore and its scheme for resettling people from offshore under a single program. The effect of this link is that each time a person is granted refugee status within Australia (onshore), one place is subtracted from the offshore component. Other countries determine a particular number of refugees to be resettled each year, depending on global needs, and meet this commitment regardless of how many people arrive in the country and seek asylum (Australian Human Rights Commission 2012).

REFLECTIVE EXERCISE 1.5
- Try to note down a couple of examples of how dominant ideologies might have influenced your perceptions. Can you identify some aspects of your identity that are privileged and some others that might be oppressed?
- Watch this four-minute YouTube clip: 'What would you do?', http://www.youtube.com/watch?v=ge7i60GuNRg&feature=player_embedded. What are your reactions to this clip? How do you explain the differential responses to the same behaviour?

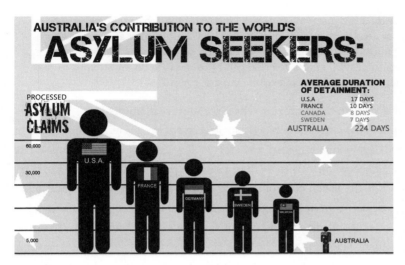

Figure 1.5 Based on data from Human Rights Watch. (Figures are averages.) Graphic is reproduced with the kind permission of WordswithMeaning.org.

Another example may be myths that blame rape victims for the sexual violence that has been perpetrated against them by focusing on what was worn, past sexual behaviour, how much alcohol was consumed, and so on – all factors that attach responsibility to the victims for the crimes committed against them, while shifting the focus away from the culpability of the offender.

Establishment or conservative social work, which is the most commonly practised form of social work in the current context, largely accepts the unequal distribution of power and resources in society and as such works to maintain the status quo and is largely uncritical towards it. Establishment social work makes concessions to the current social inequalities and oppressions, whereas critical social work exposes the problems and injustices these create and seeks to change them. We contend that all social work should in fact be critical social work. However, we also acknowledge that choosing to be a critical social worker is a more difficult path than following establishment social work. This is because most social workers practise within an institutional context that does not support the values and goals of critical social work (see, for example, Baines 2011; Healy 2000). Hence, all of us have the potential to fall into establishment practices, despite our intention to undertake critical work. Being a critical practitioner is also more demanding because it often requires the practitioner to challenge entrenched institutional and political arrangements that benefit the powerful groups (see, for example, Mullaly 2010). This invokes resistance. As Cox (1996, p. 70) puts it:

The mainstream and conservative views that control the debates are never seen as policing the system because they own it ... [They] are regarded as somehow legitimate, but radical views are not seen as needing serious attention. In an almost ridiculous contradiction, efforts for change are believed to be an attempt to take control rather than a challenge to existing implicit control.

This has much to do with the context in which social work is situated.

We agree with many other authors who suggest social work is at a crucial moment in its history and development. Indeed, as Kessl (2009) points out, social work is at risk of becoming little more than a set of techniques that are used to carry out the **social control** work of conservative governments and other powerful groups in society; it is in danger of becoming something that is still called social work, but that is quite different from the social justice ideals that social work's purpose, values and vision should be. Some have argued that this constitutes an identity crisis, concerning who social workers are, where they are going and what sorts of contributions they will make to society (Lavalette 2011). The challenges that face social work threaten to displace it, undermine its effectiveness, and reshape its very essence in terms of its role and mission as a discipline and profession (Ferguson 2008). We now need to formulate responses to these challenges. The types of responses that we develop will largely determine the sort of social work that will be carried forward into the future.

> **Social control** refers to a range of measures (both formal and informal) whereby a dominant group or institution brings other groups and individuals into conformity with its norms (Jamrozik 2009).

We have written this book with a clear and unapologetic view that social work has a fundamental role to play in advancing human rights, social justice, equity and democracy, despite the challenges presented by contemporary practice and policy contexts. We further assert that it be a critical form of social work, with its ethical commitment to creating equitable societies that will best enable practitioners to make a worthy contribution to these goals, and we develop strategies to help practitioners negotiate this challenging context creatively. We will spend considerable time thinking about the impact of the context in which social workers currently operate, and strategies for how practitioners can negotiate this context creatively.

■ Structure of this book

Following this introductory chapter, Chapter 2 will begin by exploring the significance of context, including discussing some of the key dominant social forces that create profound social inequalities and divisions in our contemporary contexts. Chapter 3 expands this discussion by outlining a number of practice strategies that enable social workers to continue to pursue a critical agenda despite the challenges created by contemporary contexts.

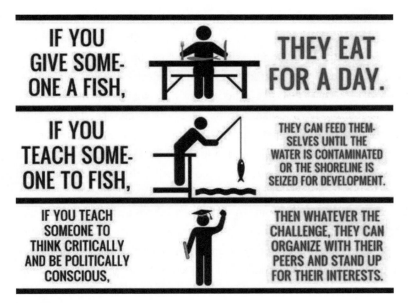

Figure 1.6
Image reproduced with kind permission of Anonymous Art of Revolution.

Chapter 4 discusses the history of the development of social work and related 'helping' professions in Western societies. It draws on research to show the problems with the various ways that the helping professions have been presented, and explores the issues that have historically and culturally informed their mission and positioning. It explores the debates in the roles and functions of social work, and particularly highlights the development of radical-emancipatory approaches that have sought to transform oppressive conditions within the history of social work.

Chapter 5 explores the concept of ethical practice from a critical perspective, beginning by examining the current codes of ethics, as well as the recent debates around the codification and limitations of professional ethics statements to guide ethical practice. It explores various approaches to decision making in relation to ethical dilemmas in practice and ways in which ethics can serve as a grounding for critical practice. You are also introduced in more detail to the notion and practice of critical reflection when we use a case example from our research to demonstrate how it can be drawn upon to inform ethical practice from a critical perspective.

Chapter 6 introduces you to the inextricable relationship between theory and practice. Specifically, we will explore the application of several theories to practice, namely: psychodynamic and cognitive psychological theories as examples of individualistic theories; systems theory as an example of a conservative social theory; and a number of critical social work theories, including radical/structural theories, Marxism, feminism, anti-oppressive approaches and some elements of poststructural thinking. You are invited to critically reflect on your own values and positioning in relation to being a practitioner who wishes to maintain the status quo, or a practitioner who wishes to be an agent of change. This chapter draws on a recent research project with first-year students to demonstrate the use of establishment social work theories (individualistic and systems theories) in relation to a case study, while comparing and contrasting these to critical social work approaches.

Chapter 7 examines how theories guide the practice methods and processes we use. It demonstrates how theory is directly linked to practice and discusses the practice methods of counselling, group work, advocacy, community development, policy development and analysis, research and social action. Examples of how critical theory informs practice are emphasised in contrast to establishment theories. It also presents a critique of the ways in which practice processes have traditionally been conceptualised and explores how critical theories can inform our approaches to practice processes. The practice processes that have been traditionally referred to as 'assessment' and 'intervention' are reviewed. We continue to explore fundamental questions about the nature and purpose of social work from a critical perspective using case studies while comparing and contrasting critical approaches with establishment approaches to practice.

Chapter 8 highlights service users' perspectives on social work and human service delivery, including the worker–client relationship and its inherent power dynamics, control of research agendas, involvement in policy development, and the privileging of professional knowledge. It also highlights the anthropocentric (human-centred) limits of traditional conceptions of the client base of social work and suggests possibilities for extending this to include a more eco-centric (nature-centred) framework that values the integrity of nature and other beings. Within this chapter, we also critically debate current approaches to working across difference, exploring how a critical approach might assist in developing anti-oppressive practice possibilities, and engage you in critical reflection on your own social and cultural location. The chapter encourages you to consider how you might productively and ethically embrace uncertainty and ongoing learning in the dynamic contexts of your practice.

Chapter 9 draws on our own and other authors' research to introduce you to a range of practice fields and some of the current debates within these fields. While historically critical practice has only been thought to be possible in community-based organisations with an explicit mandate for social change, this chapter discusses the relevance and potential for critical approaches to inform social work in all fields of practice. Fields of practice covered include mental health, aged care and child protection as examples.

Finally, Chapter 10 draws on our own and others' research to showcase examples of critical practice and highlight their importance for sustaining social work as a unique and vital contributor to individual wellbeing and social change.

■ Summary

Critical social work involves questioning our current society and trying to combat its harmful divisions and unequal power relations that result in social injustices. Social justice concerns equality of opportunity in relation to human rights, participation, access to resources, and equitable distribution of resources. Critical social work also involves critical reflection: an exploration of our own values, assumptions and social positioning with the purpose of understanding how these factors shape our view of the world and impact on our social work practice. In this chapter we have examined the differences between critical social work and more conservative approaches, which we have referred to as establishment social work. We discussed the very conservative social and political conditions that have given rise to establishment social work, highlighting the highly contested nature of social work, and the urgent need for critical social work to be further developed as a mainstream practice. We have introduced ourselves and shared our social work stories so that you have a sense of where we are coming from in writing this book. We hope that all of this has adequately introduced you to the very diverse, dynamic and exciting world of social work.

■ Review questions

- What are some of the main questions this chapter has raised for you?
- What are the things that have most surprised you? What, if anything, has intrigued you and made you want to read further?
- What does this indicate about some of the assumptions that you have made about social work and the human services?

■ Further reading

Allan, J., 2009, 'Doing critical social work' in J. Allan, L. Briskman and B. Pease, eds, *Critical Social Work: Theories and Practices for a Socially Just World*, 2nd edn, Allen & Unwin, Crows Nest, NSW.

Dominelli, L., 2009, *Introducing Social Work: Short Introductions*, Polity Press, Cambridge.

Ferguson, I., 2008, 'A profession worth fighting for?' in *Reclaiming Social Work*, Sage, London.

Fook, J., 1993, 'Can casework be radical?' in *Radical Casework: A Theory of Practice*, Allen & Unwin, St Leonards, NSW.

2

Where in the world are we? The contexts of practice

■ Introduction

I N THIS AND the following chapter we explore the importance of **context** to social work practice. Ife (2012, pp. 307–8) suggests 'context is crucial . . . it determines the way any social worker will understand an issue, and the way they will act accordingly'.

> **Context** refers to the complex layers that surround, impact upon and shape our understandings and actions.

LIFE	Is the second symbol (i.e. '**I**') in the sequences on the left a letter or a number?
0I234	Derrida (1978) makes the simple point that no symbol has an essential or final meaning. The symbol's meaning is always given by its context and its meaning will change depending on how the context frames it.

Social work does not exist in a vacuum. In this chapter, we focus on a number of powerful social forces that shape our social contexts. These include *global capitalism, neoliberalism, managerialism, globalisation, patriarchy, biomedical discourses, government* and the *law*. It is important to understand how each of these social forces operates at global, national and local levels so that we can recognise how they impact on the lives of the individuals, groups and communities with whom we work, and how they can influence our social work practice.

Australia, like other Western, developed, capitalist societies, is a changing landscape in a rapidly changing world. Some people experience this change as enabling and full of opportunities while others experience it as unsettling or even oppressive. This is because the benefits and disadvantages of social change are not evenly distributed. Our social world is characterised by significant social divisions and inequalities in **class**, **gender**,

> **Class** is a term used to refer to major social divisions that arise from the unequal distribution of economic resources in society (Van Krieken et al. 2012).
> **Gender** is the social construct related to the roles, behaviours and attitudes we expect from people based on their assignment as either male or female (Mullaly 2010, p. 212).

Ethnicity is defined as a common set of values and norms, including shared patterns of seeing, thinking and acting, that construct a group identity (Mullaly 2010, p. 96). **Race** is a problematic term often used to describe differences based on skin colour or some other outwardly apparent but biologically superficial characteristic.

Sexism refers to a set of social, economic, political and cultural beliefs, attitudes and practices that in patriarchal societies are predominantly employed to oppress women by associating a biological difference (female) with socially constructed characteristics (Mullaly 2010, p. 210). **Racism** is defined as beliefs, statements and acts that render certain groups inferior on the basis that they do not belong to the culture of origin of the dominant ethnic group within the state apparatus (Hollinsworth 1997). **Ageism** refers to negative attitudes towards elderly individuals, which associates them with degeneracy, senility and frailty, and a drain on resources as they make no contribution to a capitalist society (Mullaly 2010). **Ableism** refers to the personal prejudices, cultural expressions and social forces that marginalise people with disabilities and portray them in a negative light based on their failure to conform to the prevailing cultural definition of normality (Mullaly 2010, p. 215). **Heterosexism** is the form of oppression whereby heterosexuality is considered to be natural by society and all other alternatives are considered to be unnatural (Mullaly 2010, p. 212).

ethnicity and what some refer to as '**race**'. These divisions create multiple *oppressions*, including *socioeconomic disadvantage*, **sexism**, **racism**, **ageism**, **ableism** and **heterosexism**. These forms of oppression influence all the institutions in which we live – education, health care, the family, work, religion and government. We will now explore how they are directly linked with the dominant social forces that characterise our contemporary contexts.

■ Global capitalism

Arguably, the most powerful and defining social force that influences our contemporary context is global **capitalism**.

Economically, it turns all things into marketable **commodities**. Socially, it produces fundamental and inequitable class divisions between owners and non-owners of capital (Giddens & Sutton 2013; Marx & Engels [1848] 1969). The production of these commodities results from the labour of a working class whose members do not own the means of production, and must sell their labour for a wage, making them vulnerable to exploitation (Giddens & Sutton 2013). Capitalism became the dominant economic system of Western societies (in Europe and North America) in the 19th century, and has subsequently grown to be global. Global capitalism is therefore the extension of the capitalist system to the entire world. It is touted as free trade without restrictions and includes every aspect of our society, including our labour, health and wellbeing (Giddens & Sutton 2013).

Proponents of global capitalism claim that the common good is best served by allowing markets to operate freely. Indeed, many of us in Western societies, including the authors of this book, have benefited (and sometimes lost) from activity in the housing market, and in this sense are complicit in upholding capitalist systems.

The global capitalist **ideology** claims that consumers can look after themselves and that state attempts to protect the interests of people as a collective will interfere with the workings of the free market. This ideology has historically been referred to as **laissez faire** (literally 'let do', as in leave markets alone). Its fundamental flaw is that economic markets are inherently unstable, unsustainable and totally ill equipped to meet the social needs of all people. One author refers to this blind spot as market fundamentalism and contends that it is this 'that has rendered the global capitalist system unsound and unsustainable' (Soros 1998, p. xx). While capitalism has produced more wealth in terms of commodities and money than any other social system in history, it has simultaneously created more inequality and poverty than at any other time.

Some have argued that the more contemporary expression of global capitalism is not just in the unequal relationship between owners and non-owners of the means of capital, but also in the relationship between creditors and debtors, with debt becoming the most powerful means of exploitation of the working people by the ruling class (e.g. Lazzarato 2012). Many working-class and middle-class people spend their entire lives working to pay back interest that is accruing on their mortgage. The 'great Australian dream' of home ownership is an important part of this social context, and it combines very effectively with capitalist ideologies to bind working people into a lifetime of servicing debt. Yet the dream to own one's own home remains a distant one for the **underclass** and low-income earners struggling to survive in the private rental market. The latest Australian research shows that 4.5 million people in Australia rent, which has doubled in the last 30 years (Hulse, Miligan & Easthope 2012). One of the many problematic consequences of global capitalism, which creates wide disparities between rich and poor, is **homelessness** (for further information see Van Krieken et al. 2012, p. 240). Public housing continues to be **stigmatised**, despite people having to wait for many years to be allocated a dwelling. The cost of private rentals in Australia is among the highest in the world (Bell 2013; Yates & Berry 2011) and many people we work with as social workers will experience precarious housing and be at risk of homelessness. Groups that are particularly vulnerable are young people, people experiencing mental health issues, people solely reliant on welfare entitlements, Aboriginal and Torres Strait Islander people, criminalised people, single parent headed households and aged people (Bell 2013; Yates & Berry 2011).

Between the 1940s and 1980s, Australia had social policies that created a more equitable distribution of resources (Leigh 2013). Hence, history reminds us that governments can use social policy as a mechanism to create more equitable societies. However, since that time the financially privileged have increased their concentration of wealth: the top one per cent of Australians own roughly 20 per cent of Australia's wealth, while the bottom 50 per cent own approximately one per cent of the wealth (Van Kreiken et al. 2012, p. 193). The United Nations Development Programme (UNDP)

Capitalism is the current dominant socioeconomic system throughout the world, and is based on the private ownership of productive resources.

Commodities are anything sold on a market for profit (Giddens & Sutton 2013).

Ideology refers to a system of ideas that interprets reality in the interests of a particular social class, thus misrepresenting the interests of that class as if they were the interests of society as a whole (Van Krieken et al. 2012).

Laissez faire claims that economic systems work best when there is little government intervention (Dalton et al. 1996).

Underclass is a derogatory term used to represent a group of people with no past or future attachment to the labour market – for example, the long-term unemployed and homeless people (Mullaly 2010, p. 207).

Homelessness can be defined as:

- 'Persons who are in improvised dwellings, tents or sleeping out
- Persons in supported accommodation for the homeless
- Persons who are staying temporarily with other households
- Persons who are staying in boarding houses
- Persons in other temporary dwellings' (ABS 2011).

(2006) reported that the world's three richest men – Bill Gates, Carlos Slim and Warren Buffett – had a combined net worth of US$170 billion, which is greater than the wealth of the world's 40 poorest countries with a combined population of more than 600 million people. The richest one per cent of the population have 43 per cent of the world's wealth, whereas the bottom 80 per cent have just six per cent of the world's wealth, living on US$10 or less per day (Hickel 2013). In addition, a recent Oxfam report (2013) shows that the richest one per cent globally have increased their income by 60 per cent over the past 20 years, with the global financial crisis accelerating, rather than impeding, the growth of the wealth of the elite. The richest 300 people in the world now have more wealth than the poorest three billion people (O'Sullivan & Kersley 2012).

REFLECTIVE EXERCISE 2.1

Go to the London School of Economics and Political Science website and watch this four-minute clip detailing how wealth is divided globally: 'Global wealth inequality: What you never knew you never knew', http://blogs.lse.ac.uk/indiaatlse/2013/04/11/global-wealth-inequality-what-you-never-knew-you-never-knew/.

- What are your thoughts about the basic rules of our global economy and world trade?
- What critiques might a critical social work perspective bring to these rules and the inequalities that they create?

Now go to the Young Presidents' Organization website, http://www.ypo.org, and click the icon that invites you to join YPO.

- How many people do you know who would meet the eligibility requirements of YPO?
- What are your personal and professional reflections concerning global capitalism and wealth inequality?

Stigma refers to the socially constructed characteristics and attributes associated with marginalised groups (Mullaly 2010).

While it can feel overwhelming to be confronted with the profound inequalities of contemporary global wealth distribution, the point of critical theory, as Karl Marx ([1845] 1888) stated, is not simply to interpret the world but to change it. History tells us that inequality can be reduced. From 1915 to the 1970s, the wealth share of the top 1 per cent of the population in Australia fell from 34 per cent to 15 per cent, indicating that policies that aim to equalise the distribution of resources can be extremely effective (Leigh 2013; Van Krieken et al. 2012). This provides hope for a more socially just future, but it requires an engaged and robust critique of neoliberal approaches to policy, which will be discussed next.

■ Neoliberalism/economic rationalism and managerialism

You will recall we briefly referred to neoliberalism (sometimes called *economic rationalism*) in Chapter 1. While capitalism refers to the systems and institutions of our economic structure, neoliberalism is the **discourse** of global capitalism. Neoliberalism justifies the extension of global capitalism into every sphere of social life. It therefore creates massive societal power imbalances between rich and poor by validating global capitalism as an economic system controlled by corporate elites (such as transnational corporations and banks). Neoliberalism, or economic rationalism, leads governments to prioritise capital accumulation strategies over social concerns (Holscher & Sewpaul 2006). Directly related to these concepts is **managerialism**, which refers to principles, practices and techniques that implement neoliberal goals within organisational settings. Managerialism defines all problems in the world (including social problems) in economic and strategic terms. From this perspective, all solutions should therefore concern preserving governments' budgets, which means cutting funding to human services organisations while practitioners are expected to do more with less (Holscher & Sewpaul 2006).

For several decades, in the political context of many Western nations, including Australia, we have seen the economic management of our resources dominate social justice issues. These **economic reforms**, which began in the 1980s and 1990s, have included an emphasis on introducing business principles into the welfare sector. Such principles have resulted in 'small government' or reducing government funds being used to resource the public service sector, including the areas of health, education and welfare. This shrinking of the **welfare state** has coincided with practices of **competitive tendering** whereby different organisations compete with each other by submitting tenders (proposals) to the government to run a particular service most efficiently (inexpensively) (Healy 2005). (See Chapter 5 for an example showing some of the problems of this practice.) Two of the key assumptions underpinning all of these changes are that (1) curbing government spending on people, particularly socially

Discourse is a poststructuralist term referring to a set of ideas or language about a particular topic with shared meanings and assumptions that reflect and reinforce particular power relations (Fook 2012).

Managerialism defines all problems in the world (including social problems) in economic terms. It assumes that managers should be in control of all organisations (including human services) and that these should be run in line with business principles.

Economic reforms comprise various measures 'designed to stabilise the economy . . . and improve the financial position of the state' (Bresser-Pereira, Maravall & Przeworski 1994, p. 184).

Welfare state is the means by which governments, through social and economic policies, facilitate or restrict access to resources and opportunities that assist people to live independent and meaningful lives. (Jamrozik 2009; O'Connor et al. 2008).

Competitive tendering encourages non-government organisations (NGOs) to compete with each other to be providers of services that are deemed appropriate in the 'market' created by the state (McDonald et al. 2011, p. 52).

disadvantaged people, is the ultimate goal of government; and (2) individuals, rather than the state, should take responsibility for meeting their own basic needs.

The cutting and withdrawal of services emerges directly from the neoliberal view that people should be responsible for their own care, rather than relying on the government for support. Take Queensland, for example, where the Newman Liberal–National Government was elected in March 2012 – a staggering 14 000 public service workers were retrenched within three months as their positions in the public service were made redundant. The greatest cuts were to the health-care sector, transport and main roads, and housing and public works. Ironically, neoliberal discourses repackage the cuts as 'savings' providing a 'budget surplus', even when such cuts result in losses to essential services and jobs, and mean heavy costs to individuals and communities who are socially disadvantaged. (For more details see Taylor 2012.)

These severe cuts to the community and the welfare state have created a culture of fear in the public sector, forced people into poverty, and have been carried out with the explicit goals of saving money and reducing Queensland's debt. The notion that state debt is problematic is another ideologically driven discourse to justify the cuts. Relative to the size of our economy, Australia's national debt is historically low compared with other Organisation of Economic Co-operation and Development (OECD) countries (Di Marco, Pirie & Au-Yeung 2011). In fact, our private household debt is much higher than our public debt (Soos 2013). Part of the Australian private debt is from credit cards, the use of which has created debt of $50 billion (Australian Securities and Investments Commission (ASIC) 2013). The dominant discourse about national public debt reflects the values of most political parties, in which the agenda in the last few decades has always been about the budget, while social justice and human rights issues have been absent or secondary – unless they feature as economic issues, such as presenting the human rights of refugees seeking asylum in Australia as a management issue that is an economic burden on the country and a national security threat. Both major parties in Australia have been influenced by global capitalist doctrines, which makes it very difficult for voters to envisage socially just or **progressive** alternatives. Consistently, the value placed on money, and the ethic of people being responsible for their own welfare, are perpetuated in this context (despite the system's creation of the injustices that people experience and the consequences of these injustices).

Progressive is a political stance that aims to challenge the existing social order and move it towards the goal of greater freedom and equity (see Mullaly 2007.)

Neoliberal values and managerial techniques hold direct implications for how social work and human services practitioners operate in the field. Madhu (2011, p. 6) suggests management practices and administrative tools have started to 'define' professional social work. This has resulted in pressures on practitioners to increase their productivity and efficiency – for example, through downsizing of the organisation, managing larger caseloads, reducing the costs associated with offering services and providing fewer resources to those in need. At the same time there is an increased emphasis on accountability; this is often in the form of more paper-work, surveillance of work practices, performance monitoring and, increasingly, **technicist** practices that minimise the ethical and philo-sophical dimensions of practice (Hughes & Wearing 2013; Jarman-Rohde et al. 1997; McDonald et al. 2011). Some have argued that as we become focused on technical and administrative procedures, our work

> **Technicism** is the over-reliance on techniques, skills and competencies.

starts to lose its purpose and meaning. Within this context, the needs of the individuals, groups and communities with whom we work seem to be diminished in comparison to governments' budgets and the protection of the agency, while the substance of an assessment or report appears to be less important than the format in which it is presented, or its completion by the deadline (Ferguson 2008). Commenting on similar experiences in the United Kingdom one author states: 'Being a care manager is very different from being a social worker as I had always thought of it. Care management is all about budgets and paperwork and the financial implications for the authority, whereas social work is about people. That's the crucial difference' (Jones 2005).

As part of a neoliberal and managerialist agenda, social workers are also faced with organisational change and restructuring on a regular basis. From a managerialist perspective, any problems with organisational outcomes can be dealt with by changes to the structure of the organisation. Restructuring an organisation can also be a way of making it appear as if 'something is being done' to rectify a problem that is receiving public attention (Ife 2012), such as failures in the child protection system. However, constant organisational change can be destabilising to both workers and clients.

The neoliberal and managerial context has left many practitioners feeling over-whelmed and disillusioned with their capacity to make a difference in the lives of vulnerable people. As the radical manifesto of the Social Work Action Network states: 'We didn't come into social work for this' (Lavelette 2011). However, while neoliberal-ism and managerialism may limit our freedoms, they do not do so totally, but instead operate to ensure our work is directed towards economic interest and state control (Marginson 2006). This requires a pretence of certainty and replicable efficacy of methods that has never actually been possi-ble in social work due to the complexity, diversity and fluidity of its contexts. Social workers are both victims of this situation, and simul-taneously perpetrators of it, as mainstream establishment social work concerns fitting into and surviving in a neoliberal context in ways that try to promote the '**evidence-based** social work enterprise', (Meagher &

> **Evidence-based** practice is based on scientific presumptions that a service user has a condition or problem that can be treated, monitored and evaluated (McDonald et al. 2011).

Parton 2004, pp. 10–11) and conform to the neoliberal (conservative) definition of the professional worker. This means that contemporary practice context rewards and validates workers who abandon critical social work ideals, including goals for emancipatory social change.

REFLECTIVE EXERCISE 2.2
- How comfortable do you feel with the values of neoliberalism and managerial practice?
- Can you imagine some of the implications of these contextual factors for practice?
- Make a list of some of the criticisms that critical social work might have of neoliberalism and managerialism.

One of the major difficulties with reducing services and resources to an economic value is that this results in denying the intrinsic social value of social work practice. How can we put a price on something like social justice or suicide prevention? Social goals simply recognise the inherent value and worth in everyone having access to education, health care, human rights, and so on. The costs to society of having populations that do not have these basic entitlements are far greater in terms of social wellbeing rather than savings made to governments' budgets (Wilkinson & Pickett 2010). For example, the countries that have the greatest economic inequality tend to also have the highest incidence of social problems, including high crime rates, physical and mental health problems, suicide rates, teenage pregnancy and obesity. By contrast, the countries that have a more just and equitable distribution of resources are more integrated and report far lower rates of these social problems (Wilkinson & Pickett 2010).

Can you imagine how macro social forces (such as global capitalism, neoliberal policy and managerial practices) might impact on something like the Australian education system, the health of various population groups or income distribution? As social workers, it is important to have an understanding of how these global social conditions impact at national and local levels because we will be working with many people who are collectively disadvantaged by them. Make a list of some of the ways you think these global social forces might impact on your clients or your own practice. (At first, it can be daunting and difficult to make the connections between the local and the global. This will become easier as you continue to learn and immerse yourself in the critiques of the dominant discourses.) You will remember in Chapter 1 that we discussed social myths. Like social myths, dominant discourses ensure that certain ways of thinking and talking about social issues become **normalised** and accepted as 'truth' (ways that protect the wealthy and elite and marginalise those with less access to formal power). (For further information on the impact of economic inequality on health, lifespan and trust, watch the TED talk 'How economic inequality harms societies' (Wilkinson 2011).)

> **Normalised** refers to the process whereby many oppressed people will internalise guilt, shame and blame for their oppressive experiences because they have accepted the dominant messages that they are responsible for causing the social problems they are experiencing (Mullaly 2010, p. 238).

■ Social inequality and the Australian education system

Research throughout Western societies has consistently demonstrated a strong relationship between socioeconomic class (rather than individual ability) and educational achievement (Caro 2009; Gratz 1988; Sirin 2005). It is well established that people from higher socioeconomic (class) backgrounds are more likely to succeed academically in secondary school and proceed to post-secondary education and enter well-paid jobs than students from low socioeconomic backgrounds; such students are more likely to struggle to maintain adequate employment and secure income, based on being disadvantaged in the education system (see, for example, Van Kreiken et al. 2012, p. 118).

The policies that governments introduce can either significantly reduce the impact of class background on educational achievement (which we have seen historically) or increase this inequality. Among the OECD countries, the relationship between social class and educational success is weakest in Finland (a country with low inequity in distribution of resources), but very strong in countries such as the United States (where there are large inequities in the distribution of resources), with Australia more closely aligned to the situation in the United States than to Finland (Thompson et al. 2011).

In Australia, after World War 2 (from the late 1940s through to the 1970s), governments and policymakers held a general consensus that education should be a vehicle for social equality (Wadham, Pudsey & Boyd 2007). Hence, policies sought to create an equal opportunity for all students to gain educational success based on ability, regardless of their socioeconomic background. Such policies extended secondary education to include the working class and substantially increased access to post-secondary education for people from lower socioeconomic backgrounds. However, in the 1980s the equity component in education policy was overtaken by the neoliberal agenda that treats education as a commodity for both individuals and economic growth generally. The main idea driving this policy is that school competition and choice create a quality system for all. However, there is a strong class division in the current context of education that is reinforced by an unusual dual system of educational organisation and funding that favours the wealthy to the detriment of children from poorer households. There are two streams of funding: first, there are the so-called private schools, which in Australia are government (taxpayer) subsidised schools but can operate as private businesses (often with additional investment and endowment income streams) and have the right to select and exclude students on a user-pays basis. Second, there are the state schools, which must accommodate all students within their geographical zone, and which cannot make profits or invest. The private school system is therefore at a significant advantage because it has multiple sources of funding. In addition, the elite private schools can charge fees that can be higher than a low-income family's yearly income while still receiving government support from taxpayers, 70 per cent of whom could never afford to send their own children to these schools. The richest private schools in Victoria recorded profits of up to $14 million in 2009, of which taxpayers contributed more than half (Craig 2010).

In 2012 the average annual minimum wage before tax was $31 500. The annual cost of enrolling a year 12 student at Geelong Grammar is $32 400, while other expenses, such as camps, music lessons and uniforms, are additional to these fees (Topsfield 2012).

The benefits of competition and 'choice' are supposed to be enhanced by publicly subsidising private schooling and ranking the performance of schools in 'league tables'. However, this overlooks the preferential treatment and funding that students attending private schools experience. Using Tasmania as an example, ostensibly a $20 million 'school of choice' policy claims that all parents can theoretically send their children to any school in Tasmania served by government-sponsored private transport. However, in practice, the neoliberal and managerial context means that private transport operators will underservice or not service an area that is unprofitable. Hence, this policy functions predominantly to enable children from wealthy families to be collected from and delivered to elite private schools (to which the poor have no access) at taxpayers' expense, while students in rural, regional and remote areas of the state have limited access to this government-sponsored private transport because it is not profitable to provide a service to distant and isolated areas. The results of the social and economic inequalities created by global capitalism, neoliberal policies and managerial practices in the context of education speak for themselves. Recent research has revealed that half of the Tasmanian population between the ages of 15–74 are **functionally illiterate** and more than half are **functionally innumerate** (Australian Bureau of Statistics 2012b). The national Australian average is not much better, with dysfunctional literacy at a rate of 47 per cent (Badham 2013).

> **Functionally illiterate** means having reading and writing skills that are inadequate to function on a daily basis and maintain employment that requires more than basic levels (Schlecty 2004).

The response to the educational crisis in Tasmania of neoliberal policymakers is to close the smaller schools that service outlying communities and expect students at these schools to transfer to bigger schools with literacy specialists. However, in devising such a solution, far more profound and basic inequalities are overlooked. In an equitable system, the funding would be directed to the poorer students to enable them to access education (appoint literacy specialists in smaller schools rather than closing them down). Instead, the policy to close smaller schools only serves to further disadvantage those children and their families who subsequently have to negotiate travel and geographical access barriers in addition to struggling at school.

> **Functionally innumerate** is the inability to apply reason and comprehend basic numeracy skills. This can have a negative effect on career, health and economic choices (Reyna et al. 2009).

The key point is that neoliberal policy that supports the objectives of capitalism is currently functioning to maintain rather than reduce inequality. Education research shows that between 1996 and 2006 there was a substantial movement of high-income students out of state schools, and a proportionate movement of students with low-socioeconomic backgrounds out of private schooling and into the public education system (Bonner 2011). Indeed, the proportion of low-income students enrolling in state schools has doubled in the past 25 years (Ferrari 2013). The gap between public and private schools is not just economic as socioeconomic disadvantage for low-income background students is compounded by attending schools that are poorly resourced and where expectations of student success and progression towards higher education may be minimal. Research demonstrates that an average 15-year-old student of a low-socioeconomic background in a severely disadvantaged school is about three and a half years behind a peer of a high socioeconomic background in a private school (Bonner 2011). Moreover, only 15 per cent of university places go to the people from low-socioeconomic backgrounds and this has remained unchanged for years (Universities Australia 2008). The neoliberal agenda threatens both the quality and the equity of not only Australian schooling, but also the fabric of Australian society generally. According to international data (Thompson et al. 2011), between 2000 and 2009 there was a substantial drop in Australia's educational performance across the board compared with other OECD nations, despite a 40 per cent funding increase in that period (because the funding is being used to support the dual system, which favours the wealthy). The same international research shows that successful school systems are generally those that show above-average social equity (Thompson et al. 2011).

REFLECTIVE EXERCISE 2.4

Now visit the Programme for International Student Assessment (PISA) website, http://www.oecd.org/pisa/. Go also to the Tasmanian Government Department of Infrastructure, Energy and Resources website, which hosts this document: *Core Passenger Service Review – Final Report* (2007), http://www.stategrowth.tas.gov.au/passenger/reviews/review-services.

Make a list of some of the features of this policy on rural school bus services that serve to further disadvantage already vulnerable populations.

- What are some more socially just alternatives?
- How would these be different from existing policies?
- What principles might inform these alternatives?

■ Globalisation

Globalisation refers to large-scale changes that bring together previously separate societies into a global network, predominantly through the development of global technologies and global economies.

Global capitalism is made possible by **globalisation**. From an economic point of view, globalisation simply means integration into the world economy, which is seen as the only means for poorer nations to develop. It is a term that is used to refer to the way in which the world is 'shrinking' as new technologies, means of communication, and political and economic systems enable connectedness across the globe. (For further information see Van Krieken et al. 2012.)

The term 'globalisation' arose in the 1980s, becoming part of popular language and signifying an important change taking place in the world (Baylis & Smith 1997). Globalisation can be thought of in a number of different ways:

- *internationalisation* – the development of international institutions transcending national borders
- *liberalisation* – the spread of the 'free market' in the world economy
- *universalisation* – the imposition of the same images and ideas across the world
- *modernisation* – the modern state, bureaucracy, and so on
- *deterritorialisation* – processes whereby social space becomes more global, not located in a particular place (Scholte 2000, cited in Dower 2003, pp. 42–3).

Globalisation is manifested in mass and social media, the internationalisation of corporations that treat the whole planet as their sphere of activity, global environmental changes, world stock markets and globalised economies, global weaponry and worldwide military coalitions, and everyday thinking.

What does globalisation have to do with social work?

It is important first to acknowledge some of the ways in which globalisation and developments in information and communication technology have enhanced our capacity to practise critically. Global and instantaneous communication creates a wealth of possibilities that include opportunities to develop new insights, share knowledge and form partnerships; the formation of global coalitions to challenge social issues that transcend borders; the creation of international conventions on social, political and economic rights; and the enrichment of the diversity of **nation states** through the **migration** and movement of peoples across the world.

Nation states are a type of state that emerged around 200 years ago, in which the government claims exclusive right to sovereign power (Giddens & Sutton 2013).

At the same time, globalisation has intensified the power of dominant social forces by making them, and the oppressive ideologies that support them, global. In short, globalisation has led to the internationalisation of social problems, which now transcend the borders of a particular nation. For example, the inequalities created by capitalism that increase the gap between rich and poor now extend throughout the world. Natural resources (such as oil, forests, uranium, coal, gold and natural gas) are exploited by the demands of global markets, enriching a global elite and creating huge wealth disparities and massive environmental destruction worldwide.

Migration refers to the movement of people between nation states that accompanies the movement of commodities and capital, made easier in recent times by better transportation and communication technologies (Castles & Miller 2003).

> This YouTube video explores the inequities of natural resources exploitation: 'Exploiting West Papua', http://www.youtube.com/watch?v=KWepsOYr6iw.

The commercial mass media is also owned and perpetuated by a global elite, who can shape our 'news' and provide a view of the world that supports the dominant interests.

> The 2013 Australian federal election provides an example of the mass media taking a powerful role in creating dominant discourses and influencing the outcome of an election (particularly through editorial policy and opinion). There is no longer a pretence of neutrality in how the mass media reports the 'news'. The purpose of government is to coordinate society, not to make a profit, and yet somehow the media convinced a great many people, including those who are most vulnerable and adversely affected, to vote against their own interests and security. This is now an important part of our social context.

Individualism refers to an increasingly individualist emphasis within society; this has been created by economic and social changes that have removed a mechanism of socialisation within which collectivist ideas and attitudes were once generated. Changes in the nature of the workplace, the employment relationship and management styles have all contributed to increasing individualism (Giddens & Sutton 2013).

Consumerism refers to the increasing affluence in Western countries, which has resulted in a greater emphasis on consumption and leisure. Opportunities to consume have massively increased and are promoted extensively through the media and the internet (Giddens & Sutton 2013).

At the same time, the media bombards and saturates us with advertising images that create global cultures of **individualism** and **consumerism**, undermining local communities and indigenous diversity. Those who are left out of the global technological revolution may experience new forms of inequality as social justice is undermined by global capitalism. The West's monopoly of financial, natural and weaponry resources has caused war and terrorism. This, combined with global-scale natural disasters caused by extreme weather events due to global warming that many argue are linked to our unsustainable Western lifestyles, has begun to create major displacements of people (climate-change refugees), thus generating hopelessness, fear and tragedy (Rowe et al. 2000). Indeed, the ease and pace of international travel created by globalisation has certainly increased the prospects for global epidemics of infectious diseases (Tatem, Rogers & Hay 2006).

Sometimes it can be difficult to imagine how globalisation affects life at a local level but with some effort you can see the connections. One of the authors of this textbook lives in a regional centre where the closure of local car-manufacturing plants has profoundly impacted the livelihood of relatively large numbers of residents, as the manufacture is moved offshore to take advantage of cheaper labour and production costs. Similarly, in the rural areas surrounding this

The 2700 island residents of the Carteret Islands, seven tiny coral atolls in the Pacific, have become climate-change refugees. It is believed that rising sea levels due to global warming have increased the sinking of a volcano that supports the atolls. Worsening storm surges and spring tides inundated the islands' fresh water supply and ruined the islands' crops. The residents have relocated 80 km south to Bougainville (Morton 2009).

regional setting, farmers have moved off the land in increasing numbers as global agribusiness has taken over the traditional family farm. At the national level, we hear discussions about basic services (such as water boards and electricity companies) being bought out by foreign interests, and of course the mining industry, fuelled by multinational corporations, extracts considerable wealth from Australia and impacts on local communities in myriad ways.

■ Government and the law

While globalisation highlights the limitations and diminishing significance of national boundaries, most of us will live out our lives within the borders and be subject to the government and **laws** of particular nation states. Nation states are a type of state that emerged around 200 years ago in which the government claims exclusive right to **sovereign power** over a clearly defined territory and group of citizens (e.g. Australia, France, Canada, Sweden). Often used interchangeably with the geographical term 'country', nation state refers to a social and political entity (Giddens & Sutton 2013).

Law encompasses a systematic collection of principles and rules that define rights and duties, and the set of institutions which enforce them (Swain 2002).

The modern nation state remains a defining feature of our contemporary practice context because the entire legal basis for the welfare state is underpinned by the power of the nation state. The nation state is the basic law-making institution in modern society and the basis of our identity as citizens with certain rights and responsibilities. 'Social workers need to understand legal discourse ... because the law often defines our key responsibilities to employing agencies and service users' (Healy 2005, p. 38). This is particularly important for workers employed by government organisations who work with involuntary (statutory) clients (such as in child protection), but is relevant to all practitioners in terms of thinking about responsibilities such as **duty of care**, **duty to disclose**, **informed consent**, **relative** versus **absolute notions of confidentiality**.

As social workers we need to be aware of the dual nature of the law: both as an instrument of advocacy for service users' rights and social

Sovereign power has traditionally been understood as the unlimited rule by a state over a territory and the people in it for political, social and economic ends (Dalton et al. 1996).

Duty of care is 'The obligation to take reasonable care to avoid acts or omissions which one can reasonably foresee would be likely to injure another; also, the duty of people in particular circumstances and occupations to protect and control others' (AASW 2002, p. 26). **Duty to disclose** refers to the release of confidential information in particular situations if, for example, a client may be at risk of harm (Swain & Rice 2009).

change, but also as a vehicle for social control that can undermine justice (Healy 2005). One of the inherent contradictions of the law is that it is simultaneously caught between the pressures of **democracy** and **bureaucracy**.

As with other powerful social forces that shape our contemporary contexts, the law and government are contested and at times highly problematic. We will explore this further in Chapter 5 when we discuss the intersection of law and ethics.

■ Patriarchy

Patriarchy literally means 'rule of the father' (Ferguson 1999, p. 1048).

All known societies are patriarchal to some extent, albeit to varying degrees (Giddens & Sutton 2013). While patriarchy is a system that accords economic, social and political privileges to men, the unequal distribution of power harms both men and women. Hence, it is in the interests of both men and women to challenge the harmful effects of patriarchy. Mullender (1997, cited in Thompson 2001, p. 42) contends:

> It is not possible to understand the personal or social world without taking a **gendered perspective**. We are not able as professionals to intervene appropriately or justly in people's lives unless we perceive the ways in which women are disadvantaged by an unequal dispersal of power, and in which both men and women are constrained by over-rigid and falsely dichotomised role and relationship expectations.

This inequality is based on socially constructed gender roles, and not simply biology. As Thompson (2001, p. 45) states: 'Our conceptions of normality are "gendered".'

Information disseminated by the United Nations Development Programme (UNDP) shows the impact of patriarchy on women in

---

[1] 'In general, for [informed] consent to be considered valid six standards must be met: (1) coercion and undue influence must not have played a role in the client's decision; (2) clients must be mentally capable of providing consent; (3) clients must consent to specific procedures or actions; (4) the consent forms and procedures must be valid; (5) clients must have the right to refuse or withdraw consent; and (6) clients' decisions must be based on adequate information' (Reamer 2006, pp. 167, 168).

a global sense is profound. Women contribute 66 per cent of all the world's working hours and produce half of the world's food, yet earn only 10 per cent of the world's income and own less than one per cent of the world's property (UNDP 2011). Indeed, 60 per cent of the world's 1.3 billion people living in **extreme** (or **absolute**) **poverty** (UNDP 2011) are women (UNDP 1995, p. 4).

Historical research shows that violence against women is global and cross-cultural; the relations between women and men in workplaces are characterised by hierarchical gender relations and inequality in wages (Bell & Klein 1996). Recent research does little to paint a more hopeful picture. While domestic violence has been made illegal in 125 nations, 603 million women still live in countries where domestic violence is not regarded as a crime (UN Women 2011).

Rape in marriage has been criminalised in 52 countries; however, 2.6 billion women live in countries where marital rape is still not illegal. Approximately 68 000 women die from unsafe abortions each year, comprising one in seven of all maternal deaths worldwide. Annually, there are approximately 20 million unsafe abortions due to prohibitions of abortion in nations throughout the developing world (UN Women 2011). Half a million women die annually from pregnancy and childbirth (Millennium Campaign 2007). In 2009, women represented 53 per cent in developing countries and 21 per cent in developed countries of the 33.3 million people living with HIV. Most HIV-positive women were infected by their husbands or long-term

A **gendered perspective** refers to the fact that most major systems in Western societies are hierarchically organised and male-dominated (Mullaly 2010), and this is considered natural or inevitable, perpetuating and sustaining power relations between genders.

Femininity refers to the socially constructed characteristics of being female, including passivity, emotionality, natural caregiving, irrationality and weakness (Mullaly 2010).

Masculinity refers to the socially constructed characteristics of being male, including strength, aggression and competitiveness (Mullaly 2010).

partners, and in India, 90 per cent of women with HIV contracted the disease in a long-term relationship, indicating that women's lack of decision-making power in relationships may increase their risk of infection. Women continue to be under-represented in ministerial positions, with 30 per cent being the highest representation of women in any country (UN Women 2011).

In the Australian context, women have made considerable gains in recent decades; however, they still face considerable gender inequalities. Women's workforce participation, for example, has increased significantly over the last 20 years and in 2008, 54.2 per cent of women were in paid employment. However, this historically high rate is still 19 per cent less than the male employment rate and in 2005–06 women had only a 37 per cent share of total income (Cassells et al. 2009). There is also a persistent gap in the average incomes of women and men, despite the fact that women's pay rates have been legally the same as men's rates for equivalent work since the early 1970s, which was enshrined in the *Sex Discrimination Act 1986* (Cth). In 2012, Australian men were paid on average 17.6 per cent more than women, which over an average working lifetime would mean the average woman worker earns $1 million less than a man (Cassells et al. 2009). At the same time, the average weekly earnings figure for full-time working women was $1228, whereas for men it was $1489 – a gap of $261.60 per week (Australian Bureau of Statistics 2012a). What is most disturbing for women is that the gap has grown since 2004 (by 14.9%), corresponding with the introduction of the 'WorkChoices' legislation in 2005 by the Howard Government.

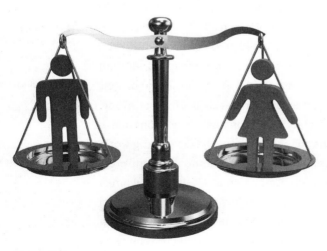

Figure 2.1

> The WorkChoices legislation placed considerable power in the hands of the employers, removing protections for workers such as unfair dismissal, and severely restricting the role of unions to protect the rights of workers.

Despite the abolishment of WorkChoices, its legacy remains: currently the gap between men's and women's wages is 17 per cent – that is, still larger than it was in the early 1990s (Workplace Gender Equality Agency (WGEA) 2013, p. 1). According to WGEA, part of the reason for this difference is that women tend to be concentrated in lower paid occupations and under-represented in the higher paid ones. In the community and disability care sector, for example, there are 150 000 workers, of whom 120 000 are women who earn on average $46 000 per year, which is $12 000 below the average wage (Coorey 2011). This is clearly a sector whose care-based skills are demonstrably undervalued by a patriarchal and capitalist economy. Women's careers are also more likely to be broken by motherhood and their taking part-time or casual work. However, part of the gap eludes any other explanation than *covert discrimination* by employers (WGEA 2013).

Social work and the human services professions are also dominated by patriarchy. Women are over-represented as women and clients, while men are over-represented as managers (O'Connor et al. 2008). Australian women also continue to have low representation in the legal system and even lower representation in the political system. Indeed, the Australian Prime Minister's cabinet is currently comprised entirely of white, middle-class men, with the exception of one white, middle-class woman. Afghanistan, a country that is widely known for human rights abuses against women, now has more women in cabinet than does Australia (Kenny 2013). Discrimination, exploitation and abuses against women are enshrined in legislation and underwritten by social policy (Morley & Macfarlane 2008). Not surprisingly, based on their disempowered societal position, women are over-represented in the mental health system as clients (Astbury 1996; Macfarlane 2009; Morley 2003b).

In addition to the harms created by patriarchy for women, research indicates that both men and women have much to gain by challenging patriarchy and replacing it with more equitable social arrangements. Research detailing the major reasons why men access social work services indicates that patriarchy causes emotional inexpressiveness, poor health, distant fathering, family breakdown, stress associated with competitiveness and overwork, the over-representation of men in substance abuse, high-risk behaviours, homelessness, suicide and criminality (Pease 2010).

■ Biomedical discourses

Biomedical discourses refer to the ideas, languages and practices used to justify the medical model (which is based on the biological sciences) as the dominant approach to health and illness (Healy 2005).

The biomedical model is another dominant social force that shapes our current context, both in terms of influencing social work practice, and in its effects on our clients. The medical model, or biomedicine, as it is sometimes referred to, is the current, dominant understanding of health and illness that derives knowledge from the biological sciences. Drawing on the work of medical sociologists, Healy (2005, pp. 20–1) adopts the term **biomedical discourse** to refer to the impact of the medical model, which she defines as 'a specific set of ideas and practices associated with a biological approach to medicine'.

Biomedical discourses powerfully construct our 'common sense' understandings of the people with whom we work, their understandings of themselves, and the nature of the services we provide (Healy 2005). For example, a strictly biomedical understanding creates the illness categories of 'schizophrenia' or 'bipolar disorder', without acknowledging how people's experiences of poverty, racism, homelessness, violence and other injustices result in what the medical model views as 'illness' and 'symptoms'. (For further information see the discussion of the case study of Sarah in Chapter 7.) Critical social work has a number of concerns about the dominance of biomedical discourses. First, because these discourses assume that illnesses or disabilities deviate from 'normal' bodily functions, it follows that a practitioner working from a biomedical perspective should aim to correct the deviation, rather than altering the environment to be more accommodating of difference (Healy 2005).

The **social model** focuses on the social construction of disability – access, stereotypes, conceptions of normality, ideas of difference and capacity are all defined by, and embedded in, the social order (Barnes & Mercer 2004).

This denies the social, political, economic and cultural dimensions that shape people's experiences of health and illness, and deflects attention from inadequate (and sometimes oppressive) societal responses. For example, is the fact that a person is confined to a wheelchair the problem? (This is the biomedical view.) Or is it the fact that the building has stairs, with no appropriate ramp or lift access that is the problem? **Social model** critiques of biomedical discourses suggest that disabilities would not necessarily be an issue if our society was more adequately responsive to accommodate, rather than **pathologise** (or problematise), difference. The problem, from a critical perspective, is not the disability, but the social problem of ableism. Ableism refers to the oppression of people in society that become marginalised based on their abilities (Wachsler 2007). It occurs when people hold **normative** assumptions about ability, and then stigmatise or discriminate against others who do not meet those expectations. A recognition of ableism is essential for critical practice that is **anti-oppressive** (Shier, Sinclair & Gault 2011).

By contrast, the focus on deficits and pathology can result in a narrative that blames the victim and is therefore not oriented towards education or social transformation (Sargent, Nilan & Winter 1997). Indeed, by invoking an **individualistic** understanding that ignores the **structural context**, biomedical discourses operate to perfectly complement neoliberal practices and policies (that also construct social problems in individual terms by focusing on individual responsibility).

A second concern about biomedical discourses is that they assume that medical practitioners have the most valuable and relevant expertise over all other disciplines and professions (Sargent, Nilan & Winter 1997). Practitioners informed by this perspective aim to conduct **assessments** using their expert knowledge, and then devise **interventions** to fix the problem (locating power and control with the practitioner and implicitly constructing the individual as the problem).

> [These] expert, pathological understandings of the problem authorise biological and psychological interventions that overlook the role that society plays (violence, poverty and other forms of oppression) in producing ill health and disease, and discounts the social patterns in health that seem to closely mirror the same patterns of social inequality (Morley 2003b).

For example, in general, people from higher socioeconomic classes have better health than people from lower socioeconomic classes. Research indicates that morbidity and mortality rates are directly linked to social class: people on lower incomes have higher rates of illness and lower life expectancy, whereas high-income earners have much lower rates of illness and higher life expectancy (Australian Institute of Health and Welfare (AIHW) 2008, p. 65). This is further compounded for Indigenous people. For example, twice as many

To **pathologise** is to treat a perceived condition as a disease or psychologically abnormal.

Normative refers to dominant cultural understandings of what is regarded as normal (e.g. 'able-bodied) (Barnes & Mercer 2004).

Anti-oppressive social work 'is a form of social work practice which addresses social divisions and structural inequalities in the work that is done with "clients"' (Dominelli 1998, p. 24).

Individualistic approaches are part of mainstream or establishment social work that understands the issue as a deficit within the individual (Mullaly 2010, p. 275).

Structural context is the way in which social institutions, laws, policies and practices allocate goods and services while restricting the access of marginalised groups (Mullaly 2010, p. 150).

Assessment involves 'making a professional judgement about the problematic aspects of a situation' (Fook 2012, p. 132).

Intervention refers to a method of practice applied after a professional judgement has been made, and is used to achieve 'measurable results using available resources in the most effective way' (Ife 1996, p. 52).

Objectivism is a paradigm that assumes there is an objective reality (that is knowable or known) and that it exists independently from the knower, and therefore it is possible and desirable to remove the subjective and intuitive dimensions of knowledge from our understandings (Meinert, Pardeck & Kreuger 2000; Sarantakos 2005a).

A **paradigm** is a set of assumptions, concepts, values and practices that provide a way of understanding the world and how it operates.

Culture is a term that aims to describe the complex and 'distinctive ways of life and shared values, beliefs and meanings common to groups of people . . . the understandings and expectations which guide actions and interactions with others' (Quinn 2009, pp. 97–8).

Aboriginal and Torres Strait Islander people report mental illness, compared to non-Indigenous Australians. Moreover, the life expectancy of Indigenous Australians is 59 years for men and 65 years for women, compared to non-Indigenous averages of 77 for men and 82 for women. Hospitalisation for dialysis is 14 times higher for Aboriginal and Torres Strait Islander people than for the rest of the population (AIHW 2008).

A third concern is that, within biomedical assessment processes, there is an assumption that all problems are logical and resolvable if we just apply the right technical solution. This is based on an **objectivist paradigm** that assumes the scientific knowledge created by these assessments, and the subsequent interventions, are objective, unbiased and universal (that is, they can be applied to entire populations regardless of **culture**, gender, socioeconomic status, and so on) (see, for example, Ife 2012). From an objectivist view, it is believed possible knowledge can be known independently from the knower, and therefore it is assumed possible to remove the subjective and intuitive dimensions of knowledge from our understandings (Meinert, Pardeck & Kreuger 2000a; Sarantakos 2005). This means that research and assessments are undertaken using ostensibly objective means in order to find the evidence and the 'truth' about social phenomena (Humphries 2008; Loftus, Higgs & Trede 2011). In practice, these sorts of assumptions translate into the use of *risk assessment* tools and the quest for evidence-based social work to guide practice. Within the current context, these attempts to make social work practice more scientific and certain are linked with aspirations of professional legitimacy and competence (Morley 2003a). Establishment social work has long had a fascination with the medical sciences and has sought ways to embrace the practices of the medical profession as well as aligning with the power and prestige it accords (ironically, from a social justice perspective). The social diagnosis framework developed by Mary Richmond in 1917 is one example (Healy 2005) that demonstrates social work's historical commitment to align with the medical model. 'Claiming to be a science-based profession with an important role in the monitoring and control of problematic populations at risk', as establishment social work claims to do in the current context, is a more contemporary example (Davies & Leonard 2004, p. x).

The ongoing neoliberal cuts to services since the 1980s have resulted in many fields of practice, including child protection, being overwhelmed by the demands placed on the services. While this in part has contributed to the rise in the development and implementation of risk assessment tools (Dutton & Kropp 2000; Walsh & Weeks 2004; Webb 2006), it also further distracts from lobbying political systems for urgently needed resources (Goddard et al. 1999) and perpetuates a managerial agenda that aims to measure and quantify all social phenomena in scientific terms, thus reinforcing the neoliberal logic of auditing and accountancy. Indeed, conducting risk assessments may actually have more to do with protecting the agency, rather than improving practice or increasing accountability of services for clients (Morley 2003a).

Likewise, the current, mainstream obsession with *evidence-based practice* has arisen from the need to control uncertainty and reduce complexity by quantifying it. Originally drawn from evidence-based medicine, in which it arguably had more relevant application due to dealing with the natural sciences where there are more observable regularities, evidence-based practice has colonised the human services. Indeed, in the context of promoting health and treating illness, evidence-based research is assumed to inform 'best practice' (Madhu 2011). Despite this, critical social workers find some of the assumptions underpinning evidence-based practice quite objectionable.

Evidence-based practice is based on the principles that one 'finds' the evidence, critically evaluates it, devises the most appropriate intervention based on the evidence and implements this course of action. However, this simplistic, **linear** model of knowledge creation has been critiqued for not being sophisticated enough to respond to the complexities and uncertainties inherent in social work practice (Plath 2013). The notion that evidence can be found as an objective process is robustly contested, especially when we consider multiple sources of knowledge outside the purely scientific paradigms, such as **reflexivity**.

> **Linear** models, processes or frameworks contain a number of chronological steps leading to a definitive conclusion.

An implicit assumption is that 'some evidence is stronger or better than other evidence' (Plath 2013, p. 230), and as we have noted throughout this chapter, dominant social forces, and the discourses they perpetuate, privilege some knowledge as evidence and exclude other forms of knowledge – not because the ideas are superior or more true, but because it serves the interests of those in power for them to be perceived as truth. Evidence-based practice does not sit outside power structures, values or politics and so the pretence of objectively finding 'truth' using scientific means sits uncomfortably with critical social work that aims to critically reflect on (rather than deny the existence of) our values and assumptions and how they shape our production, and our interpretation, of knowledge.

> **Reflexivity** involves (1) 'the ability of individuals to process information and create knowledge to guide life choices; (2) an individual's self-critical approach that questions how knowledge is generated and how relations of power operate in this process; and (3) a concern with the part that emotions play in social work practice' (D'Cruz, Gillingham & Melendez 2007, p. 75).

■ The (inter)connections of dominant social forces

A further element in understanding the contemporary contexts is the interrelatedness of the dominant social forces. Rather than operating as separate entities, they often work in partnership to reinforce and strengthen the dominance and power of each other. For example, some social commentators have argued that the biomedical discourses (and the practices that have emerged from them, including risk assessment and evidence-based practices) have achieved their powerful position in society and in service delivery by fulfilling the needs of other dominant social forces. Undeniably, the *objectivist paradigm*, on which biomedical discourses are based, is fortified by global capitalism and patriarchy, and vice versa. For example, constructing women's mental health issues as a medical problem or disease simultaneously serves the interests of both neoliberal capitalism and patriarchy. Denying the social context in a psychiatric (biomedical) assessment individualises and pathologises the problem, and in doing so serves the interests of neoliberalism that deny social context and ascribe individual responsibility. At the same time, constructing women's mental health issues as a medical problem **medicalises** the harmful consequences of our patriarchal society that creates women's distress in the first place (the role of violence, poverty, low status, poorly paid work, and so on) (Astbury 1996).

> **Medicalisation** refers to the process of redefining normal human bodily experiences as medical problems. In other words, physical experiences that were historically seen as unproblematic suddenly become, through the intervention of the medical profession and a renaming of the experience, a problem (Holmes, Hughes & Julian 2012, p. 203).

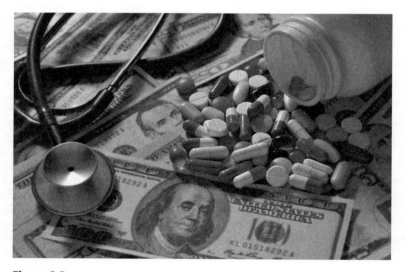

Figure 2.2

The assessment and treatment of mental health problems, according to biomedical discourses, involves prescribing an assortment of addictive tranquilising drugs to help women cope with the injustices they experience through gendered inequalities. This reinforces a patriarchal society, and at the same time meets the needs of capitalism by creating a market for pharmaceutical industries to exploit (Bainbridge 1999). For example, in the United States alone the expenditure on pharmaceutical drugs has reached US$307 billion per year (Stringer 2011).

In addition, the law and government are used to enforce certain types of treatment (psychiatric) and authorise particular practitioners and expertise (medical) to define and treat the problem to the exclusion of all others. The same intersection of social forces comes into play if we examine the Western health 'crisis' of obesity. In addressing this issue, government policies consistently target individual behaviour change as the answer to the problem, and sanction medical treatment of the issue; however, this focus on the individual overlooks key economic and social (or structural factors underlying obesity (Alvaro et al. 2010).

Another example of the intersections between the dominant social forces is evident in the way neoliberal discourse endorses the presumably objective and rational character of the ostensibly 'free' market to maximise profit, and in doing so treats the world as a finite set of resources to be exploited. It, therefore, objectifies nature in order to turn it into a set of economic commodities and tries to extract as much profit as possible using rational, objectifying procedures at minimum cost. For example, a beautiful forest that provides shade and a home for many varieties of animal and bird life, and that purifies our air by producing oxygen, seems to have no real value from an economic perspective, until it is turned into woodchips that are sold on the market. Being able to objectify and commodify nature in this way, where the only value that is acknowledged is economic value, is useful for achieving the neoliberal goals of capital accumulation.

The *objectivist* view, therefore, supports the people who are in power within society; those who own and control the means of capital. At the same time, objectivism also marginalises other (potentially discordant, dissenting) voices that are not as useful for maximising commercial gain/profit and those critical voices who favour social or environmental concerns over economic ones – unless, of course, these critical voices can be turned into a commodity! One of the perversities of the capitalism system, for example, is the amorality of the market. All that is regarded as good, virtuous and desirable within this neoliberal context is associated with profit and economic growth. Hence, even commodities that attack the system, such as Michael Moore's series of critical films, are valued by the system, provided they contribute to capital growth (see http://michaelmoore.com).

While the dominant discourses work together to support each other, we are not suggesting that they are all equally powerful or that there will not be times when they may be competing or in conflict. We are again reminded of the importance of context in understanding the impact of these social forces. Global capitalism, for example, will certainly not be the most powerful or influential discourse at a conference on climate change, where the excesses of Western lifestyles are implicated in destroying our planet. And while medical perspectives may be more dominant than critical perspectives in hospital settings, managerialist practices can undermine medical power and patient care through the same cost-cutting measures that have eroded the welfare state in the human services sector.

REFLECTIVE EXERCISE 2.7

For a concrete example of how scientific research and medical advances can be undermined by neoliberal capitalism, watch this short YouTube clip: 'Cancer cured in Canada, but Big Pharma says NO WAY!, https://www.youtube.com/watch?v=Y3x-Uj4yAMY.

The clip reports a potential cure for breast and other cancers and claims it cannot be patented because the pharmaceutical companies won't make it available, since they don't stand to make a profit from marketing it. What are your responses to this?

■ Summary

Australia, like other Western capitalist countries, is impacted by dominant social forces, including global capitalism, economic rationalism/neoliberalism, managerialism, globalisation, patriarchy, biomedical discourses, government and the law, which create major social inequalities and divisions in class, gender and ethnicity in terms of access to power and distribution of resources. These social forces that shape our contemporary contexts have direct implications for how we operate in the field as we are challenged by increasing pressures to work within managerial structures and protocols within neoliberal discourses that work to fulfil the functions of global capitalism. One of the key elements that critical social work offers us as practitioners is a critical analysis of how these social forces operate at global, national and local levels, so that we can recognise and resist their impact on the lives of the individuals, groups and communities with whom we work, and on our social work practice.

When first introduced to a critical analysis of society many students and practitioners can understandably feel quite overwhelmed and disempowered. It can be confronting to think about the magnitude of social injustices in our contemporary contexts and the experiences of marginalisation and oppression that these create. Despite the social problems created by the contemporary contexts, social work and the human services professions are in a powerful position to challenge these and work towards change. In the continuation of the discussion of social contexts in the next chapter, we explore some of the practice strategies that social workers use to respond critically and creatively to the contextual factors outlined in this chapter.

■ Review questions

* What are some of the main questions this chapter has raised for you?
* How do you feel about the information presented in this chapter? (Have you experienced an emotional response to it? What implications might this have for your practice?)
* Where do you fit in the contemporary social contexts? Are you able to identify ways that you are disadvantaged by some aspects of the dominant social forces?
* Are there ways in which you are privileged by aspects of the dominant social forces?
* How does having an understanding of the contemporary social contexts influence your decision to be a critical practitioner or an establishment practitioner? Why?

■ Further reading

Ferguson, K., 1999, 'Patriarchy' in H. Tierney, ed, *Women's Studies Encyclopedia*, vol. 2, Greenwood Publishing, New York, p. 1048.

Jamrozik, A., 2009, 'Social policy in a "free market economy"' in *Social Policy in the Post-Welfare State: Australian Society in a Changing World*, 3rd edn, Pearson Education Australia, Frenchs Forest, NSW.

McDonald, C., Craik, C., Hawkins, L. and Williams, J., 2011, 'Scoping the context' in *Professional Practice in Human Service Organisations*, Allen & Unwin, Crows Nest, NSW.

Moghadan, V., 2005, 'The feminization of poverty' and women's human rights', SAH Papers in Women's Studies Gender Research, No. 2, *Social and Human Sciences*, pp. 1–40.

3

What can we do? A critical response to social contexts

■ Introduction

CHAPTER 2 EXPLORED some of the dominant social forces that shape our contemporary contexts, including global capitalism, economic rationalism/neoliberalism, managerialism, globalisation, patriarchy, biomedical discourses, government and the law. It also outlined some of the vast social inequalities created by these macro contextual factors along the lines of class, gender and ethnicity. Following on directly from this discussion, this chapter addresses the ways in which social work and human services practitioners respond in critical and creative ways to these challenges created by the contemporary contexts.

> **Social research**, from a critical perspective, is a practice that involves generating new knowledge to contribute to the building of a more just, participatory and sustainable world.

Significantly, the theory and practices of critical social work help us to devise ways to contest and resist the harms created by dominant social forces. Developing a critical analysis of dominant social forces is an essential first step in devising creative practice responses. In exploring possibilities for critical practice within contemporary contexts we will highlight various strategies, including critical analysis of dominant discourses; analysis and development of social policy; engaging in community development, social activism and social movements; undertaking critical practice in organisations; and undertaking **social research** as a means of finding discretionary spaces to work towards social justice and **emancipatory** aims.

> **Emancipatory** literally means 'freedom promoting' and refers to an activist or social change orientation in which practice is focused on transforming processes and structures that perpetuate domination and exploitation (Healy 2005, p. 3).

■ Responding to challenges posed by contemporary contexts

The profession and practice of social work, as well as the theories and assumptions that guide it, emerged and continue to develop within multiple layers of events, influences and interactions, often referred to as *context*. The notion of context captures an acknowledgement that social work practice is constantly changing as we respond to dynamic social, cultural, economic and political contexts, as well as the local and organisational issues that influence our work. This situation provides both challenges and opportunities for ethical practitioners informed by a critical perspective. While our discussion thus far has focused on the challenges, we will be now shifting our attention to the opportunities to resist the harmful effects of dominant social forces and to develop critical practice responses.

Social work can be ideally placed to respond to the complexities of locating individual and social issues – as well as our practice – within broader contexts; in fact this is our stock in trade. The changing and responsive nature of our practice is part of what makes our profession unique. We are not afraid to reconsider past understandings and practice while we remain unapologetic about our commitment to social justice endeavours. Our hopefulness about a better world is underpinned by awareness of the ways in which the most powerful and oppressive discourses can shift and how even small actions at the level of organisational and relational practice contribute to social change. As critical social workers, our understanding and analysis of the complex contextual layers surrounding ourselves, our practice and the lives of those we work with is one of the most important parts of our contribution to a better social world. When we consider the ways in which the dominant social forces impact not only at global but also at national and local levels, we also need to consider the ways in which this process can be reversed; that is, how we can impact at the local level in ways that have implications at the global level. Thus, the actions of workers, although humble, may engender more anti-oppressive organisational processes; the actions of one organisation or a network of organisations may impact on public policy for the nation; and the actions of one community may have an impact on saving the environment of a continent.

Critical social work proceeds from an understanding of social change – to challenge the power divisions and inequalities produced by society. It questions the specific social, cultural and historical conditions that shape social institutions and individual lives to identify how things might be otherwise and how we might contribute to changing things for the better (see, for example, Healy 2000). It may be our ability to work critically with/in a range of contexts that is the hallmark of social work (Fook 2012; Healy 2000); that is, we bring our values, theories and critical perspective to whatever setting we work in. As critical social workers, attempting to understand and act in ways that engender personal and social change, we are committed to an in-depth analysis of how individual problems are shaped by *structural contexts*.

CASE STUDY

Peter

Peter has been unemployed for six months. He had worked for more than 30 years in a car-manufacturing plant but was recently made redundant because the company he had worked for was downsizing. Peter has never had to go through a formal job interview process. He is in his fifties. He has recently applied for more than 100 jobs but has not been successful in moving past the application stage. Peter says he feels ashamed. He never thought he would end up being a 'dole bludger' and he has now started taking antidepressants that were prescribed by his GP (general practitioner).

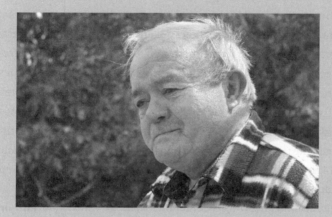

Figure 3.1

REFLECTIVE EXERCISE 3.1

- What is your understanding of what is happening for Peter?
- Make a list of the factors that you think are involved in him not being able to get another job.
- Have you tended to focus on *individualised* characteristics about Peter? (These include his age; his limited experience in preparing for successful job applications; his limited capacity to transfer to other work due to being with the one company for so long; and/or perhaps other individualised factors that separate Peter from his social context, such as his attitude, motivation, personality type and ability to sell himself in his résumé).
- How do you understand Peter's experience of depression? Is this a separate issue (medical problem) that will impact on Peter's capacity to gain employment?

An individualised analysis of Peter's story ignores contextual factors that are impacting on his experience.

- If Peter were your client and you only considered these individualised factors, how would this inform your work with him?
- Who or what would need to change in order for Peter to find work?
- From this individualised lens, who or what is the problem?
- How might the organisational context influence whether you privilege individualistic or structural analyses and what might you need to do within a conservative organisational context to maintain a structural analysis? (Might the organisation itself need to change?)

Notice whether you focused on changing Peter (*establishment social work* approach) or whether you have focused more on addressing contextual factors and changing society (progressive goal that *critical social work* approaches aim to achieve).

- How might *context* shape Peter's situation?
- What are the *structural* factors that have influenced Peter's situation and opportunities?

Hint: you might want to consider how social, political and economic structures create the societal conditions for unemployment, and the dominant responses to mental health. Regarding unemployment, for example, when economic rationalism dominates, government policies will seek to deregulate markets to be internationally competitive, resulting in the outsourcing of manufacturing to exploited overseas workers who provide cheaper offshore labour.

- How does the economic context directly influence Peter's former employer's decision to cut jobs?
- If economies are structured in such a way that approximately 5–6 per cent of the Australian population at any one time is to be unemployed, how does that contribute to Peter's unemployment?
- How might we understand Peter's sense of shame and how might this be linked to his mental health?

You may have also considered the impact of *dominant ideologies* on Peter's experience. In Australia the neoliberal policy context has created a harsh and punitive culture towards those who are not working. Not surprisingly, the unemployed often blame themselves, despite the fact that there have simply not been enough jobs created in the labour market to provide people with a dignified existence. In fact, over the past three decades there has been a shrinkage in the number of full-time well-paid, semi-skilled and unskilled jobs due to labour market reform, industrial restructuring and the rise of technology (Brynjolfsson & McAfee 2011; Rifkin 2004).

Context matters: if Peter lived in Sweden and found that he was losing his job as a result of restructuring, the Swedish Government would require Peter's employer to negotiate a redundancy package directly with his trade union, and give both Peter and the government several months' notice (a minimum of six months given that he has worked there for more than 10 years). He would have a right to re-employment in the company if its financial position improved, and he would be provided with vocational education and training as well as financial and training assistance. While retraining, his income would be covered by collective redundancy insurance up to an amount agreed by his union, which would be no less than 70 per cent of his previous income (Cook 2008). And given that Peter's age is over 40, this amount would be supplemented by the government (EIROnline 2013). The Employment Protection Act (1982) would require his employer to provide a social plan. Swedish society would see that it has a moral obligation to support him, rather than scapegoating and blaming him for the misfortune he is experiencing. Examining context would therefore assure Peter that he is not at fault because there are complex social, political and economic factors operating outside of his control.

Consider the impact of contextual technological changes (such as digital photography and the internet) on Kodak, the leading photographic company in the world in the 20th century. At the height of its success, Kodak employed more than 140 000 people and was worth US$28 billion. In 2012 Kodak became bankrupt for failing to adapt to the digital photography revolution. The leading exponent of digital photography today, Instagram, now employs 13 people and was sold to Facebook for US$1 billion in 2012, wiping out thousands of middle-class jobs in the early 2000s (Timberg 2013).

Prejudices refer to deeply held individual beliefs or negative evaluations about others based on their membership of non-dominant groups constructed around gender, class, age, ability, religion, sexuality, ethnicity or religion (Mullaly 2010).

In addition, Peter's employment history indicates he is clearly able to work, but **prejudices** about Peter's age may mean that employers opt for younger applicants. This sort of discrimination is an example of ageism, and all of these factors are relevant in a critical assessment of Peter's circumstances.

Individualist theories attempt to assist Peter to find work so that he is not dependent on welfare benefits. Workers using this theory to inform their practice would regard Peter's unemployment as a product of his personal attributes and try to enhance these so his employability can be increased (establishment social work approach). By contrast, a critical approach that emphasises an analysis of social context would encourage Peter to maximise the social benefits and services that might be available to him while supporting him to retrain. Examining social context would seek to help Peter develop an understanding of the factors that are beyond his control and how these have influenced his situation in an attempt to challenge his self-blaming perception of being a 'dole bludger'.

- How might *capitalist* and *patriarchal ideologies* impact on Peter's mental health?
- How might a **structural analysis** that takes account of context consider Peter's experience of depression as connected with his unemployment?
- If your understanding of Peter's situation included an analysis of the structural context in which his experience of unemployment has occurred, how might your work with him be different than if you purely focused on individualised factors?
- What would you miss if your understanding did not consider the importance of context?

A critical approach would expose the myths of the dole bludger and highlight the social processes and power relations that lead to people being labelled and stigmatised in negative ways. Thinking about gender as an important part of Peter's identity, an analysis of social context points to the need to consider social expectations about masculinity and how this may impact on Peter.

And what if Peter were a much younger unemployed man – in his late teens or early twenties? How might his experience be different?

On the one hand, Peter as a younger man may be regarded as more employable than his older counterpart, but on the other, *ageist discourses* can also work against young people. The dominant discourse around unemployment may categorise the unemployed young person as deficient and defective. This same young person may have grown up in a context where his local state school has been underfunded, housing has been inadequate, and a university education and the jobs associated with it seem beyond his own, his family's and his teachers' expectations. Bottrell and Armstrong (2007, p. 367) argue that social positioning significantly influences whether transitions from youth to adulthood are framed in terms of 'flexibility or precarity' and that when *marginalised* youth are positioned outside legitimate places, their potential is interpreted primarily as potential 'for harm, disorder and misbehaviour'. Thus, the global context combines with historical shifts and dominant discourses of the day to impact on local neighbourhoods and communities and the individuals within them. Some communities may become increasingly isolated and stigmatised in terms of winners and losers – messages that are then internalised by those who reside in, or come from, these marginalised areas. Therefore, a key element of the critical social worker's task is to resist co-option into 'lopsided' emphases on individual lifestyles,

> **Structural analysis**
> recognises that there are structural explanations (rather than individual explanations) for social issues and that some groups are excluded from, marginalised within, or exploited by social, economic and political power. Poor people did not invent poverty; people of colour did not create racism – these are structural problems that can only be resolved by structural change (Mullaly 2010, p. 276).

which direct attention from the social, cultural, political and economic contexts within which people live their lives (Alvaro et al. 2010, p. 91).

Many practitioners who use critical approaches remain hopeful about the possibilities for social work and human services practitioners to formulate emancipatory responses to the challenges created by the contemporary contexts in which we work. In addition to employing critical analysis of society as a form of resistance to dominant social forces, a number of prominent writers suggest that social workers have the creativity, ethical framework, knowledge and skills to work constructively with and within our contemporary contexts using a variety of strategies (Allan, Briskman & Pease 2009; Ferguson 2008; Fook 2012; Holscher & Sewpaul 2006; Lavalette 2011; Madhu 2011; Mullaly 2010). These strategies will be discussed below.

■ Responding at global and local levels

As critical social workers we need to be mindful of the effects of globalisation in our local and national contexts and the ways in which we can use global networks and information and communication technology to advance social justice aims. Our value base of human rights and respect for diversity maintains our focus on public interests rather than private greed or profit (Ife 2013) and we can use our social work skills to explore what social justice means to different people in different contexts (Fook 2012).

In responding to the oppressive and/or liberating elements of globalisation, critical social workers can continue to represent the interests and perspectives of marginalised people and consider the social justice implications of new trends and developments worldwide. Globalisation is complex and multifaceted, and different people in different settings may experience its ripple effects differently; critical social work will continually develop as new complexities and issues arise. The International

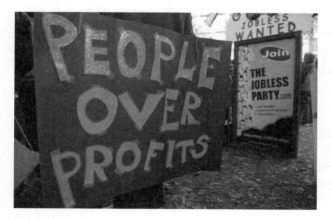

Figure 3.2

Federation of Social Workers website (http://ifsw.org) is an example of a resource for globalised social workers.

REFLECTIVE EXERCISE 3.3

Look in a newspaper or on a news link to see how and in what way the term 'global' is used.

- What are the implications of the particular news story you looked at for social justice or everyday experiences?
- In what ways does globalisation engender empowerment or oppression in specific contexts?

■ Social policy as a vehicle to respond to contextual challenges

Communities, organisations and individuals are embedded in the context of social policy. Social policies are the result of decisions made by government about the distribution of resources. They are the result of political processes in which interpretations of problems and their solutions are made and resisted. All of us are affected by these decisions, in terms of health care, access to education, housing, welfare benefits, transportation and most other aspects of our lives (Jamrozik 2009).

REFLECTIVE EXERCISE 3.4

Think about how your own life is affected by social policies. This may seem difficult and abstract initially so here are some hints about things that might affect you or your family: whether or not your local GP bulk bills for medical services; whether or not you are eligible to receive Austudy benefits; the frequency and quality of public transport in your area; the level of subsidies for childcare; changes to the sole parent pension; and so on.

Some other resources you might find useful to help you with this in thinking about the Australian context include:

- Australian Policy Online, http://apo.org.au
- More Than Luck: Ideas Australia Needs Now, http://morethanluck.cpd.org.au
- Inside Story: Current Affairs and Culture from Australia and Beyond, http://inside.org.au
- Centre for Policy Development (Australian progressive policy think tank), http://cpd.org.au.

As explored above, social policy decisions in recent years have been dominated by *neoliberal discourses* that operate to justify the goals of global capitalism, although these goals and values may not always be stated overtly (Jamrozik 2009). As critical social workers we are mindful of how social policies, power and discourse intertwine at the local level to engender both privilege and opportunity. We are sometimes able to have input into the development of policy, through consultations and advocacy; however, we are just as likely to be among those at ground level who are implementing policies that have been devised by policymakers at the federal or state level. Through the use of **professional autonomy/discretion** social workers are able to work flexibly within policy parameters in the best interests of their clients, and, at the same time, advocate for more socially just policies to be considered.

Professional autonomy/discretion describes the ability of social workers to work discreetly within managerialist, organisational policies and practices, while simultaneously advancing their clients' interests (Evans 2010).

One of the ways in which this can happen is through policy-relevant research based on values aligned with critical social work, which identifies inequities, gaps in services, deficiencies in programs, unnecessary hardships or bureaucratic indifference or incompetence (Jamrozik 2009).

REFLECTIVE EXERCISE 3.5
- While professional discretion can be a tool of emancipation, can you imagine times when professional discretion can be dangerous and potentially lead to unethical practices? (An example could be when a worker's personal biases lead to favouritism of some clients.)
- How might critical reflection be necessary for our accountable use of professional discretion?
- What might be some of the limitations of professional discretion? (An example could be an organisation's contexts that appear to be hostile and punitive to suggestions for alternative practice.)
- How might the preceding discussion about policy be relevant to our case study of Peter?

One of the most useful critical models for engaging with social policy has been provided by Bacchi (2009), who proposes a 'what's the problem represented to be?' approach. She peels back the layers to uncover how specific policies aim at 'fixing' a problem, by asking how the problem itself has been constructed and what effects and actions flow from this representation. The construction of a problem in a particular way will often flow from the values, belief systems, cultural norms and concepts that predominate at the time. Our discussion of the case study of Peter demonstrates the importance of critically analysing problem construction when discussing the social issues of unemployment and mental health and how these can be constructed as individual problems or as social problems.

It is illustrative to look at the 'problem' of the illicit use of drugs by young people. (While we use this example here, we are not suggesting that substance abuse is an issue that only affects young people. Constructions of this problem in the policy realm lead to actions made at ground level to reduce the problem, such as drug education in schools. Stanton (2005, pp. 50–1) suggests that drug education programs in schools are primarily founded on a *deficits-based model*, assuming youth are 'inept and inadequate in their understanding of drugs' and that they need to make better informed lifestyle decisions based on *normative* values around the meaning of quality of life. While individual lifestyle decisions or ignorance about the effects of drugs may be part of the problem, as critical social workers we might ask: what does this construction miss? Research conducted by Spooner, Hall and Lynskey (2001, cited in Stanton 2005), in a report commissioned by the Australian National Council on Drugs, made connections between drug use and the sense of isolation and hopelessness of some young people in today's context of widening gaps of dis/advantage and futile attempts to transition into the paid workforce. From this perspective, students might be encouraged to understand that their setbacks and crises are not totally due to their own shortcomings but include structural matters, such as marginalisation and unemployment or employment in mind-numbing jobs. Added to this is the possibility that drug use is pleasurable and relaxing in a stressful world that emphasises individual productivity and responsibility without acknowledging the structural barriers faced by some young people (Stanton 2005).

REFLECTIVE EXERCISE 3.6

What sorts of policies and programs would Stanton's version of the 'problem of illicit drug use' engender?

Now view the 'Rat Park' comic by Stuart McMillen at http://www.stuartmcmillen. com/comics_en/rat-park/.

What are the social and contextual implications of this research for our understandings of the dominant construction of 'addiction?'

From a critical perspective, rather than relying on the assumption that illicit drug use stems from a lack of individual knowledge about drugs or a failure of individual values, we would consider the contexts in which individual drug use takes place. Young people are part of wider and more complex contexts than simply those of the school or family environment: disadvantaged communities often have high levels of drug use (Stanton 2005), and as we have discussed, these disadvantages are as much a product of social, political and economic structures as personal deficits. Stanton (2005) argues that money that is currently spent on individualised approaches to drug education would be better spent on developing improved resources and supportive communities for young people. Furthermore, the 'Rat Park' comic shows that addiction is directly related to one's social context. Drug education programs in schools need to be guided by the experiences and insights of young people and their real world lives, while aiming to engender in young people an understanding of the structural factors that impact on individual experiences of alienation and frustration and their capacity for social and personal agency.

■ Participation in social movements

While the work of social workers continues to be heavily influenced by current social policy agendas – for better or worse – the role of social movements in influencing the evolution of critical social work must be equally acknowledged. Social movements are a large collectivity of people who aim to either maintain or challenge the existing social order (Giddens & Sutton 2013). While not all social movements are progressive (e.g. the National Front in Australia, the Tea Party in the United States, the anti-abortion movement) it is progressive social movements that aim to expand the scope of social justice, human rights and environmental sustainability that hold relevance for critical social work. The primary stalwart of 'old' social movements in Australia was the labour movement, which was centred around workers' rights in a capitalist system. 'New' social movements (including the women's movement, the gay/lesbian movement, the consumer/recovery movement, civil, human and land rights movements, anti-global capitalism movements, animal rights movements and the environment movement) have been based on a wide range of challenges to dominant social forces and subjected these to questioning.

The key features of progressive social movements are that they consist of a group of people who are consciously trying to promote social change, making demands of the state and bringing issues to public attention. These movements challenge the 'norms' of society that create inequality, such as patriarchy, destruction of environment, heterosexism and colonialism (Mitra, Bhatia & Chatterjee 2013). Social movements provide an outlet for collective expression by those traditionally considered non-powerful to challenge the values and institutions of society. They create new discourses and language to describe social reality and create new meanings – for example, black is beautiful, gay pride, Indigenous land rights, human need not corporate greed, women have the right to be safe.

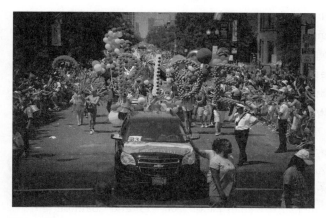

Figure 3.3

Social movements have impacted greatly on our capacity to approach social work from critical perspectives. They have raised conservative, traditional, white middle-class social workers' consciousness around diversity – challenging our moralising around what is normal and decent. At the same time, our awareness of various forms of oppression has been enlightened – for instance, social workers were involved in social control functions in both psychiatric social work (see, for example, Morley 2003b) and in child welfare policy in relation to the removal of Aboriginal and Torres

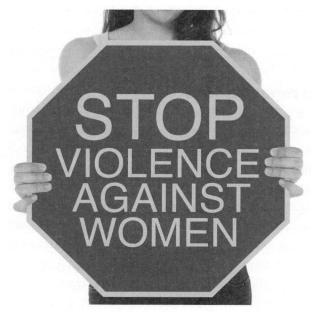

Figure 3.4

Strait Islander children from their families (Briskman 2014; Menzies & Gilbert 2013). Social movements have provided social workers with new ways of seeing the role of the professional, not as expert but as listener, facilitator, ally and skill sharer. And, importantly, social movements have helped social workers develop and extend their structural perspective, looking at how wider oppressive social discourses and institutions shape personal experience (Maddison & Scalmer 2006).

REFLECTIVE EXERCISE 3.7

- Which particular social movements do you think have influenced your own (or your parents') outlook on life?
- Can you see how social movements may have influenced the practice of critical social work?
- Now have a look at the following progressive social movement websites. Think about some of the ways social workers might interact with and contribute to these sites.
  - GetUp!: Action for Australia, https://www.getup.org.au
  - MoveOn.org: Democracy in Action (USA), http://front.moveon.org/
  - ResPublica (UK), http://www.respublica.org.uk
  - Avaaz.org: The World in Action http://www.avaaz.org/en/about.php
  - Progressive Podcast Australia: Promoting Social Justice, Political Music and Progressive Causes in Australia and Worldwide, http://progressivepodcastaustralia.com/about
  - 'Remy's Occupy Wall Street Protest Song', http://www.youtube.com/watch?v=4QTfNEDgusQ

■ Critical practice in organisations

Another way in which practitioners challenge dominant social forces is through everyday practices within the organisations in which they work. Most social workers' practice occurs in an organisation of some sort; often these are referred to as welfare or **human services organisations**.

Human services organisations 'nominate as their primary purpose the promotion of the care and well-being of people experiencing difficulties in their lives because of poverty, disability, illness, or some other life hazard' (McDonald et al. 2011, p. 4).

It is within an organisational context that most meetings between social workers and clients take place. In fact, it is within the organisational context that the roles of 'worker' and 'client' are created. At times social workers are frustrated with the constraints their organisation places on their interactions with clients and the way services are delivered. While managerialist pressures may reduce a social worker's capacity to act from their professional value and theory base, thus limiting their professional autonomy, it is also evident that critical social workers make use of professional discretion to work creatively 'within' organisational guidelines and attempt to turn organisational challenges into possibilities for change. Our capacity to engage critically in **organisational practice** is an important element of this work. Organisations, as McDonald et al. (2011, p. 3) put it simply, 'create the rules of the game'. Ultimately, individual practitioners will need to make decisions about the roles, responsibilities and actual practices that they undertake. Organisations may be government departments or community-based agencies across a wide range of fields of practice, from criminal justice, housing and aged care to mental health, domestic violence and working with youth.

> **Organisational practice**
> refers to our professional purpose, which is shaped by service users' needs and expectations, our institutional context (e.g. statutory or community-based) and our professional practice base (Healy 2012, p. 4).

Ife (2012, p. 248) suggests that:

> the capacity of a social worker to help a person or family is determined far more by that social worker's ability to work in organisational systems, to operate in team meetings, to advocate with a range of community services, and to build strong community supports than it is by his/her capacity to work interpersonal magic in a counselling interview.

Every day politics is being played out in the organisational context, in the relationships between people and the implementation of policies and procedures that may or may not be in the best interests of our clients or our social change mission. **Organisational culture** is a term used to refer to the assumptions and beliefs, conscious or unconscious, that:

> **Organisational culture**
> refers to the 'attitudes, beliefs, personal and cultural values shared by people and groups in an organisation that significantly impact on the way people interact with each other and with others outside of the organisation' (McDonald et al. 2011, p. 63).

> represent the nature of the organisation and its relationship with the environment ... expressed in rituals, formal written statements, standards, rules and policies, artefacts and formal and informal stories told about the organisation by its members (McDonald et al. 2011, pp. 8–9).

An organisation's culture is transmitted to workers and clients both formally and informally. For critical social workers, it is important to be able to 'read' the cultural climate of organisational contexts in order to practise strategically within them and engage in conscious efforts to create positive change, even in simple acts, such as how we relate to and communicate with clients and colleagues (Fook 2012).

McDonald et al. (2011) encourage us to think *about* how we can exercise leadership in improving the quality of services we provide and our own satisfaction as critical

Think of an organisation you have worked in, or in which you have been a client.
- How would you describe the organisational culture?
- Do/did you feel valued, empowered and listened to? If you thought of an organisation in which you were a worker, how do you think the clients of the organisation would describe its culture (for example, how they are treated)?
- How might you initiate even small changes to aspects of the organisational culture that may be experienced as oppressive or disempowering?

social workers. Whether or not we are in an identified leadership position, such as that of a team manager, McDonald et al. (2011) affirm that we can initiate action or show leadership in interpreting and responding to issues at hand from a critical social work perspective. Others affirm this:

> For social workers to be effective organisational operators, they not only need to be able to work competently within existing arrangements, but they also need to be able to critique these arrangements, and be able – and willing – to work strategically and tactically to change them (Hughes & Wearing 2013, p. 3).

For example, we may be able to encourage or initiate practices whereby clients are more able to participate in decision-making processes or in which the voices of all team members can be equally heard and valued, despite hierarchical positioning of various disciplines. Craig (2002, p. 679) suggests that:

> social workers should reposition themselves not as the agents of endless top-down government initiatives but as those working more explicitly with and for the excluded and deprived, that is, to find an appropriate and critical political distance from a position of being merely agents of change driven by government objectives. This would require, inter alia, relearning the skills of community development, focusing on the increasingly submerged social work values of empowerment and advocacy, and becoming even more actively engaged in promoting user involvement within the range of local initiatives. Within the organisational context, practitioners position themselves 'in and against the state', that is, working within the state mechanisms in the production and delivery of welfare, but maintaining a radical and critical position in relation to its policies and goals.

Multidisciplinary teams 'involve different professions working together by performing different roles in line with their own discipline' (Hughes & Wearing 2013, p. 93).

Another aspect of working within organisational contexts, which presents both challenges and opportunities, is that of working within **multidisciplinary teams** and in the wider sphere of inter-agency collaboration (Hughes & Wearing 2013). As social workers we often work with colleagues from a range of professional backgrounds; workers from other professions (and indeed within social work) may have different ideological and theoretical backgrounds and be focused on achieving different outcomes (McDonald et al. 2011). McDonald et al. (2011) suggest that by looking for the strengths associated with diversity among professionals and interagency coalitions we can respond more holistically to the needs of clients. This is sometimes more challenging than it would appear: how do we negotiate processes and desired outcomes among 'helpers' from a diverse range of disciplines and organisational contexts? The use of exclusionary professional jargon, variations in how values are weighed up and confusion over the roles of different players can all pose barriers to effective collaboration (Hughes & Wearing 2013). Berthoin and Friedman (2003, p. 21) suggest that action strategies combining high 'advocacy' – clearly expressing and standing up for what one believes – and high 'inquiry' – exploring and questioning both one's own reasoning and the reasoning of others – can be effective.

Fook, Ryan and Hawkins (2000) suggest that critical social workers consider the whole organisation and its culture of service delivery as their client and make conscious efforts to change oppressive organisational culture, initiating new ways of relating between management and staff, and informing policies and practices based on social work knowledge, skills and values. In this case emancipatory social work organisations would be flexible, collegial and community-based (Ife 2012, p. 313) and would engage in genuine consultation with service users. Rees (1999) coined the term 'humanitarian' to describe a style of organisational management that contrasted with managerialism and was more aligned with social work values and approaches. The essence of the *humanitarian approach* spans three interrelated elements: relationships, culture and language. In such an organisation the quality of relationships is seen as crucial to the quality of the service; the aim is to create vibrant workplace culture and conditions that enhance social justice and humanity; and a language of rights, duties and partnerships is encouraged in the creation of socially just culture and worker–client relationships. While such visions may seem like a far cry from many of the organisations we work in or with, they provide ideals to which we can aspire even in our small day-to-day actions, and fuel the imagination of critical social workers, inspiring them to be part of redefining and reorienting organisational objectives (Ife 2012, pp. 281–2). As **reflective practitioners**, we are constantly learning and mindful of how we contribute to the organisational culture of our workplace (Hughes & Wearing 2013, pp. 196–9).

> A **reflective practitioner** is one who is able to reflect on 'assumptions (hidden theory) embedded in practice, and to expose these for examination, in order to improve practice' (Fook 2012, p. 196).

■ Community development

Given the dominance of global capitalism and neoliberalist discourses that focus profoundly on the individual, some social commentators argue that today's world, generally, is becoming privatised. *Privatisation* refers to a declining sense of community, whether for the rich or poor, in that notions of society are dominated by private individuals, private spaces and private institutions (see Fisher & Karger 1997). Fisher and Karger suggest that this trend towards the privatisation of life has been assisted by new information and communication technology, new levels of obsession with security, suburban settings where people mix less with one another, the decline of the public sector, dominant discourses of individual achievement, and worth being measured in relation to market values. However, Fisher and Karger (1997) suggest that it is possible for individuals to be empowered public citizens even in contexts that value independent and autonomous private consumers. Communities, they point out, are free spaces with dynamic members who are constantly living out alternative discourses in small and large ways: the exchange of garden produce over the backyard fence, organising a walking group to the local primary school, coming together at neighbourhood centres and town meetings, and engaging in social movements. Furthermore, they suggest that social work can be at the heart of contemporary struggles not only to work with and facilitate the revitalisation of communities, but also to listen to and learn from community members. Community development is a method of practice aimed at establishing or re-establishing social life and relations within the structure of a human community, drawing on the wisdom, expertise and resources of the community itself (Ife 2013). This method of practice will be discussed further in Chapter 7.

REFLECTIVE EXERCISE 3.10

To understand the importance of community development and the changes it can achieve, watch this YouTube video: 'The power of community: How Cuba survived peak oil crisis', http://www.youtube.com/watch?v=tgqn3bTekFA.

■ Undertaking social research

Undertaking social research is another practice strategy that can be used to critique and challenge dominant social forces and promote progressive social change. '[R]estructuring of welfare services has left social work research vulnerable to reduced quality and accountability for work undertaken by independent researchers' (Gibbs 2001, p. 694) and the neoliberal context has tried to ensure 'that agency based research agendas are now firmly focused upon effectiveness, evaluation and monitoring', reducing research to 'tick-box style surveys, quality control or the gathering of units of costed information' (Gibbs 2001, p. 693). This has led to social workers creating mechanisms of resistance by developing different sorts of research designs and using different methodologies to counteract the dominant discourses. As Gibbs (2001, p. 698) explains:

> Researchers have obligations towards, and are accountable to, the wide range of participants, respondents, subjects, co-collaborators and service users, from whom they are seeking information, or with whom they are developing strategies for change ... It is clearly a value-based position to argue that social work research should have an orientation towards the empowerment of participants. Additionally, social work researchers are challenged to draw upon ethical and social justice principles when making their choices about research projects.

Similarly, Healy (2000, p. 146) aptly puts it: 'much more critical practice research is needed into the local contexts of social work practices ... at the very least [to create] respect for the complexities inherent in the local contexts of social work practices'. Local, practice-based research may also be a way to challenge **grand narratives** and universalised solutions to problems and issues that are historically and locally situated.

Grand narratives are abstract ideas that explain historical knowledge and experiences intended to legitimise the truth (Nola & Irzik 2005).

- How might our understanding of, and response to, Peter be informed by research?
- What would guide our approach to researching the situation of Peter and others who find themselves unemployed?

■ Summary

Critically analysing the contemporary contexts of social work practice and understanding the impact of dominant social forces in shaping our contexts is vital information for critical social workers. While the enormity of social problems highlighted by a structural analysis can sometimes makes us feel overwhelmed or alienated from the means of change, in this chapter we have contended that social work and related professions are in a powerful position to enact emancipatory practice aimed at championing human rights (Ife 2012). One of the key elements that critical social work offers us as practitioners is a critical analysis of how these social forces operate at global, national and local levels, so that we can recognise and resist their impact on the lives of the individuals, groups and communities with whom we work, and on our social work practice. By no means are we suggesting that this is easy. It is not. Many experienced practitioners, if they are honest, will admit the fear and anxiety invoked at challenging conservative politics, especially in their own employing organisations. However, it is a struggle that is worth engaging with as part of our lifelong learning and development as critical social workers. In addition to the critical analysis of dominant discourses, some of the strategies we have explored as practices of resistance and progressive change include the analysis and development of social policy; engaging in community development and social movements; undertaking critical practice in organisations; and undertaking social research.

■ Review questions

- What are some of the main questions this chapter has raised for you?
- What does a critical analysis of society offer you as a social worker concerned about social inequality and injustice?
- What might be some additional practices that you could engage in to challenge dominant social forces and their consequences?

■ Further reading

Deepak, A., 2012, 'Globalisation, power and resistance: Postcolonial and transnational feminist perspectives for social work practice', *International Social Work*, 55 (6): 779–93.

Ferguson, I. and Lavalette, M., 2006, 'Globalisation and global justice: Towards a social work of resistance', *International Social Work*, 49 (3), 309–18.

Gardner, F., 2006, 'Working actively within the organisation' in *Working with Human Service Organisations*, Oxford University Press, South Melbourne.

Ife, J., 2013, 'The organisational context' in *Community Development in an Uncertain World: Vision, Analysis and Practice*, Cambridge University Press, Port Melbourne.

Noble, C., 2007, 'Social work, collective action and social movements' in L. Dominelli, ed, *Revitalising Communities in a Globalising World*, Ashgate, Aldershot, UK.

Social Dialogue, free online magazine of the International Association of Schools of Social Work, http://www.social-dialogue.com.

4

How did we get here? The history of critical social work

■ Introduction

SOCIAL WORK AND the problems it addresses are products of the modern world. These problems are neither eternal nor innate to human nature, but come into being at particular points in history as a result of people's actions and the way they organise power in society. Looking at these issues historically enables us to see the way that social problems (such as poverty, racism, sexism, violence and marginality) have been constructed and, more importantly, may provide us with clues as to how people might *un-make* those problems and do something better. This historical perspective is vital for practice today because it locates critical social work as part of a much wider and ongoing struggle for social justice and human rights. Unfortunately, not all social work has supported these struggles. As we have said, the dominant tradition of establishment social work has been, and continues to be, narrowly focused on dealing with individuals' 'inadequacies' and adjusting them to fit the social order. What this chapter shows, however, is that there is another tradition, what Ferguson (2008, p. 88) calls the *radical tradition* that has developed for over a century. It is founded on social justice and continues to animate critical social work today.

It should be noted that this chapter emphasises Western notions of social justice. This is because social work began in the West but we also acknowledge that many other cultures have similar yet distinctive ideas, including Asian, African and indigenous cultures. The ancient, Indian concept of *dharma* (Prasad 1995) and the ancient Chinese notion of yi (Yang 1997), for example, can be seen as related to Western understandings of social justice and we have much to learn from these. The following list of quotes concerning social justice from different civilisations should give a sense of the diverse views on social justice.

Quotes on social justice from different cultures and religions in history

- The orphan was not sacrificed to the rich man; the widow was not sacrificed to the mighty man; the poor man was not delivered up to the man of wealth (Code of Ur-Namu – Sumer, 2100 BCE) (Gurney & Kramer 1965, p. 16).
- Do not rob the poor person of their goods; one whom you know is weak. For the breath of the poor is their property, and he who seizes it suffocates them (Book of Khunanpu – Egypt, 2100 BCE) (Karenga 2004, p. 332).
- That the strong might not oppress the weak (Hammurabi's Laws – Babylon, 1780 BCE) (Darling 2013, p. 15).
- Is not this the fast that I choose: to loose the bonds of injustice, to undo the thongs of the yoke, to let the oppressed go free, and to break every yoke? Is it not to share your bread with the hungry, and bring the homeless poor into your house; when you see the naked, to cover them . . .? (Book of Isaiah 58: 3–24 – Israel/Babylon, 600 BCE).
- In his dealings with things under heaven the noble person is not invariably for or against anything. He just does what is just (Analects of Confucius – China, 551–479 BCE) (translated in Yang 1997, p. 521).
- Just as I seek the welfare and happiness of my own children in this world and the next, I seek the same things for all men [sic] (Ashoka, Buddhist emperor – India, 304–232 BCE) (Braybrooke 2009, p. 106).
- More cruel than a murderer is the ruler who oppresses his people and acts unjustly (Thiruvalluvar, Hindu sage – Sri Lanka, 200 BCE) (Pope et al. [1886] 1982, p. 68).
- Jesus said to the rich young man, 'If you would be perfect, go, sell what you possess, give it to the poor, and follow me – then you shall have riches in Heaven' (Gospel of Mark 10: 21 – Palestine, c. 30 CE)
- You are not making a gift of your possessions to the poor person. You are handing over to them what is theirs (St Ambrose on Charity, Archbishop of Milan – Italy, 340–97 CE) (Cort 1988, p. 46).
- Do you know who really rejects the faith? The one who mistreats the orphan and does not advocate the feeding of the poor. And, woe to those who observe their prayers – who are totally heedless of the prayers of the poor (The Quran [107: 1–7] – Arabia, 609–32 CE).
- The social pact, far from destroying natural equality, substitutes, on the contrary, a moral and lawful equality for whatever physical inequality that nature may have imposed on humankind; so that however unequal in strength and intelligence, men become equal by covenant and by right (Jean-Jacques Rousseau [1762] (2012), Enlightenment philosopher – France).
- In Communism . . . only then can . . . society inscribe on its banners: From each according to his ability, to each according to his needs! (Karl Marx [1875] (1970), socialist revolutionary – Britain).
- The good we secure for ourselves is precarious and uncertain until it is secured for all of us and incorporated into our common life (Jane Addams 1912, p. 113, social work founder, feminist and Nobel Peace Prize laureate – United States, 1860–1935).
- In a civilised community, although it may be composed of self-reliant individuals, there will be some persons who will be unable at some period of their lives to

look after themselves, and the question of what is to happen to them may be solved in three ways – they may be neglected, they may be cared for by the organised community as of right, or they may be left to the goodwill of individuals in the community. The first way is intolerable, and as for the third: Charity is only possible without loss of dignity between equals. A right established by law, such as that to an old age pension, is less galling than an allowance made by a rich man to a poor one, dependent on his view of the recipient's character, and terminable at his caprice (Clement Attlee 1920, p. 30, social worker and Labour Prime Minister – Britain, 1893–1967).

- We are concerned with how to create mass organizations to seize power and give it to the people; to realize the democratic dream of equality, justice, peace, cooperation, equal and full opportunities for education, full and useful employment, health, and the creation of those circumstances in which man can have the chance to live by values that give meaning to life (Saul Alinsky 1971, p.3, radical community organiser – United States, 1909–72).

- There is no other way but to redefine 'modernity' and the goals of development, to widen it to a sustainable, just society based on harmonious, non-exploitative relationships between human beings and between people and nature (Medha Patkar 1991, social worker and founder of the 'Save the Narmada River Movement' (Namarda Bachao Andolan) – India, 1954–).

REFLECTIVE EXERCISE 4.1

In your own words note down a few sentences on what you consider to be the key tenets of social justice.

■ Historical perspectives on social justice

There was a time when there was no social work or any need for it. Let us consider that for most of human history (over 100 000 years), human beings have lived in small groups of nomadic hunter-gatherers. Archeologists and anthropologists tell us that our hunter-gatherer ancestors had to be very cooperative to survive, shared their resources, dealt with conflicts through avoidance rather than warfare and had no capacity for accumulating material wealth (Flannery & Marcus 2012; Sahlins 2004). In such a context, it makes no sense to talk of 'poverty'. They also had sustainable impacts on their environments. Compared to modern society, these societies were relatively egalitarian (economically equal) (see Beilharz & Hogan 2012) and power was more evenly shared, although they did exhibit important divisions of gender and age. Community elders were respected, and what we now call 'health-care issues' were dealt with by elders who were ritual specialists and holders of knowledge. While life was often harsh, our hunter-gatherer ancestors coped successfully with their personal and social problems. Their limited wants were generally met by the means at their disposal (Gowdy 1997). Prior to colonisation, Aboriginal Australians lived in this manner for at least 50 000 years (Stockton & Nanson 2004), in harmony with their surrounds. This reminder of social origins stands in marked contrast to the social problems that began to emerge with the so-called **birth of civilisation**.

Major social inequalities, disparities in power and oppressive practices, such as slavery, appear with the development of settled agriculture around 10 000 years ago. These divisions increased with the establishment of large-scale settlements from around 6000 BCE[1] and were justified by religious beliefs endorsing hierarchy and inequality. Ancient cities produced social categories that we would be familiar with today, such as prisoners, soldiers, priests, sex workers, criminal gangs and divisions between rich and poor, which had not existed in hunter-gatherer communities. Interestingly, with the emergence of social inequalities, we also see the birth of struggles for social justice. These often began as struggles by particular groups to redress their exclusion or economic grievances within a given society, even to the point of revolt.

The **birth of civilisation** refers to the period around 6000 BCE when towns and urban centres emerged alongside villages in what is now the Middle East. Specialised food crop cultivation allowed surplus food production to sustain urbanisation, new technologies for the manufacture of metal tools and weapons were developed, commodities such as pottery and textiles were mass produced, social classes began to develop as those who controlled resources or had political power grew personal wealth, and writing became the dominant means of communication and record keeping (Nagle 2010).

However, more inclusive notions of social justice, as an ethical norm of how the society *ought* to be, began to emerge in the ancient religious teachings of Judaism, Hinduism, Buddhism, Confucianism, Islam and Christianity. A basic assumption in these teachings is that society and not the individual is morally accountable for the undeserved suffering of poverty and other extreme forms of inequality. Therefore, society as a whole was seen as responsible for relieving such suffering and providing the means for a just distribution of goods; thereby redeeming its members from destitution and providing a livelihood that prevented poverty (Irani & Silver 1995).

Beyond this, there were quite diverse views on justice. Ancient Greek philosophers such as Plato and Aristotle sought to define social justice in terms of general principles, which they associated with notions of wellbeing and social harmony regulated by law, with each member of society accorded their due even though their positions may be unequal (e.g. masters and slaves). The Hebrew Bible, by contrast, had a more egalitarian view (in relative terms) of social justice (*tzedakah*), which declared every seventh

---

[1] We have adopted the Before the Common Era/Common Era historical dating system, BCE/CE, rather than the Christian BC/AD system.

year a 'Jubilee' in which all debts were forgiven and all slaves freed; and every fiftieth year land was returned to its original owners (Reisch 2002). The proponents of such radical visions of justice were prophets and sages, who would criticise the community, particularly the rich and powerful, for not being just to the poor. This latter view of social justice is associated with notions of equity rather than harmony or legality, and requires society (including its laws) to change in order to meet this ideal.

The collapse of the Roman Empire in the fifth century saw the division of Europe into feudal kingdoms, creating new forms of inequality between land-owning lords (the aristocracy) and peasant farmers. Social values were strongly influenced by the Catholic Church and what we might now call 'social services' were provided by religious figures and institutions throughout the Middle Ages until at least the 17th century (Moulin 1978, cited in Horner 2012, p. 19). Paradoxically, the medieval Church had contradictory positions on social justice. On the one hand, the Church ministered to the poor and sick, emphasised the spiritual virtue of poverty over greed, forbade interest (usury) on loans and even defended peasants' land rights (Cullum 1992). On the other hand, the Church itself became one of the wealthiest landowners in Europe; its leaders were part of the nobility and provided religious justifications for a system of inherited hierarchy and privilege that often persecuted the poor. The Church was also patriarchal, reinforcing the subordination of women to men in society at large.

Feudalism refers to a hierarchal social and political system based on land ownership, with a king and his lords at the top and peasant farmers and the landless at the bottom. The latter would work their lord's land in exchange for certain rights and protection (Hunt 2003).

As **feudalism** declined in the 15th century, peasants were driven off their land and drifted to the towns, swelling their impoverished populations. Governments, fearing social unrest, began to take over from the Church the regulation of the poor and vagrants. In England, for example, a series of Poor Laws were enacted between 1536 and 1601 under the Tudor monarchy, which distinguished between 'deserving' (disabled, sick, orphaned, elderly) and 'undeserving' (able-bodied but unemployed or criminal) poor. The former received relief in money and goods from the parishes derived from local taxes, whereas the latter were punitively disciplined (Horner 2012, p. 19). This discipline aimed to restrict the movement of the unemployed poor and could involve forcible return to their home parish. As cities grew, the Poor Laws were revised in 1834 to further centralise state control and reduce costs by virtually abolishing direct relief. Instead, a system of workhouses was established for all those who could not find work and the inmates were paid (**in-door relief**) below minimum wages. These institutions were neither charitable nor just. They were designed to deter applications for relief and confine the poor from the rest of society. There was also a growing belief that the poor were largely responsible for their

In-door relief relates to compensation for labouring in factories as opposed to 'out-door relief', which was public aid to the poor outside of institutions, such as soup kitchens and the supply of alms (Bremner 1988).

own suffering due to a lack of individual morals rather than poverty being caused by social injustices (Horner 2012, p. 24).

REFLECTIVE EXERCISE 4.2

Think of some of the dominant discourses that define our contemporary context. Can you identify some of the historical legacies that are still alive in understanding poverty and social inequality?

■ Social justice and modernity

These shifts in attitudes to poverty and justice were part of much broader social changes underway at the time: revolutionary changes that gave rise to our modern society or what social scientists call **modernity**.

It may be characterised as the product of three interrelated 'revolutions' that began in Europe in the 17th century and that are now global in impact. These were (1) the Scientific Revolution and '**Enlightenment**', (2) the Political Revolution and (3) the Industrial Capitalist Revolution. (For further information see Van Krieken et al. 2012.)

The Scientific Revolution refers to the intellectual transformation that began in Europe in the 16th century through the work of Galileo, Copernicus and Isaac Newton, whose use of rational observation, testing, measurement and precise calculation (without reference to the supernatural) changed the way people understood the universe. Science and reason rather than 'religion and the Bible' became the basis for reliable knowledge (Wadham, Pudsey & Boyd 2007, p. 39).

The Enlightenment promoted an optimistic belief in secular humanism and rationalism (Beilharz & Hogan 2012). Secular humanism is the belief that human beings can direct their own *progress* towards greater freedom and equality, without religion. Rationalism holds that individuals are rational creatures and that reason, supported by observation and experiment, is the surest guide to human emancipation (Wadham, Pudsey & Boyd 2007). In modernity, secular-rational (non-religious) solutions to social problems carry the most authority, and we can see examples of this in the so-called **scientific philanthropy** of the 19th century and notions of evidence-based practice in social work today.

Modernity refers to both a period in time and a set of social forms that are radically different from traditional or pre-modern societies.

In the 17th- and 18th-century **Enlightenment** movement, the scientific methods that proved so successful in gaining control over physical nature were applied to humanity.

Scientific philanthropy was the belief that public aid to the poor outside of institutions was undesirable and unnecessary and that charity should be organised and administered in order to compel would-be paupers to become self-supporting. This belief was based on the understanding that more consideration should be given to *who* received assistance (scientific assessment) and more attention paid to *what* types of assistance were given (application of scientific method to social problems) (Bremner 1988).

Critical social work shares the Enlightenment ideals of freedom and equality. However, it seriously questions claims that there is a universal rational method for realising these ideals, independent of social context or power relations.

The Political Revolution that followed the Enlightenment was strongly influenced by its ideals. If people could reason for themselves, it followed that they could govern themselves (the ideal of democracy) (see, for example, Ritzer & Stepnisky 2014). This had particular appeal for the educated, merchant classes of Europe and America who began to agitate for popular representative government, against aristocratic privilege and monarchy. This process erupted first in the American (1775) and French (1789) revolutions establishing new governments based on principles of individual liberty, equal citizenship rights and democratic representation. However, the right to vote and participate in government was initially restricted to men of property and was only gradually (often against violent resistance) conceded to workers, the poor, women and non-Europeans over the next two centuries (Tilley 2003). Nevertheless, the idea of being able to change society for the better through democracy remains a powerful, yet contested ideal. In the late 19th century this contest was often conducted between those advocating liberal and socialist political ideologies. Liberals are those who favour an *individualist* approach to social problems, arguing that poverty is mainly the result of poor choices and that the only way out of it is for individuals to work hard and be as free as possible from state restrictions on their market exchanges (trade) (see, for example, Horner 2012).

Social democracy is a form of democratic socialism that aims to extend social rights and a more equitable distribution of wealth through parliamentary reform, wage regulation, national planning and (historically) the nationalisation of strategic industries.

Communism is a form of socialism that aims to build a classless society, without private property, money or a state (Mullaly 2007, p. 115).

Socialists, by contrast, favour more *collective* approaches to problems such as poverty, which they see arising from unjust social structures. Consequently, they favour regulation of markets and public provision to promote social justice and counter inequality. While all socialists seek the transformation of capitalism (outlined below), some are reformist, attempting to gradually change the system by promoting equality or improvements from within (such as the **social democrats** of Scandinavia). Others are revolutionary, seeking the complete overthrow of capitalism and its replacement by a socialist society (as attempted by the **communists** of China, Cuba and Vietnam). Regardless, liberal philosophy has been dominant in most Western societies, such as Australia, despite concessions by the 20th-century welfare state to the provision of certain basic services, pensions and wage regulations. Liberalism's resurgence as neoliberalism since the late 1970s has had major consequences for social work practice and reminds us to what extent our work is always politically contested.

The third major 'revolution' under discussion is the **Industrial Capitalist Revolution**.

Capitalism, as we saw in Chapter 2, is a socioeconomic system of commodity production for market exchange geared to maximising profit. It is based on private ownership of capital (assets, money, machines, property), which can be invested to produce and sell commodities for profit and reinvestment. This capital accumulation is driven by market competition rather than meeting human needs or any other consideration (Mullaly 2007). Even capitalism's severest 19th-century critics, Karl Marx and Frederick Engels (1848), could see that by combining industrial technology with a specialised division of labour in factories, capitalism had produced more wealth than any other system in history and there was no going back to an **agrarian** past. Simultaneously, however, industrial capitalism has produced more inequality and a higher proportion of poor people than any previous society. This is because the social divisions between the owners (capitalists) and non-owners of capital distribute the wealth unequally. The capitalist class has replaced the **hereditary aristocracies** of the past as the ruling elite in society, exercising more influence over government than any other group. The non-owners, by contrast, have to sell their labour or skills as commodities for wages, or risk extreme hardship (including starvation in many places). Unskilled workers and the unemployed are the most likely to experience economic injustice and poverty, and on a global scale the inequalities are extreme. The system also exploits the natural environment more intensely than at any time in history and this is unsustainable. Nevertheless, those adversely affected by capitalism may organise and mobilise to resist exploitation, and some seek to transform capitalism itself in a more socialistic and sustainable direction. Critical social workers have always been associated with these movements of resistance and change (Mullaly 2007).

Industrial Capitalist Revolution refers to the emergence, initially in Britain in the late 18th century, of mechanised, factory-based production that replaced agriculture as the main means of production and ran on a capitalist basis (Giddens & Sutton 2013).

Agrarian refers to an economy based on the farming of land in small communities using human and/or animal labour.

Hereditary aristocracies refers to the dominant social class emerging within feudal or agrarian societies, in which the dominance is based on the ownership of land that is inherited. Aristocratic rank is often bestowed by a monarch and enshrined in law (Hunt 2003).

> **Universal truths** refers to knowledge that seeks to provide explanation and understanding about human behaviour and society that will apply to everyone, no matter what culture or society they live in (Payne & Askeland 2008).

The world that has emerged from these three revolutions is totally unlike that in which human beings lived for the thousands of years preceding them. First, modernity has given us a *modernist* way of thinking derived from the Enlightenment that is secular, rational and claims to establish **universal truths** (in grand narratives) about our society's problems and how we deal with them (see Van Krieken et al. 2012). Second, modernity presents us with the problem of what role democratic government should play in providing for social justice. Finally, it presents us with new and historically unprecedented social problems: extreme disparities in wealth and power on a global scale; mass migrations of war-torn populations; life-threatening pollution and destruction of our environment; rapidly transmitted global pandemics and health system crises; and violence between and within nation states, to name but the most obvious issues that critical social workers must navigate. (See, for example, Ife 2013; see also Chapter 2 for a more in-depth discussion of dominant social forces in our contemporary contexts.)

■ Social work origins

As noted earlier, there were no social workers in early 19th-century Britain (or anywhere). The dominant response to the increasing social misery of industrial capitalism was *liberal* – that is, it opposed government intervention and emphasised individual responsibility. The Poor Laws, enacted by the wealthy, were justified on the basis of the liberal utilitarian philosophy of Jeremy Bentham (1748–1832), who advocated the principle of 'the greatest good for the greatest number' (Bentham [1776] 1977, p. 393). (See also Chapter 5 for a discussion of consequentialist, or teleological, ethics.) His followers argued that direct payments to the poor outside the workhouse (commonly known as 'out-door relief') would lower ordinary workers' wages because it would interfere with the free-market principle of supply and demand in wage determination. They also feared that direct welfare payments would erode the work ethic of the able-bodied poor. So, workhouses were designed to pay less than the lowest paid workers' wages and to make relief an 'object of wholesome horror' (Spicker 2008). This system was soon beset with major problems. The general destitution of the English working class (Engels [1887] 2009) in the 1840s made it virtually impossible to create institutions worse than life in the 'real world'. The system was also met with considerable resistance not just from the poor themselves (in protest there was the formation of radical and socialist movements, **trade unionism** and mutual aid societies) but also from other middle-class liberals who found the consequences (if not the rationale) of the policy inhumane. While the former working-class-based movements eventually produced the long-term social reforms needed to uplift the economic conditions of the poor, thus expanding social justice in Western societies in the 20th century, most histories of social work trace its lineage to the liberal tradition and its efforts to provide charitable solutions that excluded state aid.

> **Trade unions** are organisations formed by employees in a particular trade or industry to collectively negotiate and advance the working conditions and income security of their members.

We suggest that social work is a mixed tradition emerging out of the clash between the *liberal individualist* and *social transformationist* (social change) approaches to inequality – a clash that has never been fully resolved. Critical social work shares the social transformationist vision that the major problems confronting individuals are rooted in unjust power relations and that both collective and personal action are required to change these (Healy 2000, p. 24). This vision, while never dominant in the profession, has been a powerful voice from the beginning; for example, the early social work educator John MacCunn (1911, p. 19) publicly declared in 1910 that the goal of social work was to 'emancipate fellow citizens' from poverty and oppression. However, as we shall see below, not all social workers would agree with this goal and/or many have been mixed in their responses about the best ways in which to approach it.

REFLECTIVE EXERCISE 4.5
- In the light of historical evidence, do you think social inequality is just part of human nature or is it socially constructed?
- Why might it be important to have an historical view of both social justice and social work?

REFLECTIVE EXERCISE 4.6
Make a few notes about why social work as a distinct profession is found only in modern and not pre-modern societies. Why is this significant for us to think about as critical social workers?

■ Charitable Organisation Societies (COSs)

The *individual casework* aspect of social work can be traced to the activities of middle- and upper-class missionary and charitable workers of the early 19th century in the form of the **Charitable Organisation Societies (COSs)**.

These 'friendly visitors' were usually middle-class white women who volunteered to visit the poor in their homes to assess their eligibility (deserving or undeserving) and needs for assistance (Horner 2012, p. 24). Many were motivated by religious convictions and some lobbied for reform. However, they all worked within the prevailing individualistic, moral framework that located the cause of poverty in the character of the poor themselves and sought to combat it through the reformation of behaviour, encouraging thrift, sobriety and self-help rather than material aid, unless the client was literally starving in their presence (Ferguson 2008, p. 90). This individual self-help ethos was central to the charitable organisations that started forming in the 1840s and became coordinated under an umbrella Charitable Organisation Society (COS) in Britain (1869) and the United States (1877) to avoid duplication (double-dipping) and to ration philanthropic efforts (Horner 2012, pp. 24–5).

> **Charitable Organisation Societies (COSs)**, which began in England in the 1840s, were funded by philanthropists and run by volunteers to provide direct service to people in need. COSs used scientific means to assess, measure and administer relief to those who were the 'deserving' poor. Data was collected and used to analyse social problems (Chenoweth & McAuliffe 2012, p. 35).

The COS opposition to direct 'out-door' relief and state aid hardened in the 1870s under the influence of Social Darwinist doctrines. These took Charles Darwin's (1859) theory of 'natural selection' for explaining biological evolution and misapplied it to competition between social groups and individuals (rich and poor, black and white) in which 'the strong' survive and thrive but 'the weak' die out. Invoking science, the COS and its patrons believed that direct relief or state aid would not only distort markets but also artificially preserve the 'unfit' and be contrary to progress (Woodside & McClam 2011, p. 35). Consequently, the COS was explicitly **anti-socialist** and fought all state assistance, including free school lunches, age pensions and national insurance. As former COS social worker and future Labour Prime Minister Clement Attlee (1883–1967) would point out, by locating the cause of poverty in moral failure and resisting social reform, the COS effectively defended class inequalities (Ferguson 2008, p. 91).

> **Anti-socialist** means being opposed to the theoretical and political positions within socialism, which include communism, Marxism and social democracy (Mullaly 2007).

The 'scientific philanthropy' of the COSs employed statistical surveys, intensive interviews and case files, gathering and classifying data about the poor ostensibly to streamline and professionalise

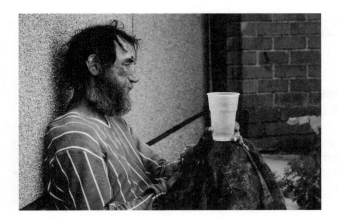

Figure 4.1

services. These rational-objectivist principles, however, were used to prevent what the COSs saw as the 'indiscriminate charity' of voluntary workers. One of the founders of modern social work (social casework) in the United States and a COS leader, Mary Richmond (1861–1928), strongly advocated professional training and what she called 'Social Diagnosis' to screen, typify and treat the poor on a case-by-case basis. She also helped establish the New York School of Philanthropy in 1898 (which became the Columbia University School of Social Work in 1963) – the first academic institution in the United States to teach social work (Bremner 1988).

The COS was transplanted to colonial Australia in 1887, where it prospered in Melbourne (but not Sydney where the Benevolent Society had secured some state assistance since 1813). However, the COS laissez-faire self-help ideology was discredited by the 1890s depression when its leader had to appeal to London for financial aid (Peel 2008). It later served as a training ground for hospital **almoners** in the professionalisation (becoming a socially recognised profession) of social work in Melbourne (1920–40). Fortunately, the profession has expanded beyond the moralising framework of the COS, but the tendency to privilege individual problems in isolation from social analysis and change is a persistent and prevailing feature of establishment social work, even in contemporary contexts. Moreover, Australia still has widespread cultural stereotypes fostered by the COS concerning the 'undeserving poor', who must be strictly tested and regulated – for example, malingerers, 'dole bludgers' and other 'welfare cheats'. Interestingly, critical opposition to the COS approach came partly from within: as the case of Attlee shows, practitioners, informed by major poverty surveys in the early 1900s and their own

> **Almoners** were chaplains or church officers in charge of distributing money (alms) to the 'deserving poor'; their positions were later filled by hospital social workers (Gleeson 2006).

experience of the slums, came to see that private charity alone could not cope with the magnitude of the social problem.

REFLECTIVE EXERCISE 4.7
Think about your experience, or the experience of someone you know, as a recipient of a service or resource.
- Were there elements of this experience that reflected the assumptions and the establishment approach exemplified by the COS?
- How helpful did you find these aspects? How might a critical perspective suggest a different approach?

■ The settlement movement: reformers and revolutionaries?

The settlement movement was a breakaway group from the COS, which developed an alternative social model for combating poverty while sowing the seeds for the group work, community development, social policy and political advocacy aspects of social work (see, for example, Ferguson 2008). They established a large 'settlement house' at Toynbee Hall in London in 1884. The idea was for university-educated, middle-class visitors to live among the poor in their communities, and learn from them, while participating in community-based education, cultural and livelihood projects. This broke with the **paternalistic** attempts of COS workers to manage the personal lives of the poor. The settlement leaders employed a social analysis for the causes of poverty. Their interpretation was that any moral failure was that of society in allowing poverty to arise, and not the fault of individual victims (Webb [1926] 1980, p. 207). This meant they also saw the solutions to poverty being social in nature, both locally and nationally. The political theorist Marion Sawer (2003, p. 19) says Toynbee Hall pioneered municipal socialism, that is, 'public enterprises at the local government level' as well as the 'establishment of public parks, museums, libraries, bathhouses, working class housing and allotments'.

A **paternalistic** approach relates to a way of working with people that provides for their needs without considering their rights or responsibilities. This form of activity is seen by some social workers as 'necessary' for those unable to take responsibility for themselves, and recipients are expected to show gratitude (Mullaly 2007, p. 82).

Settlements spread rapidly. The Women's University Settlement with the COS School of Sociology ran the first social work training course in 1903 in the United Kingdom, which was incorporated into the London School of Economics in 1912 (Pierson 2011, p. 43).

In Australia the settlement movement was modest. Former Toynbee residents and the Sydney University Women's Society propagated the model in 1891, working in the Sydney slums. They established a house in 1908, moving to their current hall in Darlington in 1925 and in 1928 proposed that social work be taught at the University. The settlement house continues to operate today as a neighbourhood community centre, which 'directs its efforts to groups within the local community who are disadvantaged and marginalised … [using] strategies that promote community development and empowerment' (Sydney University Settlement 2008).

The settlement movement had enormous impact in the United States, when the social work pioneer Jane Addams (1860–1935) took the model back home and founded Hull House in Chicago in 1889. Hull House became a community centre for social research, crisis accommodation, health care, direct relief, adult education, cultural exhibitions, childcare, preschooling, employment and housing referral, and for advocacy for legislative reforms concerning labour, migrants, women and children's rights at all levels of government. The residents of Hull House engaged in community development work, organising unions, protesting child labour, joining picket lines and often getting arrested. As Ferguson (2008, p. 94) says, the 'Settlement movement in the United States is one of the best examples of social work as a social movement', and by 1910 there were 400 of them nationwide agitating for social reform.

The movement's founder, Jane Addams, was the first woman president of the National Social Work Conference (1910), an **anti-imperialist** and a **suffragette**, labour campaigner, philosopher and peace activist of national and international standing.

> An **anti-imperialist** is one who is opposed to the ideas and beliefs of imperial (territorial) expansion of a country beyond its established borders, including wars to conquer and subjugate people of different cultures (Ife 2013).

As a critical intellectual concerned with how theory should inform action for change, Addams helped Graham Taylor and other settlement leaders found the Chicago School of Civics and Philanthropy in 1908, later incorporated into Chicago University (1920), to train social workers. As an activist Addams built numerous alliances for social reform but her opposition to America's entry into World War 1 earned her the designation of 'most dangerous woman in America' and investigation by the future Federal Bureau of Investigation (FBI) Director, J. Edgar Hoover. However, being awarded the Nobel Peace Prize in 1931 vindicated Addams and her life's work. Her vision of social work as a

> The **suffragettes** were activists who campaigned for women's right to vote.

non-violent movement for social justice shattered the 'friendly visitor' model and still challenges us to think about the possibilities for critical social work today (Weinocur & Reisch 1989).

The radical tradition initiated by Addams and her colleagues, with its social approach to people's problems, continued into the 1930s when a new generation of

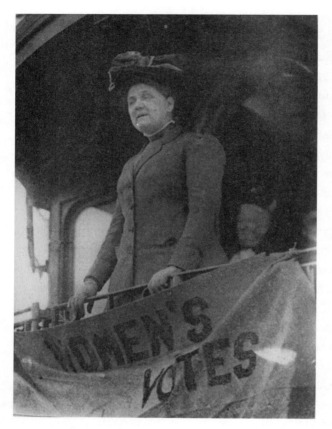

Figure 4.2 Jane Addams
Image reproduced with kind permission of Swarthmore College Peace Collection, USA.

The **Great Depression**
(1929–38) was the extreme
worldwide economic crisis
that began with the collapse
of the New York Stock
Exchange in 1929. Its
consequences were socially
disastrous, rapidly creating
record unemployment, mass
poverty and civil unrest.

social workers confronted the capitalist crisis of the **Great Depression**. These social workers formed the Rank and File Movement within the new welfare institutions created by the 'New Deal' administration of President Roosevelt (1933–45) to cope with the crisis. At one point the Rank-and-Filers outnumbered the membership of the professional social work association (Weinocur & Reisch 1989). In the context of the Depression, they were more militant in their attack on American capitalism than was Addams. They drew explicitly on Marxist theory and were open to revolutionary change more sweeping than that of the governments; identifying themselves with their clients as fellow workers, they aligned with the labour movement, left-wing parties (including communists) and the anti-racist struggles of the day. The Rank and File Movement also organised welfare workers into unions and took strike action in support of workers' rights (Reisch & Andrews 2001).

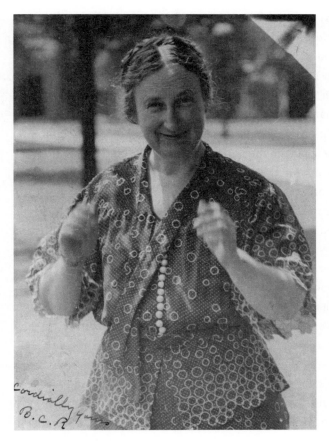

Figure 4.3 Bertha Capen Reynolds
Image reproduced with kind permission of Sophia Smith Collection, Five College.

The movement was eventually suppressed by the repressive anti-communist campaigns that preceded the Cold War (the conflict between Soviet Russia and the United States) in the late 1940s.

REFLECTIVE EXERCISE 4.8
Do you think social workers today would be more likely than in the past to align themselves with clients as fellow workers? Why or why not?

The key leader in this movement, Bertha Capen Reynolds (1887–1978), was the most widely published American social worker of the 1930s (Ferguson 2008, p. 95). She employed Marxist analysis to show the degree to which personal suffering was rooted in exploitative social conditions. She also sought equality in the relationship between social workers and their clients, to encourage the oppressed to organise themselves collectively, and to remind social workers that to be an effective movement for justice meant they had to form coalitions with other movements and not go it alone (Reisch 2002, p. 38): 'It is not we, a handful of social workers against a sea of human misery. It is humanity itself building a dike and we are helping in our particularly useful way.' Unfortunately, Reynold's Marxism and attempts to form a campus union led to her sacking and then (like many radicals) blacklisting from the profession. She found work with the Maritime Union but was forced into early retirement by the anti-communism of the era. However, Reynolds and her Rank and File colleagues did inspire a later generation of radicals in the 1960s and this activism is alive today in the Social Welfare Action Alliance (formerly the Bertha Capen Reynolds Society) in the United States (see http://socialwelfare actionalliance.org).

By the late 1940s, psychodynamic approaches dominated social work in the United States, and the settlement movement lost its radicalism as the professionally trained social workers it employed no longer lived in close proximity to their constituency as had Jane Addams. This is why the very successful founder of community organising, Saul Alinsky (1909–72), would draw sharp distinctions between community organisers (whom he saw as fostering local community leaders) and social workers (whom he saw as outsiders working for the establishment), even though his strategies and tactics would be used by many radical social workers in years to come (Hamington 2010).

At the same time that the Rank and File Movement battled with its government and conservative opponents in the United States, Australian social work was just emerging with very different origins, which we shall explore next.

■ Australia and social work, 1788–1970

Contemporary Australia is the product of a **colonial settler** invasion (1788) that dispossessed the original inhabitants of their land and was designed to deal with the social problems of modernity in Britain in the late 18th century. After the loss of America in the War of Independence (1783), Britain was looking for somewhere else to transport its surplus prison population. The social situation for the colonists was quite different from home. Britain's Poor Laws could not operate directly in Australia because the convict population was already under direct state control (Hirst 1984). Nor were there any church parishes or a capitalist class capable of sustaining charities

Colonial settler invasion, or 'settler colonialism', is a pattern of one people invading and occupying the territory of another people in order to establish a lasting, highly populated, society based on primary production or mining (Beilharz & Hogan 2012, p. 558).

until the early 1800s and even these required state support, as with the Sydney Benevolent Society. Catholic religious orders began to arrive in 1838 and their role, particularly that of nuns such as Mary McKillop, in building basic social services throughout the Australian colonies is often overlooked in histories of welfare (McMahon 2003, p. 86). As **settler capitalism** grew throughout the 19th century, so did the social divisions between capital and labour; however, unlike in Britain, the labour movement was relatively influential and had some early successes, as did the women's movement for the vote (South Australia, 1895; Commonwealth, 1902).

> **Settler capitalism** is a form of capitalist development imported by a colonial elite based on livestock farming that profits from exporting agricultural produce back to the home country (Beilharz & Hogan 2012).

The arrival of free workers saw the formation of 'friendly societies' by trade unions for the mutual support of their members (based on weekly contributions) in times of sickness, unemployment, disability or funerals (Nichol 1985). The male working class also benefited from the chronic labour shortages (compared to their counterparts in Europe and America), which strengthened their bargaining hand with employers over wages and conditions. This is why Australian and New Zealand workers were among the first in the world to win an eight-hour working day. The historian Stuart McIntyre (2012, p. 214) says that by the 1880s, Australia's working class 'probably enjoyed the highest standard of living in the world'. Things became harder during the 1890s depression when the union movement was defeated in the 'Great Strikes' but this setback only led to their organising politically for parliamentary representation to form the Australian Labor Party (1891). Labor initially supported progressive Liberal governments until it was strong enough to form the world's first Labor governments (Queensland, 1899; Commonwealth, 1904 and 1910), instituting such measures as the age pension (1909), invalid pension (1910), maternity allowance (1911) and compulsory arbitration of industrial disputes by an independent commission (1904). The latter set a basic wage (1907) on the basis of principles of **redistributive justice** (rather than the market), which governed wage determination for the next 70 years.

> **Redistributive justice** principles view the state as having a role in legislating a more equal sharing of the material benefits and resources of society; the state, therefore, must act independently – and often in opposition to – market forces and promote an ethic of collective benefit rather than individual interest (Mullaly 2007, p. 126).

REFLECTIVE EXERCISE 4.9

- How important do you think measures such as an age pension, an invalid pension or a maternity allowance are?
- Have these policy measures been important for social justice?
- Should they continue to be protected?

These principles created what Castles (1985) called a 'wage-earners' welfare state', where the profits of capitalism were to some extent redistributed through wage regulation and full employment. The darker side of this egalitarianism was its racial exclusion of non-whites (in the *Immigration Restriction Act 1901*), mandatory **assimilation** of Aboriginal and Torres Strait Islander people and devaluing of women's work.

As in Britain and America, Australia in the 19th century produced a number of activist forerunners to social work. Many of these were women who saw philanthropic (charitable) work as part of a broader movement for a more just and democratic society, including higher wages for workers, poverty relief and equal rights for women. Women such as Vida Goldstein (1869–1949), Mary Lee (1821–1909) and Jessie Street (1889–1970) could easily take their place alongside Jane Addams as exemplary activists and inspiration for critical social work today. Many such women joined the National Council of Women (NCW), the peak organisation for women's rights between the first and second world wars (1919–39). A handful of women in this network, including leaders of the Sydney University Settlement, advocated the creation of social work as a profession in the late 1920s (Marchant 1985; McMahon 2003, p. 89). A member of this NCW network was Norma Parker (1906–2004), an American-trained social worker involved in Catholic social justice programs for women's industrial and welfare rights in the 1930s (McMahon 2003, p. 89). Parker would become a key founder of professional social work in New South Wales, helping to develop the first Australian university course for social workers in 1940 at Sydney University, where she became an Associate Professor. She was also founding President of the Australian Social Workers Association (1946–54) and helped establish the peak, non-government welfare lobby, the Australian Council for Social Services (ACOSS), in 1956.

REFLECTIVE EXERCISE 4.10

Access the website of the Australian Council of Social Service (ACOSS), http://www.acoss.org.au. How does this organisation continue to advocate on behalf of 'marginalised' persons?

The birth of social work in Sydney had broader community input than in Melbourne (and elsewhere in Australia) where it grew exclusively out of hospital almoning, subject to medical control and COS assumptions about assessing the poor (Gleeson 2006, p. 75). In all states, however, the rise of professional social work marked the ascendency of establishment social work in Australia. Professionalisation and specialisation meant greater government or institutional control and a narrow, conservative orientation on the part of social workers themselves. Australian social workers from the 1940s to the 1960s, with a few exceptions in community work, generally embraced the individualising psychological and casework approaches to social problems predominant in America and Britain. There was, however, no Australian equivalent to the American Rank and File Movement, with its links to the labour movement and left-wing parties in the welfare sector. The handful of Australian 'industrial social workers' worked for employers (McMahon 2003, p. 90) and not unions. When a union advertised a social work position for its health clinic in 1964, no social worker applied, such was the conservatism of the profession. Mendes (2003, p. 19) says that social workers in the fifties and sixties did not want to be associated with anything 'left-wing', including the Labor Party and unions. This was why in 1965 the Victorian Branch of the AASW refused an invitation from the Labor Party to assist in developing its social policy (Mendes 2003). More recently and ironically, the AASW has attempted to lobby federal Labor governments for registration, and has been ignored.

> Social work is currently not a registered profession in Australia. The AASW is pursuing statutory regulation (registration) with the National Registration and Accreditation Scheme (NRAS) for health professionals. This would require social work practitioners to be registered with the NRAS, regardless of whether they are members of their professional body (the AASW), in order to practise in the field. A statutory model of regulation would provide a legally enforceable set of practice standards and professional development requirements, as well as a complaints investigation mechanism for client protection against unethical practice (AASW 2011).

Despite the AASW's conservatism, social work, Australia and the Western world generally all underwent major changes from the mid-1960s onwards. Globally, the Cold War intensified, with US aggression in Vietnam against communism (supported by Australia), generating a mass movement against the draft and **imperialism**.

Imperialism refers to the domination of a powerful country over other territories and peoples beyond its borders.

Elsewhere, the former colonies of Europe achieved liberation, often through armed revolution. The Universal Declaration of Human Rights sanctioned by the United Nations in 1948 developed more traction in political debates as a basis for pursuing social justice. Old movements, such as socialism and feminism, were reinvigorated and 'new' social movements, such as those for civil rights, Aboriginal land rights, disability rights, gay and lesbian rights, nuclear disarmament and environmentalism, emerged as part of the New Left. Economically, the long postwar boom reached its peak, leading a new generation to question outstanding injustices, including gaps in social provision. In Australia, there was also a 're-discovery of poverty' by ACOSS researchers, especially in relation to those people not covered by arbitration and full-employment (Mendes 2003, p. 19). The election of the social democratic Whitlam Labor Government in 1972, after 23 years of conservative rule, brought enormous changes in social legis-lation, with funding for **universally provided** (not just selectively tar-geted) welfare, such as a national health-care scheme (Medibank, resurrected by the Hawke Government in 1984 as Medicare), free ter-tiary education and the creation of new welfare institutions that employed social workers (Jamrozik 2009, pp. 80–1).

> **Universal provision** refers to social services given to everyone in society (not means-tested or targeted to a particular group), on the basis of comprehensive risk coverage, generous benefit levels, egalitarianism and full employment (Fawcett et al. 2009).

Australian social work was influenced by these changes and the critical consciousness they provoked. Calls for social work to engage as a profession with social movement activism, social policy advo-cacy and community organising grew. Consequently, by 1975 the President of the AASW, a Whitlam Government adviser and Australia's first woman professor of social work, Edna Chamberlain (1921–2005), was able to proclaim against the establishment view that 'social justice ... rather than social functioning' was the goal of social work (1975, cited in Cooper 2009). Chamberlain, though, was a moderate reformer compared with the radical social work that emerged in this period.

■ Radical social work in the 1970s

The new radicalism was inspired mainly by renewed Marxist critiques of capitalism in the broader political movements of the 1960s and 1970s. These critiques highlighted class division as the underlying source of most disadvantages experienced in health care, housing, the legal system and employment, despite the presence of the welfare state. In fact, the welfare state was problematic because, while it conceded certain hard-won benefits to the working class, it also preserved the class inequalities of capitalism. Marxists and other socialists argued for more fundamental changes to the unequal organisation of power and resources within society, advocating both reformist and revolutionary alternatives (Pritchard & Taylor 1978).

Radical social work publications appeared simultaneously in Australia (Throssell 1975), Britain (Bailey & Brake 1975; Corrigan & Leonard 1978) and North America (Galper 1975; Moreau 1979). In Australia, a group of Marxist social workers called

'Inside Welfare' formed at the University of Queensland in 1975 and spread interstate, producing a bulletin and hosting a 'Marxism and Poverty' conference in 1976 (Mendes 2009). They criticised not only social injustice but also the role of established social work in perpetuating it and called for alternative forms of practice. This was similar to an earlier British collective called 'Case Con', which published a manifesto and magazine of that name 'for revolutionary social work'. Case Con attacked traditional casework as a confidence trick, misdirecting professionals into dealing only with individual *cases*, effectively 'victim blaming' their clients for personal inadequacies rather than addressing the structural source of their problems in poverty, unemployment or oppressive practices (Weinstein 2011). Both Case Con and Inside Welfare criticised **decontextualised** casework as effectively serving the capitalist state and ruling-class interests by requiring disadvantaged clients to adapt and conform to unjust social structures, thereby controlling the underclass (Mendes 2009, p. 20). The favoured response to this analysis was to organise collectively *with* the disadvantaged to pursue reform.

> **Decontextualisation** is a process whereby problems are examined at the individual or group level while ignoring the social structural context. In this way, 'differences' between marginalised and dominant groups are identified as the problem, and strategies to 'correct' the differences in the marginal group so that they can be more like the dominant group are employed (Mullaly 2010).

The liberal individualist ideology that Inside Welfare exposed in traditional casework was also critiqued in establishment social work's notion of professionalism. Just as casework could be used to control the poor, so too, professionalism could be used to control social workers. In this view, professionalism was not primarily about educational or ethical standards but rather a device for directing social workers' efforts away from political action into concerns for personal status, career advancement and accreditation with a professional body (Hennig 1975).

The quest for professional recognition seems to be an issue that social work has struggled with throughout its history. However, history is instructive in reminding us that attempts to professionalise result in aligning with and/or seeking validation from dominant groups and discourses. Professionalisation has almost always occurred at the expense of the emancipatory values and vision of social work. Hence, attempts to professionalise social work marginalise critical social work while validating establishment roles and functions of social work.

Recently in Australia, this quest for professional legitimacy has again been led by the AASW. One example of this was the campaign to seek registration. This decision was made by the professional body because the overwhelming majority of members indicated that they see registration as a key priority for social work. This is arguably because social workers, on the whole, do not feel valued by dominant groups, and have a sense of inferiority in relation to other professions (see, for example, Morley 2014). However, it is paradoxical for social work to seek or expect to be valued by dominant groups because social work's purpose is to redress social inequalities. It, therefore, threatens the powerful and privileged position of those groups. If social workers had the same professional regard as other establishment professionals, such as psychologists, doctors and lawyers, then it would no longer be achieving its purpose and would exist in a form that would have very little in common with the social justice ideas of critical practice.

Despite this, many social workers currently believe that registration will create a solution for what they feel they lack in professional recognition, and that registration will bolster the profession generally. Critical practitioners, conversely, argue that social work needs a strong critical analysis to remain alive and relevant and make a distinctive contribution in the contemporary context – a position that is surrendered with the goal of professionalisation. Establishment social workers fail to see the contradictions between the social work values of social justice, human rights, democracy, freedom, and so on that they claim to be so important, and professionalisation, which is essentially an elitist, exclusionary tool that draws boundaries between social workers and working with the oppressed. Attempting to gain professional legitimacy by uncritically aligning with powerful social forces is equivalent to compromising the social justice of social work. As Holscher and Sewpaul (2006, p. 268) explain: 'All too often the dominant ideologies … are so entrenched that it is difficult to think outside of certain prescriptive ideological frameworks, thus our own [social workers] collude with and perpetuate "the very systems that oppress and work against us" and our clients.'

Another example of professionalisation weakening the critical impetus of social work is the introduction of the AASW mental health accredited practitioner, which means that social workers who operate as private practitioners are able to offer a Medicare rebate to clients who access psychologically focused counselling services.

REFLECTIVE EXERCISE 4.11

Access the document *AASW Requirements and Application for Accreditation as a Mental Health Social Worker*, at http://www.aasw.asn.au/document/item/2058.
- What do you notice about the language that is used? Which discourses are dominant in this document?
- Can you imagine any practices or theoretical approaches that are not mentioned that would make an important contribution to mental health practice?
Hint: you may find it useful to skip ahead to Chapter 7 (case study of Sarah) or Chapter 9, which covers mental health as a field of practice, to answer this question.

While having the federal government subsidise these services increases their accessibility to service users, it does so at the expense of allowing professional inducements such as Medicare to inappropriately drive the mission and role of social work. Historically, the radicals believed that professionalism, with its claims to expert status and knowledge, could only reinforce capitalist hierarchies and elitism, distancing social workers from other welfare workers and from their service users. A more viable form of organisation for socialists, according to Inside Welfare, was (as Bertha Reynolds once argued) trade unionism and active engagement in social movements (Thorpe & Petruchenia 1992, p. 185).

The struggle over social work's identity came to a head amid political turmoil in Australia. In 1975 the Whitlam Government, which had actively enlisted social workers in its reform programs, was dramatically dismissed by the Governor-General and there followed a period of reaction in social policy. Amid cutbacks and rising unemployment, radical social workers were determined to have a more effective organisation for pursuing progressive goals than the AASW structure allowed. They believed that professionalisation was an elitist strategy that played into the hands of state control, whereas social workers (particularly in the non-government sector) had to acknowledge their own exploitation and to unionise with their fellow workers in the welfare sector. This culminated in a split between the AASW, which henceforth dealt with professional accreditation and education, and the Australian Social Welfare Union (now the Social and Community Services (SACS) section of the Australian Services Union), which organised a broad range of welfare workers pursuing 'industrial and social action' (Thorpe & Petruchenia 1992, p. 181). Today, SACS has 24 000 members, with a history of defending various welfare programs and improving welfare workers' pay in an undervalued field, most notably in a breakthrough campaign in 2012 securing a 23–45 per cent pay increase for the largely female workforce in the community sector (Bottomly & Judge 2012).

Collective approaches such as unionism, social movement activism and community organising (Alinsky 1971) opened up new fields of practice for Australian social workers, even if they represented only a few of the possibilities for critical practice. However, in the late 1970s these approaches dominated the radical imagination and proved difficult to sustain when directly attacked by neoliberal governments and their supporters who were trying to suppress radicalism (including social work radicalism), which then declined in the 1980s and 1990s. In Australia, unlike the United States and Britain, the onset of neoliberalism was more gradual because the Hawke–Keating Labor governments (1983–96) attempted to combine an opening to global market forces and deregulation of the labour market (restraining real wages) with an expansion of social provisions in health care, aged care, childcare support, multiculturalism, gender equity and Indigenous land rights. This left a contradictory legacy for social progressives, with large numbers of manufacturing jobs destroyed and the socially marginalised distrusting both major parties. The succeeding Howard Liberal–National Party Coalition Government (1996–2007) further expanded the neo-liberal deregulation and privatisation of the economy (including social services) and cut the social wage for the disadvantaged under the banner of 'mutual obligation', with new testing, surveillance and disciplinary regimes for those seeking assistance. As the social policy analyst Adam Jamrozik (2009, p. 84) says, there was a return to 'the vision of a two tier society of the "deserving" and the "undeserving"' poor indicative of a post-welfare state. Subsequent Australian Labor (2007–13) and Coalition (2013–) governments have not fundamentally altered this trajectory. This has left an institutional setting in welfare provision that is very different from what the original radical social workers operated with in the 1970s and the welfare sector has had to change to deal with these challenges.

■ Critical social work: renewing the social justice tradition

Radical social work has evolved and this is not simply due to the neoliberal state. It has also changed through questioning itself about Marxism's primary focus on class oppression and how this overlooks other forms of oppression based on gender, disability, age, sexuality and **racialised** identity.

Racialisation 'is the process by which race is interpreted as the primary marker of a social phemonenon' (Holmes, Hughes & Julian 2012, p. 44).

The resurgence of feminism and the women's movement in the 1970s both challenged and broadened the radical agenda by targeting patriarchal oppression in addition to capitalism. A Radical Women's Group (RWG) was formed as early as 1973 by social workers in Victoria (Mendes 2009, p. 23). Linking personal experience with political structures, they questioned sexist discrimination against women within their own predominantly female profession, particularly in leadership positions, and the treatment of their largely female service users (Weeks 1994). Feminism drew attention to the patriarchal confinement of women to the domestic sphere as wives and mothers in Australian history. Key social measures such as the basic wage (1907) excluded women who were legally paid half the wages of men until the 1970s, and they were often sacked for becoming pregnant or married until such practices were outlawed in the 1980s. Feminist critiques of the disparities disadvantaging women in Australian society and addressing issues of specific concern to women (sexual assault, discrimination against pregnancy, women's health, maternity leave, childcare) were slow to filter into social work (Marchant 1985; Nichols 1977). However, by the 1980s, gender inequality was widely recognised as a major form of oppression in need of structural reforms and a distinctly feminist practice addressing women's issues emerged (Dominelli 2002b; Dominelli & McLeod 1989). Yet, this too revealed its limitations in the face of critiques from Aboriginal and Torres Strait Islander women and migrant women for its neglect of racial and ethnic discrimination. The issues of racial oppression and anti-racist practice provide ongoing challenges for social work (Bennett et al. 2013; Briskman 2003; Solomon 1976).

The recognition of differing forms of oppression has led to renovations of the radical tradition. Canadian structural social work (Moreau 1979; Mullaly 1993, 2002) has attempted to account for these differing oppressions with more inclusive lists of structural divisions in society. Others, however, have insisted on making one or more of the categories of class, gender, ethnicity, disability, sexuality or age central to their distinctive analysis. While there is a common anti-oppressive (Dalrymple & Burke 1995) and anti-discriminatory (Thompson 1992) theme in these approaches, it would be a mistake to say they are all the same or to attempt to explain and solve all forms of oppression in the same manner.

In Australian social work, the spirit of radicalism has never been entirely abandoned, even if it is overshadowed by establishment social work. Inside Welfare disbanded in the late 1970s but its members and influence moved on into diverse struggles without any peak organisation or dominant label. In the 1990s, however, there emerged in Canada (Carniol 1992; Rossiter 1996) and Australia (Ife 1996) a self-identified movement of critical social work, broadly inspired by **neo-Marxist** ideas and known as critical theory. The term 'critical theory' originated with a group of unorthodox Marxists in the 1930s in Germany known as the **Frankfurt School**.

> **Neo-Marxism** is a modified version of Marxism that incorporates diverse notions of power and culture (Germov & Poole 2011).

The members of the Frankfurt School sought to recover the critical core of Marx's theory (critical theory) in opposition to both liberal capitalism and the state-socialist regimes that claimed Marx's legacy. Critical theory (discussed in Chapter 6) has a much broader notion of oppression than orthodox Marxism's class exploitation (although it includes this). It exposes multiple forms of domination, not only in economic relations but also in politics, culture, knowledge, media, entertainment and everyday life. More than this, critical theory aims to be practical, not simply interpreting the world but provoking ways we might transform it for human freedom and social justice (Ife 1996; Salas, Soma & Segal 2010).

> The **Frankfurt School** was an influential group of unorthodox Marxist theorists whose project of 'critical theory' sought to recover the core of Marx's critique and use it to expose forces of domination in both capitalist and state-socialist societies with a view to promoting human freedom and social justice.

Postmodernism rejects the idea of a single, fixed and objective truth, and instead emphasises multiple perspectives and truths. In this view the world is not objective or mechanical, but complex, fluid, contradictory and multilayered, making it capable of different readings. Postmodernism disrupts the dominant modernist view and invites us to consider alternative voices and perspectives in understanding the world and its problems.

Critical postmodernism is a term used to describe how modernist critical theories such as feminism and structural theory (with their focus on universalised understandings of oppression and privilege) can combine with the emancipatory elements of poststructural thinking to extend critical practice.

Demystifying is a critical practice concerned with sharing power that involves taking the mystery out of social work practices. It involves explaining the organisation and the services offered through sharing information.

Many critical social workers, especially in Australia and Canada, have also combined **postmodern** and poststructural critiques with critical theory, under the banner of **critical postmodernism** (Allan, Briskman & Pease 2009; Fook 2012; Leonard 1994; Pease & Fook 1999; Rossiter 1996). They do this because they find postmodern analysis offers a more nuanced appreciation of the complex and constantly shifting power dynamics of particular and local social settings and problems. In such contexts, it may be the case that there is no clear-cut or fixed distinction between oppressors and oppressed or rather these roles may keep shifting with the unfolding context. In such situations, universal and grand narratives of liberation may be of little immediate value or risk being imposed in an unhelpful 'one-size-fits-all' solution. The critical social worker may be committed to just outcomes but they must first acknowledge the multiple readings and truths that they and their clients use in constructing a problem and the possibilities for addressing it.

Looking back at the history of social work in the context of struggles for social justice, we believe there is an enduring legacy that stems from the earliest radical traditions and now energises all forms (modernist and postmodernist) of contemporary critical social work. At its base, the radicals sought to fundamentally change the power relationship between social workers and service users, collaboratively engaging with them as equal, fellow citizens and addressing their problems with explicit acknowledgement of the social context. This radical conception of social work involved both (1) a rejection of establishment social work and (2) the construction of something new that would faithfully serve their service users' interests both individually and as part of society. This rejection meant a refusal by social workers to accept the 'top-down' expert or social control role and to help **demystify** the welfare process with their clients, pointing out the social causes of their problems (Moreau 1989, p. 15). The construction of alternatives meant attempting to find ways to counter or change these social conditions while meeting individual's immediate needs.

Viewed in this way, while very difficult, it is possible to imagine how the radical social work agenda can be pursued not just in overtly political movements, unions and community work but also in more conventional fields such as casework, group work and counselling within establishment institutions, such as hospitals, nursing homes, jails and government departments (Fook 1993; Wagner 1990, p. 23). This is why Bob Mullaly insists that any critical or structural social work can and must be conducted both 'outside and against' and 'within and against' the dominant system: 'using social work skills and techniques in such a way that we "demystify" it by discussing its origins, purpose [and] by encouraging service users to ask questions' (Mullaly 1993, p. 174). The prospects for such practices will be explored further in Chapter 9, which looks at critical practice in the fields of aged care, mental health and child protection as examples.

REFLECTIVE EXERCISE 4.12

Make a list of those aspects of the radical-critical social work movements of the past that you find attractive and those you think we should leave behind. Now, compare your list with other members of your class and provide your reasons why you have listed certain aspects as valuable or not.

■ Summary

At the outset of this book we said that social work is a mixed, indeed a contested, tradition, and the historical overview presented in this chapter has highlighted this conflict. From the birth of social work in the late 19th century there have always been those who have emphasised dealing with individuals' problems and perceived insufficiencies on a case-by-case basis, where the main aim is to adjust the individual to suit the social order. This remains the dominant tendency in establishment social work today. On the other hand, there have also been those practitioners who emphasise the impact of various social divisions and inequalities on individuals' lives and attempt to collaboratively change social conditions to meet those people's needs (Drakeford 2002, p. 294; Mendes 2009, p. 17). The latter is the approach of critical social work, which despite every attempt to marginalise and silence it, remains a powerful voice for social justice today.

■ Review questions

- Has the history related in this chapter challenged or changed your previous view of social work?
- If so, in what ways has your view changed?
- Does this affect how you would now define the main purpose and scope of social work?

- Does an historical understanding of social work give us grounds for hope or pessimism in the efforts to achieve social justice?
- Can you give some examples of successful and unsuccessful political struggles?

■ Further reading

Australian Council of Social Services, http://www.acoss.org.au

Australian Services Union (ASU) – Social and Community Services (SACS) (formerly the Australian Social Welfare Union (ASWU)), http://www.asu.asn.au/sacs

Jane Addams – Hull House Museum, http://www.uic.edu/jaddams/hull/hull_house.html

Social Welfare Action Alliance (USA: formerly The Bertha Capen Reynolds Society), http://socialwelfareactionalliance.org

SWAN – The Social Work Action Network (UK), http://www.socialworkfuture.org

The International Federation of Settlements and Neighborhood Centers (IFS), http://www.ifsnetwork.org

The Radical Social Work Group (New York), https://sites.google.com/site/radicalswg/about-us

The Rank and Filer: Political Analysis for Radical Social Service Workers (USA), http://www.rankandfiler.net

The Settlement Neighbourhood Centre, http://thesettlement.org.au/home

The Toynbee Hall, http://www.toynbeehall.org.uk

5

Values and ethics for critical practice

■ Introduction

IN THIS CHAPTER we explore in detail the concept of ethical practice from a Western perspective, beginning by familiarising you with current codes of ethics, as well as recent debates about their limitations in guiding ethical practice. We examine some of the dominant assumptions and myths about supposedly objective ways of knowing and contrast these with critical understandings of knowledge, values and ethics. We give an overview of various approaches to decision making in relation to ethical dilemmas and explore how a critical approach can ground ethical practice. We further examine the notion and practice of critical reflection and share a case study with you from our research to demonstrate how one practitioner used critical reflection to inform ethical practice.

Ethics is a domain of philosophy concerned with questions of what is right or wrong in human conduct (see, for example, McAuliffe & Chenoweth 2008). Given that social workers often work with people who are affected by poverty, unemployment, illness, violence, deprivation of liberties and other forms of social disadvantage and oppression, we are often faced with making complex ethical decisions that can affect the lives of others. These decisions may concern the safety of service users experiencing long-term depression and psychological upheaval, the **limits of confidentiality** in relation to the law, decisions about potential harm to a child within the context of their family, and decisions about professional integrity if the organisation we work for is engaged in practices that offend our social work values. Ethical evaluation involves not only describing what is the case but also raising questions about what one ought to do or how one should live. These types of moral questions involve consideration of both personal and social values that are central to critical social work, including values such as honesty, justice,

> **Limits of confidentiality** refers to the situations in which complete privacy (confidentiality) between the social worker and the client cannot be assured. Examples include when there is risk of serious harm to the client or another, when there is a legal requirement (court order) to disclose information, and when information is shared within an agency or team for the purposes of continuity of care (Banks 2012).

compassion, freedom and peaceful coexistence. Critical social work is thus an inherently value-driven enterprise that has ethics at its core. Moreover, many of us are drawn to social work because our own personal values 'fit' with the values and ethics of social work.

In Western culture, ethical thinking has two major sources: the Ancient Greeks and Jews, who still influence us today. In general, the Greeks were concerned with knowing what was good and using reason to establish the right principles that would ensure there was good in all circumstances regardless of context. Jewish thought, by contrast, was much more concerned with practice, with doing what was just or performing right actions that were consistent with a **utopian** moral vision of human worth and the good society (Barton 2003; Morgan 2011). The Greek view of ethics, which is more intellectual, has been dominant and this is where the tendency has arisen to think about ethics in terms of universal rules and principles. However, both the Greek and Judaic views influence contemporary ethics, and a critical approach to social work ethics draws something from each. From the Greeks we retain the idea of constantly questioning our values and laws but we resist their temptation to think there is only one logical solution or true answer to such questions, a temptation to which modern ethics often succumbs. From the Judaic influence, we emphasise practical ethics informed by moral visions of human worth and equality. These visions are not supplied by a religion but rather by critically reflecting upon different theoretical and moral traditions, such as Marxism, **feminism**, social democracy, **anti-racist theories** and poststructuralism, which we discuss at more length in Chapter 6.

In everyday practice situations, important decisions often need to be made; some of our values might come into conflict, and it may be difficult to see what is the most ethical course of action to take. Examples of difficult decisions include whether to remove a child from a tearful mother; whether to challenge organisational policy because you think it is unfair to service users, even though this may jeopardise your employment; whether to betray the trust of a child because you believe this may prevent risk of harm; and whether to record and share information about your contact with service users. Establishment social work attempts to resolve these dilemmas through formulating and imposing codes of ethics.

A **utopia** is an imagined future of complete wellbeing. It literally means 'no-place-land' or 'good-place-land' (More [1516] 2001) but is commonly used to refer to an ideal society.

Feminism is a body of theories that exposes women's oppression (patriarchal domination); it is associated with the women's movement and its struggles for women's emancipation.

Anti-racist theories refer to a range of theories that expose and oppose the use of race, ethnicity and culture as a basis of oppression, discrimination or exploitation.

■ Codes of ethics

Most professions require their members to practise in accordance with a code of ethics. Given that the social work and human service professions engage with some of the most vulnerable and socially disadvantaged individuals and groups in society, professional bodies consider codes of ethics to be particularly important in articulating some of the key values, ideals and purposes of the profession while providing guidance to practitioners about ethical standards associated with professional conduct. Most students and practitioners accept and aspire to follow the espoused intent of the codes of ethics.

The core values identified by the Australian Association of Social Work (AASW), the Australian Community Workers Association (ACWA) and the International Federation of Social Workers (IFSW) include social justice, professional integrity, and respecting the dignity and worth of individuals while promoting their autonomy, choices and rights. The spirit of the values of the AASW Code of Ethics is captured in statements such as this: 'Social workers will aim to empower individuals, families, groups, communities and societies in the pursuit and achievement of equitable access to social, economic, environmental and political resources and in attaining self-determination' (AASW 2010, 5.1.3c, p. 19) and 'will promote policies, practices and social conditions that uphold human rights and that seek to ensure access, equity, participation and legal protection for all' (AASW 2010, 5.1.3a, p. 19).

Consistent with a critical approach, the AASW Code of Ethics states that social workers 'will respect diversity and use anti-oppressive practice principles, seeking to prevent and eliminate negative discrimination and oppression' (AASW 2010, 5.1.3b, p. 19) and 'recognise and challenge racism and other forms of oppression experienced by a range of culturally and linguistically diverse groups, through use of anti-racist and

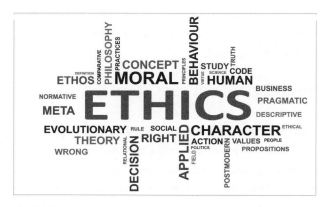

Figure 5.1

anti-oppressive practice principles' (AASW 2010, 5.1.2l, p. 18). Such principles are also central to the philosophy and practice of critical social work, and as such a critical approach finds nothing objectionable with any of the underlying sentiments of the codes of ethics as represented here.

■ A critical analysis of the codes and their limitations

Some tensions arise between the codes of ethics and a critical approach when these broad ethical principles are presumed to double as prescriptions 'that hold members accountable for ethical practice' (AASW 2010, 2.2, p. 10). There are a number of concerns a critical analysis brings to our attention, such as (1) some aspects of the codes are not consistent with critical social work; (2) some aspects of the codes are vague about ethical practice; (3) ethics depend on context; and (4) some aspects of the codes appear to be contradictory. These problems can lead to confusion for practitioners and bring the values and purpose of social work into question.

(1) Some aspects of the codes are not consistent with critical social work

While most of the principles that are contained in codes of ethics reflect what are usually considered to be universal social work values, other statements in the codes are more contentious. An example of a principle that is challenging for critical social workers is the following: 'In exceptional circumstances, the priority of clients' interests may be outweighed by the interests of others, or the legal requirements or conditions'

(AASW 2010, 5.2.1b, p. 25). This principle is problematic because critical social work is committed to putting the interests of service users first, over and above the needs or requirements of the system. From a critical perspective, we would also be interested in how 'exceptional circumstances' are defined, and by whom, as well as how power dynamics underpin the weight and legitimacy given to the 'interests of others'.

(2) Some aspects of the codes are vague about ethical practice

Codes of ethics need to be sufficiently broad to have application beyond a specific set of circumstances, yet can consequently appear vague and open to a variety of different interpretations. For example, the AASW Code of Ethics states that following the receipt of a complaint, the redirection of a client or the refusal to offer a client a service is expected to be done on 'justifiable grounds' (AASW 2010, p. 16), yet the meaning of what is considered 'justifiable' is not self-evident. It may also be difficult for practitioners to know exactly what is meant by 'setting and maintaining clear and appropriate boundaries' (AASW 2010, 5.1.6c, p. 22). Problematically, what may be considered 'appropriate' in one context might be entirely different in another. Consider the worker's boundary-setting responsibilities in two different situations: working with children in a therapeutic counselling relationship, where critical practitioners would try to facilitate the children's control and direction over a session; and working with perpetrators of violence in a

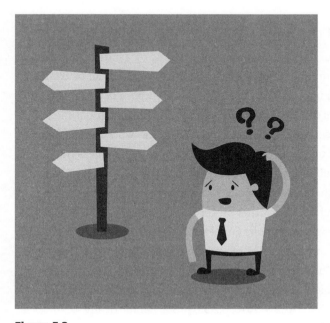

Figure 5.2

prison setting, where there is a need to maintain strict control over the purpose and direction of a session. Another example comes from the AWCA Code, which refers to the need for welfare and community workers to 'maintain proper standards of practice'. Indeed, what practitioners regard as 'proper' may vary, based on their own values, assumptions, experiences and theories that they use to inform their understanding of the world.

(3) Ethics depend on context

Another difficulty with relying on codes of ethics to guide practice is that they fail to adequately take account of context. The AASW Code acknowledges 'that practice is contextual and that many factors will influence decision-making outcomes' (AASW 2010, p. 15). Importantly, it also recognises that 'All ethical decision making occurs within the context of managing power relationships' and that 'Social workers need an understanding of the social, political and historical context in which decisions are made' (AASW 2010, p. 14). However, codes of ethics do little to address the impact of these contextual factors, which inevitably determine how the ethical standards and principles are read, interpreted and used in particular situations. In other words, ethical statements that present as if they have universal applicability and acceptance, but do not acknowledge that they can be understood in a number of different ways, are quite limited in terms of their capacity to provide practitioners with meaningful guidelines for ethical practice.

(4) Some aspects of the codes appear to be contradictory

One of the main criticisms of the codes of ethics, highlighted by a critical approach, is that they appear to have a number of contradictory principles. This can be confusing for practitioners and brings into question the values and purpose of social work. For example, the codes of ethics generally stipulate a set of principles that outline practitioners' responsibilities to service users, to colleagues, to the workplace and to the profession. However, one of the challenges of these principles in practice is that sometimes the interests of the different groups intersect in ways that are competing or oppositional. For example, the AASW Code of Ethics states that social work 'advocates change to social systems and structures that preserve inequalities and justice' (AASW 2010, 3.2, p. 13). This requires social workers (quite rightly from a critical perspective) to take sides, or to take up a value position in relation to promoting social justice. At the same time, however, the Code states that 'Reports [prepared by practitioners] will provide a professional opinion and are not to be a submission to emphasise one particular interest over another' (AASW 2010, 5.2.5c, p. 30). Paradoxically, then, social workers are positioned by the Code as both agents of value-driven change (as in the first example) and as neutral arbitrators (as in the second example). The assumption that social work can or should be neutral (remain impartial or not take sides between competing interests or values) or objective is highly problematic, from a critical perspective, as neutrality and objectivity are regarded as both impossible and dishonest. A more critical view suggests that the pretence of taking a neutral position only serves to reinforce the power of the dominant party, whose position remains unchallenged, with the end result being the maintenance of existing power relations.

Critical reflection assists practitioners to develop greater awareness of the ways they might have positioned themselves along a continuum of challenging dominant power relations and structures, or been complicit with existing injustices in the system. While some codes of ethics encourage practitioners to engage in critical reflection (see, for example, AASW 2010, p. 14), they simultaneously instruct practitioners to do the very opposite of this, by insisting that practitioners can and should be neutral and objective. Some examples of this include stating that practitioners should 'provide assistance to clients in an objective … manner' (AASW 2010, 5.1.3f, p. 19), 'exercise professional discretion and unbiased judgment' (AASW 2010, 5.1.7a, p. 23) and 'record information impartially and accurately' (AASW 2010, 5.2.5a, p. 29).

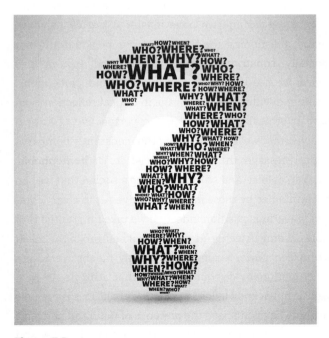

Figure 5.3

■ Leaving my values at home? An objectivist view of ethics

Some codes of ethics read as if they are written from an all-seeing, satellite view of the world that, from a neutral standpoint, represents the one and only, right way of knowing that exists outside of history and context. These 'truths' are assumed to be universally applicable, untainted and unchallengeable. A key explanation for professional bodies presenting global codes of ethics as if we operate in a vacuum can be traced to the acceptance of assumptions associated with an objectivist way of seeing the world (for further critique, see Ife 2012).

An objectivist paradigm assumes that things have a meaning in themselves, independent from the person interpreting them and the contexts in which the person or object is situated (Crotty 1998). From an objectivist point of view, it is believed that a true knowledge about reality is possible, regardless of context and interpretation (Meinert, Pardeck & Kreuger 2000a). Therefore, it is assumed that codes of ethics can be read independently and separately from context as it is thought that their principles will hold the same meaning for different people in any situation.

> **Social construction** refers to 'the socially created characteristics of human life based on the idea that people actively construct reality, meaning it is neither "natural" or inevitable. Therefore notions of normality/abnormality, right/wrong, and health/illness are subjective human creations that should not be taken for granted' (Germov & Poole 2011, p. 521).

An establishment view of social work suggests that it is desirable, ethical and possible for practitioners to be objective, unbiased and neutral in professional practice. However, one of the difficulties with this is that once we assume we have mastered a truly objective stance, we stop questioning the ways that our personal and our culturally/**socially constructed** views, values and assumptions shape the ways we see the world and influence our perceptions. This awareness and willingness to engage in critical reflection is an essential part of ethical practice from the perspective of critical social work. Given that we live in a society that constantly bombards us with powerful messages that are often racist, sexist, **homophobic**, ageist, colonialist, ableist, and so on, accepting a notion that we can somehow be untouched by these influences leaves us in a very compromised and precarious position indeed. If we take for granted that we are capable of being objective (detached and neutral) in the midst of seen and unseen power struggles, it usually means we accept uncritically the dominant discourses about that struggle. In fact, such a struggle is not acknowledged as existing at all! This is perhaps why some authors have criticised the pretence of taking an objective stance in which practitioners mistake 'pre-formulated' codes and

> **Homophobia** is an irrational fear of, or discomfort with, homosexual people that often manifests as individual violence or structural discrimination (Mullaly 2010, p. 212).

rules for a more nuanced form of ethical practice. Rather than encouraging critical reflection, ethical practice that aims to be objective actively opposes it through simplifying the messiness and complexity of social work practice (Meagher & Parton 2004, pp. 10–11).

PRACTITIONER'S PERSPECTIVE

Consider the following case study, drawn from our research (Morley, unpub). The practitioner we interviewed gave what she said was a factual description of what happened in a critical exchange between herself and the service user. The role of the agency that she works within is to provide material assistance and referral to people experiencing financial hardship, poverty and homelessness.

A male and female with one child in a pram came into welfare and asked for an appointment to see me today. A volunteer came and asked me if I wanted to see them. I went out to reception and asked what was happening for them. He replied, 'I don't have any food for my kids and I would like some.' I reminded him that he has had a lot of help from us in the past years, and he was asked to go to budget counselling because I was not able to keep helping him. He said he went and the lady helped him with the electricity bill and nothing else. He said he's been waiting to see the budget lady, but no one has called him. He now says that he is falling behind in rent. He has debts to repay to Cash Converters, fines to pay, and can't buy food to feed his family. I asked why he keeps going to Cash Converters for loans. He believes it's my fault because I don't give him grocery cards! He says if I just gave him $30 he wouldn't have to go to Cash Converters and get a loan of $100 (being the lowest amount Cash Converters will lend). He says it's not his fault that the budget worker hasn't phoned. I asked him how long this problem of food and debts, etc. had been going for. He said since he had kids.

Meanwhile his partner said nothing. I looked at her to join her in conversation. She rolled her eyes. I explained I cannot keep giving them things until they learn how to take responsibility for this situation and get help to sort this out. Our agency has a rule that we are only supposed to help people in emergency situations, for a maximum of twice per year, and he has already exceeded the limit. I asked him again, 'So tell me how far back you can remember when you were not in debt, paying fines and can't find enough money to feed yourself?' He replied, 'I don't know, wherever I go this has always happened to me.' He then stood up and said, 'You're not going to help me. You're okay letting my kids starve so I am leaving.' I then said that I would give him one last bag of food but I would require him to call our financial counsellor and make an appointment. He replied, 'I can't do that because I don't have a phone.' I then said I would make the appointment, which I did. Neither one of them turned up.

This case study raises a number of questions:
- How objective do you consider the above description of practice to be?
- What are the 'facts' that you can identify in this story?
- What are your personal reactions to this story?

- How do they compare with the worker's perspective?
- Can you recognise some of the **implicit assumptions** informing the practitioner's construction of the story?
- How might some of these assumptions compare with ethical practice that is informed by critical social work?

> **Implicit assumptions** are assumptions that we hold, but of which we are not necessarily aware (Fook 2012).

While you may find these questions difficult or challenging to respond to now, by the time we revisit the case study later in the chapter you will find it clearer.

■ Critical reflection

Critical reflection goes beyond a simple 'aware[ness] of personal beliefs and history, values, views, prejudices and preferences', with a view to 'refrain from imposing these on clients' (AASW 2010, 5.1e, p. 17). The notion that we can develop awareness of our views, yet resist imposing them on others, implies that we can avoid questioning personal views and values that may reflect and support social injustices, provided that we somehow keep them separate from our professional practice. This reduces the references to critical reflection in the codes of ethics to rhetoric. Statements such as 'Social workers will ensure all prepared reports ... include separation of fact and opinion ... and that the conclusions reached are based on fact' (AASW 2010, 5.2.5c, p. 31) reinforce the myth of objectivity as a goal for social work practice.

From a critical perspective, it is impossible to separate your personal values from your professional practice. Therefore, social workers have a professional responsibility to interrogate their values and ensure they are consistent with the ethics of the profession. Critical approaches reject the objectivist assumptions that contend it is possible (and desirable) to separate the personal from the professional. The notion that we can privately hold racist, ageist, sexist or homophobic views in our personal lives but somehow act as if we do not in the context of our professional practice with these groups is inherently flawed. The sense that we can leave our personal values at home and apply a different set of values (our professional ones) in the context of our work is simply not adequate for ethical practice. Instead, critical approaches require our personal values to be congruent (aligned with) with our professional ethics and practices. Sometimes it takes a very long time, perhaps even a lifetime, to challenge deeply entrenched mindsets to truly bring our personal values in line with critical social work values. If it is to be a real change, rather than something superficial, it can take a lot of work to develop congruence between social work values and one's own personal values. This is an intellectual as well as a potentially harrowing emotional process. Critical reflection is a useful tool we can apply to assist us with this ongoing goal.

Epistemology

One of the key issues underpinning the differences between an establishment approach to social work ethics that accepts the goal of objectivity, and a critical understanding of ethics that rejects objectivity and endorses critical reflection largely relates to epistemology. In its most basic sense, epistemology is our theory of knowledge. It addresses the question, how do we know what we know? For example, do we know through the senses? Do we know through experience? Do we know through scientific research, through all of these or something else? Epistemology has to do with what we believe is the basis of knowledge (see, for example, D'Cruz & Jones 2004).

Holscher and Sewpaul (2006) suggest that there are two distinctive epistemological positions that inform ethics in social work and related professions: the *objectivist* perspectives (which they refer to as **positivist**/modernist) and the *critically reflective/poststructural* paradigms. Mullaly (2007) has made a similar distinction, highlighting the differences between what he refers to as conservative social work and progressive social work. This mirrors our distinction between establishment and critical social work, or the ethics of social control versus the ethics of critical reflection/social change (Holscher & Sewpaul 2006). These competing theories and practices all have implications for how we understand ethics in social work.

> **Positivism** is a theory of knowledge that claims that the only reliable form of knowledge is that which can be stated in law-like propositions and is open to empirical verification (knowledge directly observed or experienced).

A critical approach to ethics

In contrast to an objectivist view of ethics, a critical perspective argues that knowledge, power, fact and values are intimately connected. In the same way that our personal values influence our professional practice, fact and opinion are not necessarily distinguishable because 'facts' are regarded as social constructions that we elevate to the status of a 'truth' based on our own values. Our understanding of any situation will never be total or holistic, but necessarily a partial representation of our experience. For example, the 'truth' about the young woman who has been diagnosed with bipolar disorder, or the family that has been labelled dysfunctional, has, at least to some extent, been created from dominant cultural and social perspectives about what is considered 'normal', productive and desirable behaviour. The information we choose to include, the information we choose to emphasise and the information we choose to leave out all shapes our construction of our 'facts', our truths and our realities. Our reasons for choosing one interpretation of 'reality' over another, or one set of 'facts' over others, has to do with the *biographical lens*, informed by our immersion in dominant discourses, from which we view the world. Our biography has to do with our own moral, social, economic, historical, geographical, cultural and gendered positioning and experiences. Critical reflection is essential to understand the impact of this lens in shaping our perceptions.

REFLECTIVE EXERCISE 5.3
- How would you describe your own biography? For example, how does the historical period that you live in shape your identity? If you find this difficult to answer, consider how you might have been different if you were born 100 years ago. How might your ideas, values, goals and aspirations have been influenced by this different historical period? Think about some of the historical changes that have happened in the last century, such as the rise of social media and new technologies, and changes to the education system. How have these impacted on you?
- How does geography impact on you? If you were born in a rural area, how has this shaped your identity? How might you have been different if you were raised in a metropolitan area, and vice versa?
- Now consider who you are in cultural and gendered terms. How does being a man or women shape how you see the world? How does your gender influence your values and views in relation to particular social issues?
- What are the other structural dimensions of your biography that shape you as a person and the values and ethics you will bring to professional practice?

A critical perspective contends that 'the personal is political' and as such our personal and professional selves are one and the same (Mullaly 2010, p. 222). The personal and professional dimensions of our lives are inevitably linked. As critical social workers, the values and ethics associated with our philosophy of practice become our way of seeing the world: a way of life, not just a way of doing things at work, but a way of being (or striving to be) in all contexts. From this perspective, every single decision we make has ethical dimensions and critical reflection is vital for ethical practice to ensure that we do not unthinkingly take on socially and culturally dominant views and allow them to infiltrate our practice by uncritically assuming ourselves to be objective. Others have similarly advocated critical reflection as a means of countering the potential for codes of ethics to promote the social control functions of social work that are fundamentally at odds with the purpose and values of critical social work (Chambon, Irving & Epstein 1999).

Ethical practice as critical practice

In addition to discouraging critical reflection, within the current contexts a commitment to objective practice can also be used to undermine the purpose and goals of ethical social work. When being objective or neutral becomes the goal of the practitioner, the value or ethic that is being favoured is the pursuit of 'truth'. However, as critical social workers who engage with *poststructuralism*, we are aware that there are many possible constructions of reality that could potentially be presented as 'truth'. Poststructuralism, with its critique of singular *grand narratives*, points to the need for us to be mindful of 'multiple' truths, perspectives and realities (Fook 2012). (We explore this in more depth in Chapter 6.) In addition, when social workers begin to privilege 'truth' over other core values (such as social justice, respect for diversity, autonomy and freedom), the possibilities for ethical practice to be co-opted and undermined are massive. This is because objectivist views uncritically reflect and reproduce the dominant views of society and therefore accommodate neoliberal values as if they are right, good and universal.

Paralleling the objectivist goal of truth, neoliberal discourses have produced a new set of values that have emerged from managerial priorities. These values can loosely be defined as economic priorities, and when combined with the quest for 'truth', other values (such as freedom, democracy, social justice and human rights) are further marginalised, and regarded as expensive, unnecessary and dispensable in the contemporary neoliberal context.

The 'ethics' of truth, efficiency and value for money include initiatives such as offering services at the lowest cost to conserve the agency's budget. Some of the ways this has been manifested in practice is to **standardise** the services offered; to adopt a 'one-size-fits-all' approach instead of aiming to cater for the individual needs of diverse populations. The value that guides practice then becomes one of saving

> **Standardisation** refers to adopting 'a one size fits all' approach instead of aiming to cater for the individual needs of diverse populations; this fits well with neoliberal management models aimed at cost-cutting and reducing the range and complexity of social work skills (Baines 2007).

money and doing more with less, rather than upholding the quality and range and services (Holscher & Sewpaul 2006).

Consider for a moment the example of a 'meals on wheels' service that has been **contracted out** to a private provider. This service delivers meals to people's residences and is offered to people who live in the community but may not have the capacity to prepare their own food. One of the ways that some funding bodies have saved money is to reduce the quality of the food, thus also reducing the essential nutritional intake for the recipients. Further, funding bodies concerned more about the bottom line have reduced the variety of available options, so everyone is offered the same meal, regardless of their dietary needs or preferences. You may be thinking about the situations in which people suffer food allergies, or request a vegetarian option. The value of saving money has been preserved, but the value of providing a quality service to people in need has been removed from the agenda in this neoliberal context.

A focus on neutrality, objectivity and truth can therefore result in codes of ethics being distorted and inappropriately reduced to rules, in a context where the rules are being mistaken for ethical practice, despite the obvious lack of moral consideration. Practitioners who work in this way follow the rules, don't question the rule book and fulfil their obligations as defined by the agency or the law, regardless of whether this practice reflects moral concerns (Banks 2012). From this objectivist perspective, ethics are mistaken for compliance with technical and managerial procedures, and by contrast, moral concerns are seen to be quite separate from, and irrelevant to, ethics (Banks 2012). From a critical perspective, social workers cannot or should not ever aim or claim to be neutral or objective, as they are part of an inherently value-driven profession with explicit core values that should not be compromised. After all, if we are not asking questions about the quality of services, thinking about the implications of cutting quality and choice for service users, and considering social issues in addition to economic ones, who else will?

Going further down the neoliberal path, funding bodies concerned with profit may decide that practitioners can offer the meals on wheels service more efficiently if, instead of waiting for the service user to open the door and chatting about their health and the weather, they just press the doorbell, leave the food and hurry to the car to deliver the next recipient's meal in the same manner. Service providers could save funding bodies a lot of money by adopting this sort of practice, which, again, meets the values of finding new, more efficient, standardised and cost-effective ways of delivering a service. This practice would be regarded as appropriate by establishment social work approaches because practitioners would have technically fulfilled their obligations to

> **Contracting out** involves the government buying the services of a non-state provider. The relationship is managed by a legally binding contract between the purchaser (government) and provider (private provider) (McDonald et al. 2011, p. 52).

the service provider, ticked the box of their service agreement and strengthened the financial viability of the organisation. However, potentially sick or injured recipients would be neglected in this process and might suffer accordingly.

To support these practices and allegedly measure the value and ethics or 'quality' of services, funding bodies will require service providers to undertake regular audits of their procedures and routines, surveillance of workloads and compliance with operational standards (Fook & Gardner 2007; Madhu 2011). Of course, quality, from this economic viewpoint, is about efficiency and saving money for the organisation. These audits are not designed to gain information about the service user's experience or level of satisfaction with the service they were offered and indeed service users may feel too vulnerable to comment honestly. In the case of the meals on wheels example they would not examine the impact of the lack of variety, the inappropriateness of absence

REFLECTIVE EXERCISE 5.4
Refer back to the case study presented earlier in the chapter.

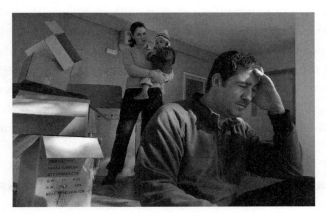

Figure 5.4

- Can you identify the ways in which dominant discourses have influenced the practitioner's perspective?
- What particular assumptions do you think might be problematic about her construction of the case scenario for ethical practice that is informed by critical perspectives? For example, who does she think is to blame? How does she see her role? Does her practice reflect more of an establishment approach to social work, or a critical response – and why?
- How else might she have interpreted the situation, the clients and her role to develop a more critical and ethical practice response?

of choice and quality of food, or the vital function of human interaction that the service also provided. Hence, the quality of such a service, as we understand it from a critical perspective, has been severely undermined. And ethics in this sense is not about helping people but managing them more efficiently and in the most cost-effective ways.

From an economic/business point of view, our service users are positioned as customers and consumers who are expected to be grateful for any service they receive because myths and dominant ideologies promote the view that they are a burden on society and taxpayers' contributions to the public budget. Efficiency is also understood as reducing cost. And social workers/human services practitioners are seen as staff who technically (uncritically) carry out tasks as defined appropriate by funding bodies (Madhu 2011).

Hence, a focus on being objective, which uncritically accepts the neoliberal agendas as 'truth', is at odds with the purpose, values and ethical concerns of critical social work. Therefore, the current context of globalised capitalism and neoliberal policies and discourses (as outlined in Chapter 2) has direct implications for how we understand social work values and engage in ethical practice. It is perhaps more important now than ever before for social work to recognise how ethical practice principles can be marginalised and co-opted by our participation in dominant discourses that have the potential to seriously undermine the values and purpose of social work as we have historically understood them (Holscher & Sewpaul 2006; Madhu 2011, Rees 1991). Resisting the imposition of economic imperatives on social work practice to instead promote the value of practices that support service users' rights and emancipation is consequently a key ingredient of ethical practice in the current socioeconomic environment.

■ Critical evaluation of ethical decision-making models

Social workers are often faced with what are commonly referred to as ethical dilemmas – situations, such as the one presented in the case study, can be challenging for practitioners when it is unclear what interpretation, decision or action is ethically 'right' or 'wrong' (see, for example, Bowles et al. 2006). For instance, should I break the organisation's rules to assist the client? Or should I follow my employer's rules and deny the client a service? Although professional codes of ethics provide some guidance, there are many situations where diverse pathways appear ethically supportable. Social workers have attempted to devise various ethical decision-making models to assist practitioners by providing systematic ways of thinking through ethical dilemmas, often based on a series of steps or questions (Bowles et al. 2006).

These models are based on particular theories or sets of ideas about the world. A model is a form of theory that 'describes what happens in practice ... in a structured form . . . which gives practice consistency . . . and helps you to structure and organise how you approach a complicated situation' (Payne 2005, p. 5). Traditional or establishment social work theories about the nature of ethical behaviour are often categorised as virtue-based, deontological or rule-based, consequence-based or care-based (Bowles et al. 2006).

Virtue ethics are premised on the notion of the virtuous practitioner: that by cultivating and enacting particular character traits or personal qualities one will inherently be guided to practise ethically. These virtues are thought to consist of open mindedness, good judgement, moral courage, capacity for reflection, empathy, commitment to social justice and the values of the profession, and tolerance (Bowles et al. 2006).

REFLECTIVE EXERCISE 5.5
- In relation to the practitioner's perspective presented earlier in this chapter, what virtues do you think the practitioner demonstrated?
- How might her practice have been different if she had demonstrated the virtues of moral courage to challenge the organisational protocols and support the client, rather than uphold unjust policy in the agency to the detriment of the client?
- Might there be difficulties in identifying what qualities are worth cultivating and how they are best expressed?

Consequentialist (or *teleological*) *ethics* emphasises the consequences of decisions or actions, suggesting that the greatest good for the greatest number of people should be pursued (sometimes called *utilitarianism*). From this perspective, by tallying up the perceived good or bad consequences we can determine what action is correct to serve the greatest good (Bowles et al. 2006).

Deontological or *duty-based ethics* infers that some acts are obligatory regardless of their consequences; that because some principles sit above others (that is, we have a duty to follow them), choices are clear and absolute. They are either right (consistent with rules) or wrong (against the rules) and the law must be followed to the letter. From a critical perspective we would question what the implications of such an approach might be. Certainly our duty to protect human rights and respect diversity can be seen as absolute and essential; however, our duty to one individual may conflict with our duty to another (for example, the right to freedom for one conflicting with duty to protect another) (Beckett & Maynard 2005). From a deontological perspective, torture of another being is wrong; no exceptions. From a consequentialist perspective, if the torture of one leads to protecting the many, the positive consequences outweigh the negative. A less extreme example might be the quarantining of welfare payments. Is this an infringement on the human rights of people struggling to make ends meet or a necessary measure to ensure taxpayers' money is being 'well spent'?

REFLECTIVE EXERCISE 5.6

- For whom should we consider 'the consequences'? Should the needs of one group be more heavily weighted than another?
- Can we know with certainty what the consequences of an action might be?
- Are there some actions that are simply intolerable even though they might lead to good for a greater number of people? (You might want to consider medical experimentation.)
- How might a consequentialist model of ethics apply to the case study?
- Was the practitioner in this case acting to protect the greatest good for the greatest number by ensuring that the family did not receive more than its fair share?
- Was she obliged to follow agency policy regardless of the consequences for the family?
- What principles has she assumed should be prioritised over others? If she valued the principle of distributing societal resources to those most in need, how might her practice have been different?

Finally, we look at *care-based ethics*, which is an action-oriented approach that focuses on nurturing, patience, relationship and connection. The ethical nature of actions is judged for their impact on the relationship between key actors, in particular worker and client (Bowles et al. 2006). From a critical perspective this approach has value: its emphasis on relationships, compassion and nurturing provides a resource for challenging managerialist and **technocratic** approaches to human service provision (Meagher & Parton 2004). However, 'care' can be seen and experienced as patronising and marginalising rather than empowering (Meagher &

Technocratic means over-reliance on technology, which poses a threat to 'professional expertise and autonomy' (Fook 2012, p. 24).

REFLECTIVE EXERCISE 5.7

- Do you think the practitioner in the case study demonstrated care-based ethics? Why or why not?
- How might the practitioner's interpretation of the family's presentation and her subsequent practice with them have been different if she was using care-based ethics to inform her practice?

Parton 2004) and may place too much emphasis on individual relationships rather than overall principles.

At this point, you may have decided that you prefer or resonate with one of these ethical approaches more than others, or you may have considered, like Bowles et al. (2006), that none of these approaches contain all the answers and that a **pluralist** approach is most desirable. Most ethical decision-making models are based on consequentialist, deontological and virtue-based ethical theories, and are linear in nature. Such models contain a number of chronological steps leading to a definitive conclusion.

Pluralist approaches seek to find ways of incorporating different visions of what is morally 'good' without arriving at a single unitary position (Hugman 2013, p. 137).

An example of such a linear model can be found in that proposed by Garcia et al. (2003, cited in Bowles et al. 2006, p. 199), whose seven-step model comprises:

1 gathering facts and identifying the problem
2 referring to a code of ethics and professional guidelines
3 determining the nature and dimension of the problem
4 considering potential consequences of all options
5 choosing the best option
6 evaluating the course of action
7 implementing the course of action.

Linear models such as this are often described as 'process models' based on logical reasoning in which actions are prioritised. A 'right' decision is made and the act is therefore justified through having followed the process. From a critical perspective, we might wonder if process models are based on assumptions that can be usefully questioned. For example: decisions should be rational, not instinctive; decisions should be based on logic and reason; objectivity is desirable and achievable; and a 'correct' decision' is achievable. Process models have benefits in terms of breaking a situation down into manageable components, challenging workers to consider values and providing a logical framework, as well as being particularly useful for inexperienced workers. However, reliance on such models can also create a false sense of security that there is a 'right' decision, and, by not allowing for intuition or consideration of the specific context or complexity of the situation, may miss important factors (Ife 2012).

Linear, process-driven models can also lead practitioners into ethical decision making that is accomplished in isolation. Other models emphasise the importance of consultation and dialogue in addressing ethical dilemmas. Cultural models of ethical decision making, for example, prioritise its cultural context, suggest consultation with cultural experts and favour its basis on consensus. Reflective ethical decision-making models also emphasise the importance of dialogue and the inclusion of clients in decision-making processes, thus tackling the issue of power in decision making. Reflective models take account of intuitive as well as rational ways of knowing, and acknowledge that emotions also play a part in decision making. Furthermore, reflective models encourage a cycle of reflection (rather than a linear model) as the decision maker moves through an increasingly deep exploration of the ethical dilemmas (McAuliffe & Chenoweth 2008). In the real world of ethical decision making, coming to a definitively 'right' conclusion is never a structured, linear process. People are not always available for consultation and may not always give good advice. Sometimes clients do not fully understand the situation they are in nor are we always able to obtain all sides of a story (Gray & Gibbons 2007, p. 222).

■ Critical reflection as ethical practice

Dialogical processes or relationships are mutual and two-way, with the participants in the dialogue each learning from and teaching each other. 'Both work together so that they can ask the questions as well as think about the answers' (Mullaly 2010, p. 240), which then will inform their actions.

As critical social workers we need to acknowledge that it is impossible to generate a complete list of options and to fully anticipate their consequences. However, by taking a **dialogical** and reflective approach to ethical decision making we open ourselves to new discoveries. By critically reflecting on our assumptions and the validity of our reasoning we can continually develop our practice and our learning about what is ethical behaviour in particular contexts (Goldstein 1987). Ife (2012, p. 179) further emphasises that ethical issues must be resolved not by a single worker acting in isolation, but by a process that involves other actors. He suggests that the first question for the worker is not 'what should I do?' but 'whom should I talk to?'. This would include not only one's supervisor, but also the client, the client's family, community members, colleagues and other professionals.

An openness to examining one's own assumptions and to valuing diverse forms and sources of knowledge is a key element of a critical approach to social work; a form of social work that Rossiter (2011, p. 980) describes as 'unsettled practice'. Rossiter encourages us to acknowledge that our *representations* (understandings/constructions) of people are always inadequate because people 'exceed representations' (2011, p. 983). As ethical practitioners we acknowledge the uniqueness of each person, rather than constructing others as an extension of our own concepts and experiences or restricting them by a singular theoretical perspective. Rossiter (2011) suggests that ethical social work is a form of practice that acknowledges the limitations of our own construction of others. While traditional or establishment concepts of professionalism value our capacity to know (and often label) the client in order to help them, Rossiter's view of ethical social work practice suggests it is our ability to be open to others – and particularly the challenges they pose to dominant and/or personally held assumptions – that is the hallmark of ethical practice, and not our ability to define others by our limited sets of theoretical concepts. Questions, rather than answers, Rossiter suggests, should be prioritised, along with interrogation of the language we use to represent clients about what opinions may be disguised as facts and how the presentation of 'facts' is a function of power.

Categorising and creating representations of clients (and even the word 'client' is a potentially oppressive representation) are necessary. We need representations to achieve our social justice aims. However, as critical and ethical social workers we are also 'committed to living on the razor's edge of the violence of representation and the necessity for justice and service' (Rossiter 2011, p. 987). In the Australian context, a striking example is the way in which Aboriginal and Torres Strait Islander people are often referred to as 'disadvantaged'. This construction potentially enables access to resources, but at the same time masks the profound historical legacy of colonisation, and the continuing oppression and marginalisation experienced by Aboriginal and Torres Strait Islander people.

REFLECTIVE EXERCISE 5.8
Rossiter's concepts about ethical practice are deep and potentially 'unsettling'. How do they fit with your understanding of social work?

Think back to the case study presented earlier in the chapter. How might the notion of 'unsettled practice' as ethical practice have assisted the practitioner to challenge dominant discourses that served to disempower both herself as the worker and the family who had approached her agency for assistance?

■ A critical reflection on practice

In your reflection on the practitioner's narrative you may have noticed the following implicit assumptions hidden in her account of her practice.

- The father should be able to 'feed his family'.
- He is in poverty because of poor budgeting in which he has not taken 'responsibility for this situation'.
- Budgeting counselling will solve the family's problems.
- The members of this family are abusing or becoming dependent on the service because they have accessed resources from the service previously.
- The poverty his family is experiencing is the father's fault because his history demonstrates that he has always been in this situation.

- The practitioner's role is to protect the resources of the agency so that one family does not receive excessive help.
- The needs of the family are completely at odds with the goals of the organisation.
- It was appropriate to use the food parcel the father was seeking for his children as leverage to manipulate him into agreeing to attend budget counselling.
  - The practitioner is clearly the expert who knows what the family needs to do.
  - The family is '**undeserving**'.
  - The parents are hopeless because they didn't 'turn up' to the appointment the practitioner had made for them.

Undeserving is a term derived from dominant discourses that is used to invalidate the needs of service users by declaring them unworthy recipients of services and/or resources.

These are some of the unconscious assumptions that the practitioner identified while using critical reflection to research her practice (Morley, unpub). Hopefully, by now you will be beginning to notice how different this response would be with a critical social work approach.

REFLECTIVE EXERCISE 5.9

Make a list of the ethical concerns that critical social work would raise about the assumptions embedded in this practice.

You may have noted that the practitioner's *individualistic* analysis of the situation seemed to blame the family while ignoring the wider social, economic and political factors that would also be impacting on this family's opportunities to access the basic resources it needs to live. You may have noted the practitioner's disapproval and judgemental attitude towards the family, which reflects the same moralistic judgements that were made by the Charitable Organisation Societies (COSs) (outlined in Chapter 4). You may have noted the practitioner's view that she knew best, or her need to protect and align with the system, which is consistent with establishment social work.

Make a list of how a critical social work approach might understand and respond to this family's situation differently.

Given that critical theory seeks to understand the impact of social structures on people's experiences, a critical practitioner views poverty as a failure of our society to adequately support its most vulnerable citizens, not the fault of the people who are socially disadvantaged. Critical practitioners understand that economic conditions and social policies determine people's life chances, create inequalities, and directly affect employment opportunities and affordable housing options. Social justice is the overall goal of a critical perspective. Resources such as food and housing are regarded as basic human rights that the state has a responsibility to provide. Hence, the role of human services organisations is to facilitate access to resources to people who need them, and the practitioner would aim to foster this process.

If we think about the impact of establishment practice on this family, and the worker's abuse of her power to protect the system and scapegoat the victims, it can make us feel quite disparaging towards the practitioner. However, what we also need to remember is that her practice has occurred within a particular (conservative) organisational culture, in a practice context dominated by neoliberal and managerial practices that support and foster establishment practice. All of us are capable of falling into similar practice responses if we do not regularly and critically reflect on our practice.

Significantly, one of the most powerful themes to emerge from this practitioner's narrative, once she reflected on it, was her own sense of powerlessness. This sense of powerlessness was one of the key determinants in leading this practitioner to practise establishment social work. As she explains:

Looking back I knew it was wrong; the way that I went about it. But, how do you cope and how do you do critical practice when you're in a corner and you've got management pushing these things onto you? I felt like the boot was being pushed into me from above ...

When I started this job, I had this beautiful relationship with my clients, and then something changed. You get bogged down and it [your practice] becomes about the rules of the organisation rather than the needs of clients, and I have been complicit in that. I can see that now ... I just adopted the confinements of the work practices [as defined by] management. I just gave up all my power and I went fine: I'll do it the way you want it done whether it's right or not. What else can I do? So, I was stuck in a place where I believed what management was saying; took it on as fact ... that I had to do it their way because I didn't have anything else to go by. So I put management on a pedestal and said to myself: 'This has to be right because who else can I trust?' And I dislike the injustice of it. I think that's why I got cranky with him [the client], because I felt I can't do anything to help this person and I was frustrated, so I took it out on him, and saw him as the problem because I didn't want to look at the injustices in the organisation or my role within that.

These feelings of frustration, fatalism and powerlessness are experienced by many critical practitioners, who at times feel challenged and overwhelmed by the system (Ferguson 2008; Fook 2004; Morley 2014). At the same time, such feelings represent a direct threat to ethical practice as understood by critical social work because they can

> **Recapitulation** is to believe that critical social workers' personal and professional lives would be easier if they just accepted the way things are as 'natural' or 'inevitable' and became mainstream or establishment social workers, letting go of their social change objectives (Mullaly 2010).

lead us to **recapitulate**. However, our research shows that critical reflection can be an important tool in assisting practitioners to resist unethical practices and reclaim their power to pursue emancipatory goals (Morley, unpub).

To use the same example again, once the practitioner in the case study realised that her practice had become captured by her management's agenda rather than her own ethical commitments, it created the 'conceptual space' (Rossiter 2005) to free her to think differently about the clients' situation and her role in assisting them. As the practitioner commented:

> *I have to unlearn that stuff [managerial practices and economic rationalist discourses] and throw it in the garbage bin. Their [management's] perspective is right if you're about defending the system, but if you're about acknowledging there are injustices in the system, then there are definitely other ways to see the situation and ways my practice could have been different.*

Using a *structural analysis* assisted the practitioner to put the family's situation into a social context, thus removing blame from the family, and enabling her to view them as worthy recipients rather than undeserving burdens. The internal question for her practice became: how can I best assist this family in meeting their needs? This was instead of: how do I manage these people? Approaching them with this understanding would have changed the sorts of questions she was asking them, and changed the nature of the interaction. As she explains:

> *You have very different sorts of conversations with clients when you start examining yourself and thinking about power and humility and all those sorts of things. And you can change the interaction that you have with people: changing the way you respond to people changes the ways that they interact with you ... Maybe they would have come back if I had just listened to them instead of trying to lecture them about what I thought they should be doing.*

Another key consideration raised by the practitioner was her concern to be able to do more critical work and maintain ethical practices, while also developing a 'space to survive in that system because I still need to keep my job'. Critical reflection enabled the practitioner to recognise that she could meet the goals of management while still preserving her social justice commitments. As she explained:

> Ultimately management too will say they want to support the client and they might not have the best understanding about how to do [it] but that's where my discretion as a professional practitioner becomes important. And so, by supporting the client, you are actually meeting the needs of management. So, the two groups don't need to be seen in opposition or competition. It's probably a bit limiting to see them in that way because it left me feeling powerless. And if I choose to see it as 'I'm doing the best I can for the organisation and management by doing the best I can for my client', then I've actually resolved the ethical dilemma of having to choose between the two options. I've actually found a mutually beneficial outcome for everyone that sits comfortably with my ethics.

This is just one practice example, but the findings from this study suggest that practitioners could use critical reflection as a way of developing a much broader understanding of ethics that more closely aligns with the values of critical social work (Morley, unpub). As Ife (2012, pp. 181–2) explains, thinking about human rights issues 'can provide a more robust framing of "practising ethically"' ... rather than a reliance on an 'externally codified morality in the form of ethics' that seem to have little relevance, given the complexity of contemporary social work practice.

Analysis of this case study indicates that critical reflection provided the practitioner with opportunities to unsettle her practice in ways that allowed her to identify how her thinking had been influenced by dominant (economic, social and political) discourses about the 'undeserving poor' that were working to disempower the family. A critical analysis of social problems was essential for ethical practice because it involved questioning the usefulness of received ideas that blame individuals for social problems that society perpetrates against them. Instead the practitioner developed *empathic solidarity*, which takes account of the social structures that create individual hardship and social disadvantage (Banks 2012, pp. 93–4). The practitioner was thus able to examine the problems associated with taking on these dominant discourses for ethical social work practice and create a discretionary space to rethink a more socially just response to the family. This process also enabled her to question the ethics of practices that created unequal power relations between herself and the family, and instead develop alternatives that worked towards resourcing and empowering the family; for example, challenging rather than upholding agency policies that were oppressive and punitive towards services users. This has been

Relational autonomy is an ethical view of human agency that seeks an optimal balance between individual freedom and the fact that people are always underpinned and shaped by their social relations and context (Mackenzie & Stoljar 2000).

referred to as **relational autonomy**, which involves social workers working with others to exercise power as 'moral agents' of progressive social change (Banks 2012, 93–4).

Finally, the practitioner recognised that she did not have to make a choice between the requirements of the organisation *or* the needs of the client, if she developed a way to think about the situation where these two objectives were not in competition with each other. For example, the purpose of the service in which she works is to assist clients with welfare support, including the provision of food parcels, so providing assistance to this family is actually meeting the objectives of the service. This closely aligns with what Banks (2012, pp. 93–4) refers to as '*situated* ethics of social justice for social work' (emphasis added), which involves working to exploit the gaps and contradictions within dominant discourses. One is 'alert to the dominance of managerialist and neoliberal agendas ... working in the spaces between the contradictions of care and control, prevention and enforcement, empathy and equity' (Banks 2012, pp. 93–4) in order to facilitate socially just outcomes for service users, despite practice contexts that might be hostile to critical emancipatory aims. As we have discussed in previous chapters, being a critical practitioner is not the easiest social work path to choose. As this practitioner commented, 'It's challenging, humbling, liberating, terrifying and exciting all at the same time', but it is definitely worth the struggle with ourselves to develop ethical practice responses.

■ Summary

Ethics, like many other important concepts in social work, is a contested domain. Ethical principles are a central concern for critical social work as an openly value-driven approach to practice. From a critical perspective, a key dimension of ethical social work practice depends on our ability to be open to others and our willingness to engage in critical self-reflection on personally held values and assumptions, rather than our ability to follow codes of ethics and ethical decision-making models as rule books, or to define others by limited sets of theoretical concepts. This requires our capacity to generate more questions, rather than develop answers, and to scrutinise the language we use, and our representations of 'facts', all of which invoke power relations.

In this chapter we have explored the use of codes of ethics and various ethical decision-making models as well as their limitations to guide ethical practice. We examined some of the problems from a critical perspective with objective ways of knowing, particularly in relation to how objectivity may be used to mask dominant ways of knowing. Emphasising the importance of context, we have contrasted establishment social work approaches with critically reflective understandings of knowledge, values and ethics through examining a case study from our research. This case study demonstrates how one practitioner used critical reflection to change her thinking and practice in ways that would create more emancipatory and socially just outcomes for service users. This is the cornerstone of ethical practice from a critical perspective.

■ Review questions

- What issues or dilemmas has the practitioner's account of her practice in the case study above raised for you?
- What questions still remain for you about ethical practice?
- How do you plan to explore these issues?

■ Further reading

Banks, S., 2012, *Practical Social Work – Ethics and Values in Social* Work, 4th edn, Palgrave Macmillan, Basingstoke.

Holscher, D. and Sewpaul, V., 2006, 'Ethics as a site of resistance: The tension between social control and critical reflection', *Research Report*, 1: 251–72.

Hugman, R., 2013, 'Pluralism and ethics is social work and human services' in *Culture, Values and Ethics in Social Work: Embracing Diversity*, Routledge, Oxford.

Rossiter, A., 2011, 'Unsettled social work: The challenge of Levinas's ethic', *British Journal of Social Work*, 41(5): 980–95.

6

||||||||||||||||||||||||||||||||||||

Theories for practice

■ Introduction

THIS CHAPTER WILL introduce you to some of the key formal social work theories that underpin practice. We begin with the *individualistic* and *systems-based theories*. As was evident in Chapter 4 on the history of social work, these establishment theories grew out of liberal philosophy and generally dominated social work, despite notable exceptions, before the emergence of critical social theories. We then shift our attention to the development of *critical theories*, such as Marxist, radical, structural, feminist and anti-oppressive perspectives, and discuss the more recent contribution of poststructural theories to the evolution of critical theories and to critical social work. The newer critical theories developed out of critiques of the older, establishment theories and so it is necessary to have a familiarity with the principles of both. Finally, we draw on research with our first-year students to demonstrate the application of theory in relation to a case study. We will contrast the *conservative* and *objectivist* approaches of establishment social work against the critical approaches so that you can begin to develop an appreciation of the differences between them and their implications for practice.

Consistent with the rest of the material presented in this book, we take an approach that invites you to critically reflect on your own values and positioning in relation to the theories. As we explore the different perspectives, we ask you to consider whether your values and preferences orientate you to be a practitioner who wishes to maintain the status quo, or a practitioner who aspires to be an agent of progressive social change. Of course, this is not a neutral presentation of theory; like everything else, theory is inherently contested and political, and it is our intention to make this transparent. We are also aware that in asking you to choose whether you are conservative or progressive in your orientation towards social work, your options are presented as if there are only two opposing choices. This reflects the sort of **binary thinking**

> **Binary thinking** (or dichotomous thinking) sees the world in terms of two mutually exclusive, often opposing categories (Fook 2012). For example, black or white, establishment or critical, male or female, able-bodied or disabled.

typical of modernist thought, which *poststructuralism* tells us is oversimplified and limited (see, for example, Fook 2012). While thinking about conservative (establishment) *or* progressive (critical) approaches may be an appropriate place to begin consideration of the differences between these theories, poststructural ideas (as you will see in this chapter) remind us that our options are more diverse than this, and that we may be influenced by both conservative and progressive theories at different times and within different contexts.

■ What is theory?

Theory is a term that often causes great anxiety and puzzlement for many students. This is because there are some popular but misleading stereotypes about theory, either because it is seen as an unproven idea, or because being *theoretical* is seen as the opposite of being *practical* (another binary construct). Both these ideas cast doubt on the usefulness of theory. However, like many popular ideas, these views are mistaken and we will demonstrate here that theory is an essential part of ethical practice for critical social workers (see, for example, Healy 2005).

> A **theory** is a 'way of looking' that helps us understand or make sense of some aspect of the world.

The word **theory** comes from the Ancient Greek word *theoria* (θεωρία), which means 'to look', and came to be associated with reflection upon what we observe and do (Phillips 2000, p. 38).

A theory interprets the things we (and others) experience that would otherwise not make sense as isolated events or observations (see, for example, Joas & Knobl 2009). For example, a young woman arrested for drug use or a man begging on the street may well be facts of contemporary urban life, but simply describing what occurs without asking how or why these things are happening is going to leave us with limited understanding and options for social work practice. A theory takes us beyond describing the immediate experience or observations and places these in a wider context of understanding.

As in the humanities and natural sciences, a theory in social work is a set of ideas (concepts) that offer a clear and ordered interpretation of what something means or how it works. In social work, much of the theory we use is shared with other social sciences (such as sociology, anthropology, politics and human geography) in dealing with social and personal life. Generally speaking, many establishment social workers tend to employ a lot more *psychological theory* that is focused on individual behaviour, rather than looking at the social sources and context of such behaviours. Critical social workers, by contrast, will look more acutely at social barriers and inequalities and so emphasise **social theory** to guide their practice (Healy 2005. p. 172). One of the first things you might

> **Social theory** examines the social sources and contexts (including social barriers and inequalities) of people's behaviours and the social changes impacting on these more broadly (Joas & Knobl 2009).

notice about the theories in social work is that there are many of them and this can be quite daunting at first.

REFLECTIVE EXERCISE 6.1
- What reactions do you have to the word 'theory'? Does it excite you? Terrify you? Bore you? Or do you have some other reaction?
- How might the assumptions that you hold about theory influence the way you read material or shape the ways that you think about practice?

Social work is not a discipline that has ever had just one dominant theory about which all of its practitioners share a high degree of consensus, as appears to be the case in the natural sciences (for example, the theory of relativity in physics or the theory of evolution in biology). This should not surprise us because social work is concerned with human beings living in society, with all our conflicts, inequalities and complex ways of behaving and constructing our lives. This is arguably more fraught than what physicists have to deal with in measuring atomic particles or what a biologist observes of cells in a micro-scope. To begin with, atoms and cells do not 'talk back' or alter their behaviour in response to what is written about them. However, people can and do respond to those who attempt to study and work with their problems.

As social workers, we belong to a society, which makes us part of what we seek to understand, and this has implications for the way we practise. Society is not simply 'out there' like an object for social workers, but also 'in here', inside our subjective experience and actions, through the processes of socialisation and acquiring language that have made us part of society since birth. This subjective experience of society is always there influencing each one of us through our social positioning (our socioeconomic class, gender, age group, nationality, ethnicity, values, customs, attitudes and language). So, we can never stand totally apart from and view these things as objects (that is, show objectivity) in quite the same way that you can view physical phenomenon without significant consequences for practice. In short, our location in society and **subjectivity** are always going to affect our view of the world and this includes our theorising. This is the main reason there are so many different theoretical approaches to understanding the human world as seen by social workers.

Not all social workers or their employers value the different theoretical perspectives in social work. Establishment social work, for

Subjectivity is the personal experience, judgements, feelings and perceptions of the world shaped by culture and language but specific to an individual person (subject). In Western thought, subjectivity is contrasted with 'objectivity', which is said to be knowledge of things (objects) independent from any individual's perception and therefore more reliable.

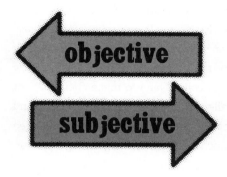

Figure 6.1

example, is impressed by the natural scientists' detached *objectivism*, their capacity for *certainty* and, consequently the *control* this yields over the natural world. They imagine that if the social worker had a theory of society like the laws of physics then they could fix all manner of social problems, from child abuse to world poverty. However, in the human world, such certainty remains elusive and control is an ethically and politically contentious goal at odds with critical social work's commitment to justice and freedom. Many of history's greatest dictators devised theories for controlling their populations rather than enabling people to determine their own lives.

> Hitler had a racist theory of Aryan superiority over all others and used this to commit genocide (mass extermination of entire human populations) (Bauman 1989).

This sort of objectivist theorising (viewing others as objects to be assessed, treated and managed) is how social workers from the 1930s to the 1970s became involved in programs such as the forced removal of Indigenous Australian children from their families, damaging thousands of people's lives because the dominant, racial assimilationist theories of the day assumed it would be better for the children to live in a white society (Van Krieken 1999).

Critical social work theorising recognises that society is both an objective and subjective reality. On the one hand, society has enduring social patterns, power divisions and institutions called 'social structures' that shape us, limiting or providing opportunities in relation to one's class, gender, ethnicity or racialised identity, and so on (see, for example, Fook 2012). We can map these structures and to some extent measure their effects in terms of income, wealth, education, employment, health status, and so on. On the other hand, people's experiences of, and within, these structures are quite different (such as the difference between a privileged upper class, white man's experience in comparison with that of an impoverished Aboriginal girl in a remote community), which gives rise to different world views or discourses that can likewise be enabling or constraining. These discourses cannot be measured with any precision but they can be interpreted by looking carefully at the language people use in explaining their particular situation. People draw upon various discourses (both as individuals and collectively) to make choices about their lives and can act to either affirm or challenge prevailing social structures and discourses. There is considerable debate about how much our actions are conditioned by social structures and discourses, and how much agency individuals and groups can exercise in consciously constructing society. Generally, critical social workers employ theories that enable an understanding of both social structures and discourses in people's experience, and their capacity to exercise agency in *reconstructing* these for a better future (see, for example, Allan, Pease & Briskman 2009; Fook 2012).

As members of society, the diversity of social divisions and discourses influences the way we theorise society and social problems, producing a variety of perspectives. For the critical social worker, this means there is no single, 'neutral' and objective God's-eye view of society (from 'the outside') that explains it all. Rather, critical social work values theoretical diversity for furthering our understanding of people's lives (Allan, Pease & Briskman 2009). However, mixing theories – a practice known as **eclecticism** – has to be done in a critical and reflective manner.

> **Eclecticism** refers to mixing theories uncritically, even if the assumptions underpinning the theories contradict each other (Plionis 2004).

This is because not all theories are equally valid (a position associated with *relativism*) or appropriate for analysing a situation. As a critical practitioner, you will need to select theories that best explain a given situation and provide insight into how practice might bring about just and autonomy-enhancing outcomes. In this respect, one theory is not as good as another. As we shall see, some theories – for example, Marxism and functionalist systems theory – contain contradictory assumptions about the basic nature of society (conflict versus consensus), which cannot be ignored without consequence.

Becoming a critical practitioner means carefully considering your theoretical framework in any given situation. In some situations, some theories may be totally inappropriate or counterproductive. It all depends on what one wishes to know and what values are informing one's understanding. In some respects, choosing an appropriate theory to understand a social situation is a bit like choosing which lens to use on a camera. In daylight, close up, an ordinary lens will do. At a distance you need a telescopic lens and at night, an infrared lens, and so on. Using the wrong theory for the wrong problem will distort rather than illuminate your vision. As you become more familiar with the different theories available, you will become more discerning as to what is the most useful theory. This is where *critical reflection* becomes important. Part of being critical practitioners means that we recognise our own personal values and preferences in selecting particular theories and constantly ask what the theory has to offer to an understanding that promotes social justice and human freedom.

■ Why is theory important for practice?

Over the years, our students have often asked us why we place such an emphasis on theory in the practice classes that we teach. There is often a sense that practice is something that workers 'do' out in the field, and by contrast, theory is something we have to learn about in the classroom that does not seem to hold much relevance for practice. Indeed, we have heard these views expressed and reinforced by field educators, while research too has shown that experienced practitioners, who are identified as experts with more than five years of experience in their particular field, cannot necessarily articulate the theoretical frameworks that inform their practice (Fook, Ryan & Hawkins 2000). This is what Garrett (2013, p. 3) calls the 'fallacy of "theoryless practice"'. He points out, however, that those who claim they have no theory or just use 'common sense' are simply subject to the implicit assumptions of an unacknowledged theory, usually one embedded in the dominant discourses of society, such as neoliberalism or biomedicine. Such implicit theories tend to reinforce the existing order and are, according to Wardhaugh and Wilding (1993, cited in Garrett 2013. p. 3), often complicit in the 'acceptance of abusive practices'.

The inescapable fact is that all practice is underpinned by theory, whether we acknowledge and are aware of it or not.

> Are we looking at a family pathology, a Freudian spider's web, a legacy of patriarchy? Theory decides whether you believe a runaway girl's story ... It shapes what you tell the tearful mother ... It determines the policy you design for the offender ... It decides whether or not you intervene at all ... (Nelson 1987, p. 97, cited in Saraga 1993, p. 75).

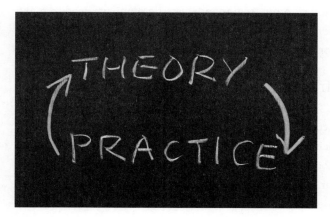

Figure 6.2

Social work is an inherently moral, political, theoretical and intellectual activity that also involves a practical dimension. Theory enables us to go beyond simply knowing how to do the practice to understanding why we would choose to do the practice in a particular way in preference to other ways, and what the social and political implications are of our practices compared with other practices. As outlined below, there are a number of important reasons why we need to be cognisant of and articulate about our use of theory in practice.

(1) Theory is embedded in our actions

Whether we like it or not, our use of theory, through our values, interpretations and assumptions, is embedded within our practice. We can never do practice without theory so we may as well be conscious and intentional about the theories we are using to inform our actions in practice (see, for example, Schon 1987; Thompson 2010).

(2) Theory is part of our professional accountability as practitioners

Knowing theoretical concepts is an essential part of practice. We need to be able to articulate our theoretical framework because we are often asked to account for the decisions we make. As practitioners, we may find ourselves in situations where we need to make an argument to funding bodies or managers about why we should offer a particular service in a particular way. We might find ourselves needing to articulate to a magistrate why we chose to remove a child from their family, or why we worked towards reunifying the family. We may find ourselves needing to justify our practice to our supervisors and external legal bodies in coronial inquests if one of our service users commits suicide, or dies in other circumstances. In short, as social workers we are accountable to society, the organisation in which we work, the people we work with, our own ethical standards and external legal mandates. Therefore, we need to make sure we have a strong theoretical base that provides a sound justification for the decisions we make and actions we take in practice (Swain & Rice 2009).

(3) Our theoretical framework differentiates us from other professions

In the current employment context, we need to be able to indicate what differentiates our unique approach to practice from other related professional groups. Some organisations no longer employ social workers as such, but rather use generic terminology such as case manager or counsellor for staff performing this role. The role is defined by the tasks that the practitioner carries out, instead of the professional background or qualifications held by the person in that role (Healy & Lonne 2010). Certainly, social workers can apply for and perform these roles, but we may find ourselves competing with other professionals, such as speech therapists, physiotherapists, nurses, occupational therapists and psychologists. This is a function of neoliberal practices, in which the values and disciplinary expertise of professionals are reduced to a generic body of technical skills (Holscher & Sewpaul 2006; Madhu 2011). Within this context it is of vital importance that critical social work–related professionals are acutely aware of having a theoretical framework that differentiates us from uncritical practitioners and managerial discourse, and that we are able to clearly articulate this (Payne 2006).

While we believe that critical approaches should be the distinguishing feature of the social work profession, not all forms of social work, or indeed social work theories, are critical. The table below chronicles the evolution of social work theories. Each of us will have our own theoretical preferences. We will naturally choose some theories over others, depending on our own value base, life experience and worldview. This is perfectly understandable, and although we are favouring a critical approach in this text because of our value base, it does not have to be yours. By now you will be aware that social work is a contested profession. There are many competing ideas about the best approach to practice and these ideas change over time. As a minimum, social workers need to engage critically with theories, be able to identify their strengths and weaknesses, and develop an awareness of the issues that they draw our attention to and those that they minimise or ignore.

Historical development of key theories in social work

Date	Theory
1890–1920	Liberal and some socialistic philosophies
1920s	Psychodynamic
1930s	Psychosocial
1960s	Systems and ecological models
1970s	Marxist/radical/structural (anti-oppressive)
1980s	Feminism (anti-oppressive; gender-sensitive)
1990s	Postmodern (social constructionist theories; narrative therapy)
2000	Critical (incorporating radical/structural, feminist and anti-oppressive ideas with postmodern critique.[1]

[1] This is a loose guide of when particular theories became prominent in social work. As with any list there are exceptions and omissions. Marxism, for example, was significant among the Rank and File social workers in the United States in the 1930s and was revived more broadly in the 1970s. Systems theory also dates back to the 1930s but only became prominent in the 1960s.

The remainder of this chapter will explore the application of several theories to practice, namely *psychodynamic* and *cognitive behavioural theories* as examples of individualistic theories; *systems theory* as an example of a conservative social theory; and a number of *critical social work theories*, including Marxism, radical and structural theories, feminism, anti-oppressive approaches and some elements of poststructural thinking. Our purpose here is to expose you to a range of theories for practice, and to apply these theories to a case scenario about a man named Giuseppe. Adopting a critical view highlights some serious problems with using individualistic and systems theories in isolation; however, it is important to have an understanding of them as they have been formative in creating intellectual debate and critique, which has led to newer, more critical developments in practice.

CASE STUDY
Giuseppe

Imagine yourself in the role of a case manager within a family services department in a regional shire. As the practitioner, you receive a telephone call from a local resident who tells you she is concerned about the wellbeing of an elderly neighbour: Giuseppe Marchesani. She tells you that Giuseppe has been living alone since his wife died five years ago.

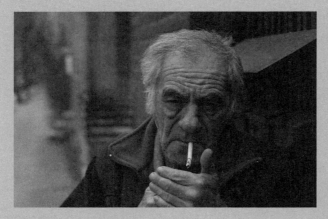

Figure 6.3

Your job requires you to investigate the situation. You and a colleague visit Giuseppe. You introduce yourself to him but discover that he does not speak much English, although he speaks proficient Italian, Spanish and French. Unfortunately, you and your colleague only speak and understand English. Nevertheless, he welcomes you into his home. You are instantly aware that Giuseppe seems to be quite unwell in that he has a very troubling cough. You find that the house is in a state of disrepair and you are shocked by the living conditions. There is old food scattered throughout the house and piles of papers, debris and washing everywhere. The furniture is covered in dog hair, and the dog appears to have urinated in the house in a couple of places. You notice an ashtray with a cigarette burning, even though Giuseppe is smoking another. Your colleague has looked into the bedroom, and she comments that there is an old heater burning brightly in one corner. Giuseppe's television continues to play very loudly and you wonder if he may be hearing-impaired. Giuseppe insists on making you a drink. You notice flies crawling over the cups. On the way to the kitchen Giuseppe trips and stumbles on a mat. You attempt to help him but he seems annoyed by this. He is shaken, although apparently not injured at all. Soon afterwards, he asks you to leave and shows you to the door. It is obvious to you that he now wants to be left alone. As you leave, you see one of the neighbours peering at you from her window across the street.

REFLECTIVE EXERCISE 6.2
- What are the three main issues you would prioritise in responding to Giuseppe?
- Why have you chosen to prioritise these particular issues?
- What do your priorities/choices indicate about your values and assumptions? Can you identify whether they indicate individualistic or social/structural factors, or a combination of both?

Numerous theoretical models exist that attempt to explain how we should respond to social issues impacting Giuseppe, including grief, poverty, social disadvantage, social isolation, illness and risk. The theories themselves will determine how we prioritise these factors, or whether we even choose to regard them as relevant issues to be addressed. The theories that we use are underpinned by various assumptions and values that have major practical implications for social work in terms of the actions we take. We will return to consider Giuseppe's situation later in this chapter.

■ Individualist theories in social work

Individualist social work theories view the object of (or the target for) change as the individual, with the worker's role at a basic level that of 'fixer' (Payne 2005, p. 45; see also Healy 2005; Howe 2009). We will examine two types of individualist

Defence mechanisms are those unconscious strategies that serve to protect the individual from emotions such as pain, anxiety and guilt. Defences arise as a reasonable response to unreasonable circumstances; however, they mask the true nature of the anxiety (Howe 2009).

Denial means negating or refusing to accept as real something that is real (for example, the death of a loved one) (Longres 1995, p. 422).
Repression means bottling up feelings of anxiety or distress (for example, saying things are okay when they're not) (Longres 1995, p. 422).
Regression involves unconsciously returning to a type of thought, feeling or behaviour associated with an earlier stage of development in order to allay fear or anxiety (for example, an older child reverting to thumb sucking when a new sibling is born) (Longres 1995, p. 422).
Projection is the imposition of unwanted feelings about oneself onto another (for example, blaming others for not keeping in contact when you don't keep in contact yourself) (Longres 1995. p. 422).
Sublimation involves converting a socially objectionable thought, feeling or behaviour into a socially acceptable one (for example, yelling at the television during a football game rather than hitting someone) (Longres 1995, p. 422).

theories – psychodynamic and cognitive behavioural – to see how they assist us in understanding Giuseppe's situation and how those understandings might shape our work with him.

Psychodynamic theories

perspectives are based on the work of Sigmund Freud (1856–1939) and his later followers. They stem from the assumption that individual behaviour comes from 'movements and interactions in the mind' (Payne 2005, p. 73). Instinctual needs, drives and feelings are thought to motivate one's behaviour, coming from processes taking place internally in the minds of individuals, often beneath the level of awareness or consciousness (Longres 1995). Early life experiences, from infancy onwards, are thought to be central to personality development; thus the adult personality, 'for better or worse, is a stable playing out of childhood patterns' (Longres 1995, p. 416). Unconscious mental activity is considered a key motivating force in human behaviour, and the task of the worker (or therapist, if we are using psychodynamic language) is to assist the person to uncover and examine childhood experiences and memories, thus gaining insight into how those early experiences are played out in adult life and, in particular, in relationships (Longres 1995). However, the individual may resist bringing unconscious memories to awareness, and may resist other anxiety-producing circumstances through the deployment of **defence mechanisms**.

From a psychodynamic perspective, defence mechanisms are not inherently bad, but they may become overly rigid and prevent us from moving forward. Defence mechanisms often function unconsciously and can manifest in **denial**, **repression**, **regression**, **projection** and **sublimation**. These notions of the unconscious and the relevance of the past to the present have been influential in social work, and have also crept into public and everyday language. You may have used them yourself in informal conversation. Another important element of psychodynamic approaches – that of the centrality of the worker or therapist–client relationship as a vehicle for change in itself – has formed one of the cornerstones of traditional and contemporary social work practice (Healy 2005).

REFLECTIVE EXERCISE 6.3

- How might some of these psychodynamic ideas be relevant to understanding Giuseppe?
- Now, think more deeply and critically about the concepts of denial and repression: how might these be shaped by dominant discourses, such as patriarchy, which tells men they must be strong and stoic and must not acknowledge 'weakness'?

Freud (1953) also developed a set of ideas about different stages of development of the child; others who followed him in this stage-based approach to personality development extended his stages beyond that of childhood through the entire life cycle. One important theorist who did this was Erik Erikson (1902–94). Erikson (1959) argued that throughout one's life, one passed through a series of stages, each with their own developmental issues and tasks, which, if not successfully resolved, immobilised the individual and did not allow for full maturation (Crain 2014).

Erikson's stages of life cycle development

Age	General stage	Successful negotiation
Birth to 18 months	Trust vs mistrust	Baby senses their caregiver/s are caring and reliable.
18 months to three	Autonomy vs shame/doubt	Child learns social behaviour but still has sense of self-determination/ own will.
Three to six	Initiative vs guilt	Child learns to check their own behaviour and channel their goals in socially acceptable ways.
Six to 11	Industry vs inferiority	Child learns to do meaningful work; danger is that they may feel inadequate and may not have completed previous stages – for example, they may feel more shame/doubt than autonomy.
Adolescence	Identity vs role confusion	Young person feels urgent need to develop their own identity (healthy self-definition).
Young adulthood	Intimacy vs isolation	Attainment of intimacy, possible only after one establishes sense of identity.
Adulthood	Generativity vs stagnation	Production of something meaningful through work or child rearing
Old age	Ego integrity vs despair and feelings of failure	Life review about worthiness of one's life; wisdom/acceptance.

REFLECTIVE EXERCISE 6.4

The table above shows what form successful negotiation of the life-cycle stage takes from a psychodynamic perspective. Can you imagine what unsuccessful negotiation might look like and how it might carry on into later life-cycle stages?

Others have extended the individual life-cycle theory to a family life cycle, suggesting that the individual is generally formed and continues to develop within a family or family-like context, and as families move through time, stress will be experienced by individuals at key transition points from one stage to another 'as families rebalance, redefine, and realign their relationships' more or less successfully (Carter & McGoldrick 2005, p. 7). Similarly to Erikson's theory, if emotional issues and developmental tasks are not successfully resolved at appropriate stages, the assumption is that they will be carried forward and hinder future transitions and relationships. The stages of the family life cycle include young adults leaving home, the joining of families through marriage or creation of new couples, couples transitioning to families with young children and then adolescents, raising children and moving on, and finally families in later life accepting shifting generational roles. The latter, which is potentially relevant to Giuseppe, includes maintaining relationships and wellbeing in the face of physiological decline, others in the family making room in the system for the wisdom and experience of the elderly, and dealing with loss of a spouse, siblings and other peers, as well as preparation for death (Carter & McGoldrick 2005, p. 2).

REFLECTIVE EXERCISE 6.5

- What relevance might the life-cycle theories hold for Giuseppe?
- How would you know or find out if these ideas were relevant to his experience?
- How would psychodynamic theories lead you to emphasise particular aspects of Giuseppe's experience as important?
- What are some of the factors or issues that psychodynamic theories might miss?

Psychodynamic theories give us a number of lenses through which to view Giuseppe and his circumstances. We might first wonder about Giuseppe's past; seeing him not just as an old man, but someone whose identity was significantly formed in childhood and through the resolution (or lack thereof) of developmental stages. We may also be wondering if part of his reluctance to engage with us may have to do with defence mechanisms that alert him to the dangers of the power we could wield to change his living situation. These defence mechanisms are understandable and we would need to be transparent about the power we have to influence his future.

Life-cycle theory, such as that of Erikson, would suggest that the developmental task Giuseppe is currently facing is that of integrity versus despair. While we might assume, from external observations about the material conditions of his life, that he is in decline, we do not know this is how Giuseppe views his life. Further, if we look at family life-cycle theory, we would be wondering how Giuseppe has negotiated the death of his partner and perhaps other peers or siblings, and how he is placed within the context of his wider family, in terms of being valued, respected and included to the extent that he wishes to be. The development of an honest, genuine and supportive worker–client relationship would be crucial to hearing more of Giuseppe's narrative.

Cognitive behavioural theories

Cognitive behavioural theories are another category of *individualist* approaches to social work practice, aimed at changing the behaviour of people by changing their thinking (see, for example, Payne 2005). Therefore, they are used to identify problem behaviours, such as those that inhibit social interaction, appear to place the individual at risk, are deemed socially unacceptable by others, or are identified by individuals themselves as problematic. Strategies are then developed that will lead to the 'extinction of unhelpful behaviour patterns' (Payne 2005, p. 120). Problems are reduced to their component parts in order to be systematically addressed. Useful behaviours are introduced, and are practised and reinforced by the worker and perhaps others in the individual's social network through a series of small steps leading to greater change. Bandura (1977, cited in Payne 2005, p. 121) suggested that most learning is gained by people's perceptions and thinking about what they experience, including the example of others around them. The assumption is that since problem behaviour has been learned, it can also be unlearned and substituted with more acceptable or desirable behaviour.

REFLECTIVE EXERCISE 6.6
- Are there behaviours that Giuseppe might be exhibiting that are cause for concern?
- For whom are they concerning?
- How else might cognitive behavioural theories shape your understanding of Giuseppe's situation?

One of our first reactions to Giuseppe's situation from a cognitive behavioural perspective may have been to identify a range of problematic behaviours that need to change. We may find ourselves caught in an ethical dilemma in terms of the person's right to *self-determination* versus our *duty of care* to protect others from harm. This leads us to the question of who should define what problem behaviour is. What does Giuseppe himself see as problems in his current life situation? As the worker, you may have identified a range of problem behaviours, from smoking and leaving cigarettes burning, to leaving the heater on, to food spoilage. His stumbling on the mat and the high volume of the television may have led you to wonder about his physical wellbeing and competence. You, as the worker, could identify all these behaviours as problematic, and devise an appropriate intervention encompassing the continuum of teaching him better living skills through to recommending he lives in supported accommodation.

REFLECTIVE EXERCISE 6.7
- What do you consider to be the strengths and limitations of the individualist theories?
- How might a critical perspective view these theories?
- What power dynamics are present in adopting and drawing upon these theories, in terms of the worker and the client?

■ Systems theory

Systems theory refers to a diverse range of theoretical approaches with a long history in social work. These perspectives are centred on the idea of a 'system', which refers to a specific set of interrelated parts that make up a larger whole (see, for example, Healy 2005). Examples of this would be the parts of a car or the organs constituting a living body and how these parts or organs function together to make the system work. This idea was explicitly developed in the 1920s by the biologist Ludwig von Bertalanffy (1968), who sought to apply 'general systems theory' to the scientific analysis of all physical, mechanical, biological and social phenomena. He saw systems as a more adequate way of understanding the complexity of the universe than simple models of cause and effect or stimulus–response mechanisms.

Functionalist theory is associated with Emile Durkheim (1858–1917), who sought to understand modern societies and the functions of institutions, and people's 'roles' within them, in terms of the metaphor of a living organism.

The idea of understanding human situations and problems as the products of 'social systems' and not simply individual behaviour has had a major impact in the social sciences. The system concept is so general that it can be applied to almost any type of social phenomenon, from small, *micro-social systems* (individuals, families, friends) to middle-range, *meso systems* (school, organisations, local institutions) and *macro-system* issues of globalisation, class inequalities and state institutions (Bronfenbrenner 1979; Healy 2005, pp. 140–1). The latter have been analysed in sociology under the banner of **functionalist theory**.

Just as the human body has to have its parts working in harmony with each part performing its proper function, so society needs to reg-

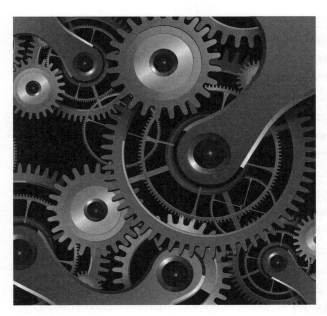

Figure 6.4

ulate the functioning of its parts, (e.g. the family, schooling, law enforcement, media, religion, social hierarchy), thus maintaining their equilibrium. If it does not do this then the implication is that society, like an organism, will become dysfunctional or fail. The pioneer of sociological systems theory, Talcott Parsons (1902–78), held that the 'proper functioning' of society and its parts (including its inequalities) is secured by an underlying consensus over social rules (norms) and values shared by the majority of its members. This is very debatable because Parsons' emphasis on normative consensus understates the role of power, force and conflict in maintaining the social order and its inequalities. By assuming that disparities of wealth and power are inevitable or normal features of society rather than injustices to be challenged or overcome, functionalist theory is politically conservative (Mills 1959, pp. 33–6). While Parsons' elaborate macro-theory was never popular with social workers, many of its key assumptions and abstract terms (such as role, function, equilibrium and feedback) influenced much social analysis and policy work up until the 1970s and beyond (see, for example, Seidman 2013).

Systems thinking was imported from sociology into social work at the micro- and meso-levels of practice in the 1930s and became very prominent from the late 1960s onwards (Healy 2005). Originally, it was employed to bolster the scientific credibility of social work and distinguish it from other human services professions. It also counter-acted the excessive psychological focus on individual problems that had dominated social work in the 1940s and 1950s. Systems theory was usually employed to understand people and their interconnectedness within their social context (a 'people in environment' perspective). This enabled social workers to encourage people to understand their issues not in terms of personality problems but as the result of social systems they were part of and how these interacted in complex ways. This had a particularly strong impact on working with families, where roles within 'family systems' and the relation of families to other systems became central to analysis. This was facilitated by the use of visual tools, such as eco-maps and genograms, to model relationships. More recently, the systems concept has been broadened in an ecological direction, encompassing interactions with both human and non-human environments (Healy 2005).

The advantage of ecological and systems approaches is that they enable practitioners and service users to understand the problems confronting them in a social context. This avoids the uncritical tendency to blame and pathologise service users for their problems, which is common in individualist approaches. However, systems theory alone is a very objectifying way of understanding human beings and their problems. Its clinical, abstract and 'neutral' sounding language positions the user of this framework as an external observer or expert, with the power to classify, judge and intervene in the service users' situation. While it is a social theory, systems approaches have mainly been conservative in social work because they typically suggest that the service users must fit in (integrate) with a dominant system, such as capitalism, rather than becoming agents for changing the system (Mullaly 2007, p. 49). In this way, systems theory can be paternalistic or managerial rather than empowering or promoting justice. However, there are some critical practitioners who argue that if systems theory is linked to other forms of analysis, which can appreciate the service user's reality and recognise destructive power relations, then a more complex, critical systems approach may be useful (Healy 2012).

PRACTITIONER'S PERSPECTIVE

Genograms and ecomaps in child protection practice

A critical approach to child protection practice promotes the use of the genogram and ecomap as tools to engage families as an alternative to analysing their situation through an individual lens. This practice rather champions the family as the expert in their own history and experiences. To work as intended, the practitioner's own framework must value that a child is best supported within their own family and the practice must focus on building the capacity of the family system. Importantly, when we focus on family it also includes extended family so if the child has experienced significant harm and cannot remain with their immediate family members, we look to the extended family but can still include the child's own family in the planning of this.

Genograms and ecomaps are tools that enable practitioners to engage with clients about their families of origin and their support systems. Genograms have had a strong foothold in family therapy, so whilst they won't identify primary power divisions that impact on the family, such as the role of patriarchy, class inequality and so on, they can identify what some have referred to as secondary institutional structures [Carniol 1992, p. 5; Moreau 1979] to define and analyse a client's intergenerational patterns and experiences. Similarly, ecomaps have derived from an ecological perspective as a way of analysing the relationship between clients and their environment. These tools are being used within contemporary child protection practice to build the capacity of frontline staff to understand social context and social connection. An isolated family will place a child at much higher risk of harm if their parents are unable to navigate assistance and support. Enabling families to develop and link with appropriate support builds capacity and self-efficacy, with the aim of reducing the need for statutory intervention. Exploring the possibility of broadening the immediate family's needs and concerns with extended family and other supportive relationships increases the protective factors for children. Gathering this information with the family through an anti-oppressive lens provides a deeper understanding of the family's narrative and develops intervention 'by design', driven by the family. *(Joanne Roff, Manager, Queensland Department of Communities, Child Safety and Disability Services)*

■ Giuseppe: what do students think?

We conducted research that surveyed more than 600 first-year students in a critical social work program about the issues that they felt were most pressing for Giuseppe. The first questionnaire asked students to respond to the same questions you considered in the first reflective exercise about Giuseppe in Chapter 6, and was completed by them at the beginning of their first semester at university (Stage 1). The same questionnaire was then repeated at the end of the semester with the same students (Stage 2), and again, with final-year students who had just completed their second field education placement (Stage 3). The following commentary reports on this research. The Stage 1 findings revealed that when students commence their studies in social work and human services, overwhelmingly their views, values and assumptions reflect those found in conservative theories that inform establishment approaches to social work. These include individualistic, psychologically orientated theories and conservative social theories, such as systems and ecological approaches (Morley & Ablett, unpub1).

This is not surprising given that the assumptions embedded within these establishment theories maintain the existing power relationships and inequalities within society, and consequently are embedded in our media, education system, socialisation processes, and institutions. It also happens that powerful groups in society, who benefit from current social arrangements, actively promote and perpetuate conservative beliefs and thinking within the fabric of our society (Mullaly 2010).

Individualist theories and students' understanding of Giuseppe

During the first stage of the research 87 per cent of students prioritised concerns about Giuseppe's health as their number one practice issue, identifying factors such as 'physical and mental conditions', 'sickness' and 'ill health', 'his cough', 'disabilities/impairments', 'his smoking' and 'his hearing' (Morley & Ablett, unpub1). This reflects an individualistic understanding of Giuseppe's situation, which does not take account of the social context in which he lives. The emphasis on his health uncritically accepts the dominance of the biomedical discourses, which were also evident in how students stated they would work with Giuseppe. Well-intended responses (such as 'organise medical attention', 'get doctor to check up on his health', 'get a doctor to look at him' and 'get a nurse in once a week to check up on him') reflect dominant ideas about risk and surveillance, positioning the practitioners as agents of social control by focusing on narrow **therapeutic interventions**.

> **Therapeutic interventions** involve working with individuals, families or small groups in order to bring about change at a personal or relational level (Chenoweth & McAuliffe 2012, p. 195).

Many students in the first stage of the research responded by indicating what they thought should happen to 'fix' Giuseppe, on the assumption that *he* is the problem. Their responses included: 'assess this elderly man's ability to look after himself'; 'take him to hospital'; and 'find out what is going on in this man's mind and find out why he is living this way' (Morley & Ablett, unpub1). These individualistic responses hide the social, political, economic and cultural factors impacting on Giuseppe's situation, reducing his circumstances to private or personal problems. Change is constructed in terms of Giuseppe coming to terms with either his unconscious feelings, which is the goal of psychodynamic practice, or changing his faulty beliefs, which is the goal of cognitive psychological approaches. Both these individualistic approaches assume that the problems are located entirely in Giuseppe's personality; therefore, he alone becomes the site for the practitioner's intervention, rather than society.

These understandings also reflect an *objectivist* paradigm that assumes a universally correct course of action and a linear problem-solving model in which the service user is seen as the problem that the practitioner 'fixes' or who is provided with solutions for their dysfunction (failure). Also evident was the adoption of a non-consultative, non-collaborative, top-down way of working, which creates unequal power relations between Giuseppe and the practitioner. After all, from an individualistic theoretical perspective, the worker sees themselves as the expert, and the service user as the empty receptacle of the worker's wisdom (Mullaly 2007).

Difficulties in engaging Giuseppe were seen as problematic by students who implicitly blamed him by referring to his 'unwillingness to receive help', 'his lack of openness to assistance' and his 'refusal of help'. Others talked about their need to 'get him to agree to get some help'. They also raised questions about his 'ability to care for self' or 'capability to look after himself', and at the more punitive end of the spectrum noted 'his obvious incapability to live alone' (Morley & Ablett, unpub1). Such responses reflect an individualistic approach in that there is a paternalistic assumption Giuseppe should comply, that he should conform to their expectations, to graciously receive the practitioner's help because he is the problem and it is irresponsible of him not to surrender himself to the practitioner's intervention.

Only a small number of our students (4.6%) thought Giuseppe's issues of grief in mourning the loss of his wife might be important (Morley & Ablett, unpub1). Grief is a key issue in a range of theories, including individualistic ones, but these understand grief as a psychological (and personal/private) problem that Giuseppe should seek to resolve through participating in counselling or mental health treatment, medicalising the issue. None of the new students mentioned any broader social, cultural or political factors that might have been relevant to Giuseppe's situation.

Systems theory and students' understanding of Giuseppe

The assumptions of systems theory were equally represented in students' initial responses to Giuseppe (Morley & Ablett, unpub1). After health, Giuseppe's 'safety' and his 'unsafe living conditions/environment' were the most cited responses (53%). Some students also made reference to conditions that they thought provoked certain risks, such as 'heater burning' and 'fire hazards' (Morley & Ablett, unpub1). Risk, from a systems perspective, is something to be identified and eliminated because it represents a potential threat to the equilibrium of the system. Others talked more specifically (and judgementally) about Giuseppe's 'unkept house' or the 'untidiness of [the] house', also questioning the 'state of his environment' and whether the 'house is acceptable for living in' (Morley & Ablett, unpub1). These responses assume a universal consensus on values about order being morally right or normal, resulting in the need to restore a healthy equilibrium (Howe 2009).

Several students stated that Giuseppe's 'living conditions need improvement' and that their goals should be to 'stabilise his physical living situation' and organise 'home help' for Giuseppe. Directly related to this, 11 per cent of students made particular reference to 'hygiene', also referred to as a 'lack of sanitary environment' and 'cleanliness of the household' (Morley & Ablett, unpub1). Consistent with systems theory, such responses seek to make minor changes within Giuseppe's existing environment, but not to address the broader social, political, economic and cultural issues that have shaped the development of the conditions in which he lives. From this perspective, there is no need to challenge any sort of injustice. Systems practitioners aim instead to assist people to adapt to their unjust conditions (Howe 2009; Mullaly 2007; Payne 2005).

Systems approaches were further evident in student quotes such as 'Need to find his friends and family and get them involved'; 'Get ACAT [Aged Care Assessment Team] involved'; 'Get someone to clean his house'; 'Get him back into society'; 'Ask a neighbour to keep an eye on him'; and 'Organise a carer to visit him regularly' (Morley & Ablett, unpub1). The aim of these practices is to help Giuseppe maintain his living situation by connecting with outside social resources in his immediate community, rather than seeking to challenge the social barriers that are creating his disadvantage.

Related to this, a further 15 per cent of students in the first stage of the research identified social isolation as an issue for Giuseppe. This was expressed in terms of his lack of 'social networks', 'community support – Italian community', 'support/social systems', 'family support', 'family/relatives – someone who can help him' and questions posed such as 'does he have family and friends?' Several responses also documented the 'remoteness' of 'living alone' (Morley & Ablett, unpub1). Again, the assumptions embedded in students' responses reflect a systems approach in trying to enhance the interconnectedness between Giuseppe and his social environment. Systems theory has a very limited view of 'society', which is assumed to be a relatively fair and stable order – a set of interrelated parts, such as one finds in an organism or a machine (Howe 2009; Payne 2005).

REFLECTIVE EXERCISE 6.8
Think back to your reading of Chapter 4. Make some notes about how some of the assumptions embedded in these establishment social work approaches may resonate with the Charitable Organisation Societies (COSs).

REFLECTIVE EXERCISE 6.9
- How did your responses to the questions about Giuseppe compare with those of students beginning their social work or human services studies who participated in our research?
- Did your responses reflect largely conservative or progressive theories? Did this surprise you? Why?
- Now, imagine yourself in Giuseppe's situation. Would you like a practitioner to make these kinds of assumptions about you and work with you in this way? Why or why not?

■ Adopting a critical lens: limitations of establishment theories

All of the establishment theories mentioned so far share two significant and related limitations:

1 political conservatism
2 commitment to scientific objectivity as the dominant way of knowing, to the exclusion of other approaches.

From a critical perspective, many establishment theories are conservative because they take *social* problems (for example, suffering as a result of unemployment, poverty, partner violence or domestic drudgery) and construct these as originating in the individual, rather than in unjust social structures. Psychological explanations of social problems, in particular, often result in 'blaming the victim', making the service user responsible for issues that have social, economic, political and cultural origins (Healy 2005). However, not all social theories are necessarily critical or progressive. As we have seen, systems theory may locate the problem in society but still accepts the basic power arrangements of society as just and so will tend towards making the service user adjust to the status quo. As critical practitioners, it is not good practice (or indeed ethical) to leave the current social order unquestioned and simply help it regulate our service users more efficiently. Such an approach positions social workers as agents of social control, and is therefore aligned with supporting the system, rather than the individuals, groups or communities with whom we work.

The second limitation of establishment theories is the way they use scientific objectivity as the most privileged way of knowing. As you will recall from Chapter 4 the scientific revolution gave rise to a new *modernist* way of thinking that seeks to establish secular, rational and universal certainties (truths). This is exemplified in the *positivist* theory of knowledge, which holds that the only reliable knowledge is that which can be expressed in scientific laws that are open to **empirical** testing. This approach to knowledge is very attractive to people who want to control situations because it offers (or so they imagine) a degree of certainty about what exists and the potential to manipulate it. The modernist thinkers of the Enlightenment, however, did not set out to serve conservative purposes. In addition to scientific theories of how the world is, they shared moral visions of how it *ought* to be. They believed that their universal truths would be liberating for all human beings, overcoming all manner of oppression and want. In a world dominated by kings, lords and a single religion, modernist ideas challenged the basis of traditional domination and were associated with the values of human freedom

> **Empiricism** refers to the principle that knowledge must be 'tested by some kind of evidence drawn from experience', preferably under controlled conditions (Abercrombie, Hill & Turner 2006, p.130).

and equality (see, for example, Beilharz & Hogan 2012; Ife 1996). In our view, this critical legacy within modernism, to which we now turn, remains a potentially liberating resource for critical social work.

◼ Critical perspectives

What is critical theory?

To appreciate critical social work, we must have an understanding of where its foundational ideas derive. In Chapter 1 we noted how the notion of 'critique', developed in Western/Enlightenment thought, moved beyond the questioning of ideas to the questioning of societal oppression and how we might overcome it. This practical intent was famously captured in Karl Marx's (1845) statement: 'philosophers have only interpreted the world, the point however, is to change it.' As mentioned in Chapter 4, the term *critical theory* was first coined by a group of unorthodox Marxists in the 1930s known as the Frankfurt School who were attempting to rescue Marx's critique from the distortions of orthodox Marxism in the communist countries and to reassert its primary goal of liberation (Kellner 1989; Bronner 2011). Since then, the term has been applied broadly but retains the core idea of exposing existing forms of oppression in order to bring about *emancipation*. What follows is a very general account of critical theory in contrast to other forms of theory. We then look briefly at how it developed out of the Marxist tradition and how this vital work of critique inspires both structural and poststructural critical social work today (Allan, Pease & Briskman 2009).

At its simplest, critical theory is based on the idea that the way the world *happens to be* (at this moment with all its oppressive divisions) is not the way it is *meant to be*, or *could be* if we acted (individually and collectively) to make it otherwise. This intuition rests on the assumption that society and social problems are largely the result of people's actions. Therefore, if people have made the social world unjust, violent, alienating and a grim struggle for survival, then we can also unmake these to build a more just, peaceful, convivial and caring society. Oppression and social inequality are not inevitable and are neither the will of a God nor laws of nature; they are *social constructions*. Although never easy, socially constructed injustices can be remedied.

Critical thought is often praised in Western philosophy but in practice it is usually marginalised by other ways of thinking. After the Enlightenment, positivist science and objectivist thought predominated in the management of human problems (Agger 2013; Ife 1996). (See Chapter 2 for further information about the way this manifests in contemporary social contexts, such as managerialism, evidence-based practice and neoliberalism.) However, many important human experiences (e.g. those of love, friendship, belonging, autonomy, wellbeing, fairness, dignity) require a broader understanding than managerial thinking. Critical thought can help us here. It suggests visions of what the world *ought* to be like – utopias or imagined futures – framed on the basis of ethical values (Feenberg, Pippin & Webel 1987). These utopias serve as the baseline for critical judgement about *what is*. For example, it is only by anticipating what a *just* society might be like (at least implicitly) that we can criticise the current organisation and distribution of resources as *unjust*. Therefore, critical theory is anti-positivist (Marcuse 1972). Understanding how society currently is and how it works is only the beginning for critical theory. This makes critical theory a profoundly hopeful basis for social work. It questions the existing conditions of each situation in the hopeful expectancy that we might contest it to achieve something much better for people.

While critical social work is as old as the profession itself, the contemporary range of critical perspectives were largely introduced from the 1970s onwards. These critical theories reject establishment approaches geared to regulating the individual behaviour and social functioning of people to fit within an unjust social order. Some of the key modernist critical perspectives in social work include the Marxist, radical, structural, feminist and anti-oppressive theories.

Marxist and radical social work theory

The early radical social workers of the late 1960s (like their predecessors in the 1930s) drew explicitly on the theories of Karl Marx (1818–83) and the various 'Marxisms' of his later followers, which constituted the major alternative to capitalist development in the 20th century. Marx was a German philosopher and revolutionary socialist whose theories contain both the objectivist-scientific and critical-emancipatory impulses of modernism. Marx challenged the exploitative impact of industrial capitalism on members of the working class and worked towards their emancipation. He questioned why the most productive societies in history (capitalist) impoverished the people; the vast majority in fact who produced the wealth. He thus had a conflict model of society and social change. This division remains a massive global problem, even though we produce enough resources (for food, clothing, housing, and so on) to meet everyone's material needs on the planet (Cheal 2005, p. 89). Marx also believed that people did not have to accept unjust social structures but had the capacity to consciously make history by combining critical theory with transformative practices (what he called **praxis**).

> **Praxis** is the term Marx used for humanity's capacity to combine theory and practice for self-reflective agency in history. Revolutionary praxis is the collective capacity to fundamentally transform oppressive social structures to further human emancipation.

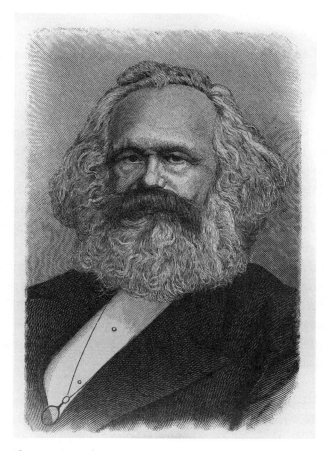

Figure 6.5 Karl Marx

Dominant ideology is a term used by Marxists to describe the ideology of the ruling / capitalist class, which misrepresents its interests as if these were in the interests of society as a whole. It is thus a political tool used by the ruling class to reinforce the subordination of workers by masking exploitation and promoting capitalism as natural and beneficial (Van Krieken et al. 2012).

Marx saw that capitalism produces an unequal and exploitative class structure that divides the owners (capitalists) and non-owners (workers) of capital. The capitalist class controlled work and kept workers' wages as low as possible to maximise profit, aided by the threat of unemployment. This class also held political sway over the state and strongly promoted its ideas (ideology), defending its interests as the dominant view of society (**dominant ideology**) through schools, the legal system, religion and the media.

By contrast, the workers' only way out of poverty and alienation according to Marx was to develop a critical class consciousness, organise collectively (in unions, political parties and movements), confront the system and fundamentally *transform* (revolutionise) its structures of ownership and power. Marx called the confrontations between workers and capitalists (or their management) 'class struggle', which he saw intensifying to the point where workers would revolt to abolish class divisions by seizing control of production and replacing capitalism with a socialist or communist society, based on public ownership and participatory democracy (Mostov 1989; Burkett 2005).

Marx's followers are diverse. For example, the unorthodox Marxists of the Frankfurt School coined the term 'critical theory' in the 1930s to renew Marx's project, critiquing oppression in both capitalist and state socialist (communist) regimes. In their view, capitalist social structures are not simply external to us, but also operate from within, *colonising* even the consciousness of the most destitute with dominant ideas justifying their own oppression (see Healy 2005, p. 173).

REFLECTIVE EXERCISE 6.10

What is the dominant ideology surrounding the unemployed?

Consider the Australian Government's Work for the Dole scheme in which people who are unemployed are forced to work in the community sector in order to receive basic entitlements (that are substantially below the minimum wage).

- How might a Marxist perspective be useful for social work practice with the long-term unemployed who are affected by this policy?
- What do you think the policy's impact on wages might be?

REFLECTIVE EXERCISE 6.11

Think of some examples of class struggle that have occurred in recent years (e.g. the London riots, Occupy Wall Street, unions striking).

- What do you notice about how the media portrays class struggle? How might Marx provide an alternative way of thinking about these issues?
- Should social workers be unionised or members of movements for political reform?
- Why might collectivisation be an integral part of critical social work practice?

Another critical Marxist who helps to explain these ideas is Antonio Gramsci (1889–1937), with his concept of *hegemony* that expands Marx's notion of *ideology*.

He shows that the acceptance of ideology is not automatic. The oppressed are not fools. Rather, the ruling class must actively win the consent of large sections of society to its dominance by presenting the system (and its inequalities) as fair, reasonable and inevitable. Hegemony, therefore, 'is the domination of one powerful group over others, such that the consensus of the subordinated groups is not achieved by physical force, but rather by convincing people it is in their interests to agree with and follow the dominant group's ideas' (Germov & Poole 2011, p. 114). Although never uncontested, hegemony is most successful when the majority accept the beliefs of the ruling class as 'common sense'. This results in subordinate groups exhibiting what Gramsci (1971, pp. 326–7) calls **contradictory consciousness**, whereby they know and resent oppression from practical experience but simultaneously express dominant ideas about the reasonableness and fairness of the system producing their oppression. To combat hegemony, according to Gramsci and social workers such as Steve Rogowski (2010, pp. 166–7), one begins by contesting the dominant ideology while organising politically around counterhegemonic values, such as social justice, economic cooperation and direct democracy.

> **Contradictory consciousness** refers to the situation whereby subordinated groups and individuals recognise their oppression from practical experience but simultaneously express dominant ideas about the reasonableness and fairness of the system producing their oppression.

Marxism and radical theory enable social workers to understand the broad structural dynamics of social inequality, poverty and economic crises, not as aberrations but as an integral part of the capitalist context in which they will meet fellow citizens and service users (Garrett 2013). The radical critique alerts us to the material needs of the people we serve and how deprivation, including poverty, is the product of a class-based society and not individual failure (Ferguson 2011). Marxism and radical theory also go some way in explaining the role of the capitalist state (which is still the main funding source and provider of social work employment), when it places the interests of business ahead of welfare, education and health. From this capitalist point of view, the expansion of market principles to every sphere of social life (including human services) makes a lot of sense. It also helps us understand why those most disadvantaged by the system may adopt a range of neoliberal beliefs, opposing measures that may assist them and even voting for parties that pass measures increasing their material disadvantage. At the same time, it gives us hope that even structural oppression is contestable, especially if we think seriously about the possibilities for collective organisation and social workers participating in progressive reform movements (Ferguson 2008).

Structural social work

Structural social work is a Canadian variant of radical social work, pioneered by Maurice Moreau (1979). It emphasises the central role of social structures, such as class, in producing personal suffering and thus advocates both personal and social change to address this. While radical social work was marginalised in neoliberal Britain in the 1980s, Canadian structural social work continued renovating itself in the face of various critiques from feminism (for neglecting gender oppression), anti-racist theory (for neglecting racial oppression) and, more recently, poststructural critiques (Mullaly 2010). In responding to these critiques, structural social work has broadened its recognition of various structural divisions and the diverse 'interweaving of oppressions' (Moreau 1989) beyond class exploitation, without automatically privileging any particular form of oppression. However, there exist other critical perspectives, working in particular contexts that continue to insist on the specificity or primary significance of the particular form of oppression they confront. As we saw in Chapter 4, the first of these to assert its distinctive critique, initially within radical social work, were the feminist perspectives.

Feminism

Feminist theories focus specifically on women's experiences and the key role of socially constructed gender inequalities in organising society (Lengermann & Niebrugge-Brantley 2014). A pioneering feminist thinker of the 20th century, Simone de Beauvoir (1908–86), pointed out that throughout history the category 'woman', despite cultural differences, had always been defined as man's 'other' in ways that disadvantaged or marginalised women ([1949] 1993). Some feminists would argue that the subordination of women is the oldest and deepest form of oppression, underpinning all 'civilised' societies, including the destructive ways

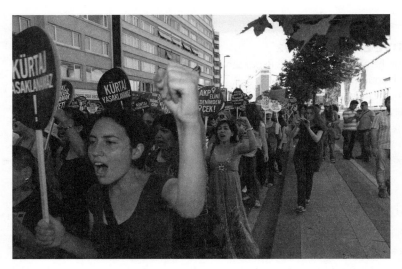

Figure 6.6

Feminist social work
'arose out of feminist social action being carried out by women working with women in their communities. Their aim has been to improve women's well-being by linking their personal predicaments and often private sorrows with their social position and status in society' (Dominelli 2012, p. 6).

patriarchal societies relate to nature (Lerner 1986). **Feminist social work** approaches link the personal to the political and focus specifically on *gender* as the most problematic part of social structures (Dominelli 2002b; Marchant & Wearing 1986; Orme 2013; Weeks 1994). In a similar vein to the Marxist identification of capitalist structures producing class exploitation, modernist feminists have identified the way patriarchal structures perpetuate the subordination of women by privileging men in most spheres of social life. While the women's movement has made great gains since the 1970s, gender equity remains elusive because the sources of male domination are multiple and capable of countering change.

Feminist analyses typically begin with the question 'and what about the women?' (Lengermann & Niebrugge-Brantley 2014, p. 440). What are women doing or how are they represented in this situation? What roles do they play and why? How are they positioned in relation to men? What is expected of women that is not expected of men and what harms arise as a result of this different positioning? These questions have major implications for social work practice and research in almost every setting, where most of our service users are women. Feminism is also a critical theory because its critique of patriarchal oppression aims to create alternatives, including establishing relations in which gender is no longer oppressive or damaging. Many feminists are wary of utopian thought but it is still implicit in the quest for reforming the structures and culture of patriarchal society. Since the 1990s, under the influence of poststructural, postmodern and postcolonial ideas, feminism has become a lot more explicit about difference *within* gendered categories (like 'woman'). The feminist theorist Judith Butler (1990) has even queried whether or not the gendered binary of man/woman is an obstacle to overcoming gendered oppression, and stresses the contextual, unstable and fluid nature of socially constructed, sexual identities (Featherstone & Green 2013). Feminism, confronted by women of colour, women with different sexualities and women in the developing world, has had therefore, to re-examine universal (one-size-fits-all), modernist analyses of patriarchy and liberation, not because they are useless but because these ideas can mean quite different things, and may require radically different strategies, in different contexts (Morley & Macfarlane 2012).

REFLECTIVE EXERCISE 6.13

Refer back to page 142 and reread the case study of Giuseppe.
- In the light of structural and feminist social work, what do you imagine are some of the key social structures giving rise to Giuseppe's situation and the issues he faces?
- How might the issues highlighted from a structural social work or feminist social work analysis be different from the establishment approaches presented earlier in the chapter?

Anti-oppressive social work

The response of modernist critical theories (such as Marxism and structural social work) to critiques of their failure to appreciate diversity and multiple forms of oppression have generally been inclusive and positive. Bob Mullaly's (2010) 'new structural social work', for example, has included feminist, anti-racist and poststructural concerns about difference. However, some social workers believe an undue focus on social structures diminishes recognition of the subjective 'lived experience' of oppressed identities and prefer the term 'anti-oppressive social work' (Dalrymple & Burke 1995; Dominelli 1998, 2002a; Campbell 2002). They use this as an umbrella term for radical, Marxist, structural and feminist perspectives. We have used the term *critical* in a similar inclusive spirit. We do this not to enforce particular concepts or solutions but to recognise that what all of these theories have in common is an emphasis on patterns of inequality in society: the underlying social structures of class, race, ethnicity, age, gender, (dis)ability, sexual orientation and the adverse experiences arising from these (see, for example, Fook 1993). Furthermore, all of these approaches seek some form of transformation of the sources of oppression while bringing relief to immediate suffering.

Postmodernism/poststructuralism

In this book, the critical approach that we are presenting draws on both the modernist critical theories, and the potentially emancipatory aspects of poststructural thinking and analysis. Poststructuralism originated in France in the 1970s and is generally regarded as the intellectual movement of postmodernism, which is usually seen as a much broader cultural movement, although some writers will use the terms interchangeably. Poststructuralism literally means 'after structuralism' and refers to theories that reject the idea that all human activities can be totally explained as the outcome of a definite set of underlying 'social structures' in a simple cause-and-effect manner. Both poststructuralists and postmodernists reject the idea of there being a singular, objective or complete 'truth' (black-and-white view) about the world and its problems. In their view, the world is not mechanistic but complex, fluid, contradictory and multilayered, making it capable of different readings. In fact, we inhabit a world of competing interpretations expressed in competing discourses and, for poststructuralists, these discourses are what make the universe and our identities within it. Therefore, modernism is just one more narrative or discourse alongside others in a world of multiple perspectives and multiple 'truths', whose validity depends on context. Art and poetry, for example, present us with different truths that many people find more compelling than science in making sense of their lives at particular moments. Moreover, differences in culture, gender, age, socioeconomic background and context are going to construct different narratives (and different worlds) than say a predominantly Western, middle-class, male, academic narrative. (For further information see Cuff, Sharrock & Francis 2006; Seidman 2013.)

A leading poststructuralist thinker, Michel Foucault (1926–84) was concerned with the way that knowledge and power mutually reinforce each other. Unlike Marxists, he didn't think power is mainly concentrated in a ruling class or the capitalist state and its repressive agencies. Power, for Foucault (1977, 1980), is present as a set of fluid forces in every social relationship and distributed throughout society in many forms and locations. Different groups in society are able to exercise power by promoting a particular discourse or truth, and knowledge of this discourse gives them power (Cuff, Sharrock & Francis 2006, pp. 264–5). Medical practitioners, for example, have power over their patients because they have knowledge that their patients lack, but usually accept, in defining their conditions. Social workers can also use this sort of power/knowledge with their 'clients' when they know the institutional rules of the welfare system and its

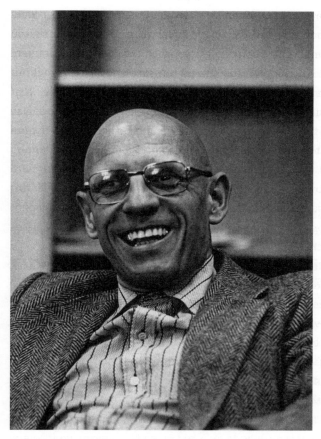

Figure 6.7 Michel Foucault
Reproduced with kind permission of the Bettmann Archive, Corbis Images.

various categories. Foucault believed these were instances of a new type of power, peculiar to modernity, namely 'bio-power', which, unlike 'state power' in the past, seeks to increasingly measure and regulate the 'personal lives' of citizens through schools, nursing homes, hospitals, employment agencies and welfare institutions (Powell 2013). This power is not so much exercised 'over' people (as domination) but rather 'through' them as discourses shaping our identity and actions.

Foucault's analysis draws attention to the surveillance and control aspect of the neoliberal welfare state, alerting us to the arbitrary use of power in institutions and local settings not normally seen as 'political'. However, Foucault also assures us that where there is power there is also resistance, although he refuses to elaborate on a grand narrative of liberation. Rather than pinning our hopes on emancipatory grand narratives, which too often unintentionally produce their opposite, Foucault urges us to be attentive to the little 'practices of freedom' that may be possible through critical reflection in the micro-settings of daily life. So, social workers employing a poststructural (or Foucauldian) lens will ask questions such as which discourses are present in the language used by this person, organisation, document or media form? Is there a recognisable dominant discourse? How does this discourse construct the world or situation as presented? What experiences does this discourse make visible and what is excluded? How might this discourse bolster or channel power? Is it possible to empower another discourse that aims at a more inclusive, democratic and/or just use of power? (Fook 2012; Chambon, Irving & Epstein 1999).

REFLECTIVE EXERCISE 6.14

How might these poststructural questions assist us to understand how Giuseppe's situation has been constructed?

Poststructural and postmodern insights disrupt modernist attempts to provide a complete and universal account of reality. Instead, they invite us to take other voices and narratives (those normally dismissed as perhaps anecdotal, foreign, mythical, 'unscientific' or 'merely personal') just as seriously in understanding the world and its problems. However, in valuing multiple views and theories, we are mindful of the problem of **relativism**.

Relativism is the idea that truth depends entirely on context, that what is true for one group may not be true for another, because there are no universal criteria for settling truth claims (Cuff, Sharrock & Francis 2006, p. 117).

If 'truth' is relative, however, then the question arises as to why anyone should give credence to social workers, whether structural or poststructural, critical or establishment? This is where we believe it is important to distinguish between critical and uncritical, poststructural (or postmodern) positions. Coming to poststructural insights out of critical social theory, we do not accept that all values are the same. We have taken an ethical stand that social work must treat each and every person as being of unique dignity and worth. We cannot (and do not seek to) prove this ethical conviction with science; however, we know from our diverse practice experiences, and that of many others, that critical social work can make a powerful difference for the better in people's lives.

From a critical perspective we believe it is possible to embrace the way poststructuralism draws our attention to diversity, the multiplicity of truths, the power of discourse to construct individual and social lives, and the fluid and complex nature of identity (Fook 2012). It also enables us to combine structural and poststructural analyses. Structural/feminist analyses, for example, assist us to understand the institutional dimensions of power (Mullaly 2010; Morley & Macfarlane 2012), whereas poststructural theories assist us by highlighting that oppressive power relations are maintained through the acceptance of various dominant discourses, which we have the agency to deconstruct and resist (Fook 2012; Fook & Morley 2005).

In view of the above, we argue that critical social work must draw on the critical values of modernism, its exposure of domination and oppression, and its advocacy of human rights and social justice. However, we also believe that critical social work in promoting these values today must combine them with the humility of postmodernism's capacity to entertain multiple perspectives, multiple realities and multiple truths. In other words, we believe that critical social work today has to cultivate a *critical* (*modernist* and *postmodern*) view of theory and practice (see, for example, Allan, Pease & Briskman 2009; Fook 2012).

◾ Developing a critical response to Giuseppe

So, what does the development of a critical approach look like in practice? For many first-year students who had completed the first semester of critical social work studies, there was a subtle, yet significant, variation between their pre-test (Stage 1) and post-test (Stage 2) responses. This was expressed more in the ways in which they would respond to the priorities rather than a change in the identification of priorities. For example, 70 per cent of students continued to view health as the number one priority in the Stage 2 questionnaire, while 50 per cent maintained their preoccupation with Giuseppe's safety in relation to his living conditions as one of their three concerns. Thirty-seven per cent of students indicated arranging access to an interpreter as one of their three priorities, 15 per cent identified grief and loss, and approximately 11 per cent indicated social isolation was a significant concern.

However, some important differences emerged with reference to *processes* that involved students working *with* Giuseppe, rather than doing things *for* or *to* him. In relation to health, for example, instead of intervening to invoke a range of invasive measures to be implemented, one student stated that 'the important thing about Giuseppe's health is for him to be consulted about his options'. Consistent with a critical approach, this reflects a commitment to working in partnership with Giuseppe, respecting his autonomy and rights to make decisions about his level of care and life in general. Similarly, in identifying the need for an interpreter, one student wrote: 'Assist him to find a translator (if he wants one) that he feels comfortable with.' Again, students identified the need to consult with Giuseppe about his options, rather than assuming his wants and imposing interventions in a top-down way, representing a more equal and democratic power relationship. This reflects a more critical approach to practice than in Stage 1, where responses were more closely aligned with establishment approaches.

In contrast to the policing/social control role that was evident in Stage 1 in respect of students' perceptions of the safety risks involved in Giuseppe's living conditions, the Stage 2 responses instead made reference to 'talking to Giuseppe about assisting him with support to maintain independent living', or finding out whether Giuseppe is 'interested in accessing supported accommodation'. Several first-year students also explicitly referred to poverty in the Stage 2 data, indicating the use of a *structural analysis*, rather than simply relying on risk or blame/pathology discourses. And, of those who identified social isolation as a priority for Giuseppe, this was articulated in more critical ways than at Stage 1. For example, one student suggested that they 'explore with Giuseppe if he wants to connect with community resources'.

Such statements are more reflective of a critical response as they indicate a shift to thinking about Giuseppe's situation in its social context and with an awareness of power relations. The Stage 2 data indicates that 61 per cent of students made statements that were reflective of this shift in thinking. A number of students expressed this by making reference to building a relationship with Giuseppe, in terms such as the following:

- making Giuseppe feel comfortable with your presence
- explaining your role as social worker
- building rapport
- having an ability to develop a respectful relationship with Giuseppe
- getting to know Giuseppe a little more and building a relationship.

Others talked about positioning Giuseppe as a partner or resource in their work with him to value what he might bring to the interaction. For example, they referred to:

- talking to him to find out what's happening from his perspective
- connecting with him and understand how he feels.

Some first-year students referred to more empowering aspects of work with Giuseppe that are more reflective of a critical approach. These included:

- respecting Giuseppe's right to privacy and confidentiality
- advocacy for just treatment
- Giuseppe's self-determination and autonomy
- understanding Italian culture and customs.

Generally, the Stage 2 data indicates there was far less certainty from students about what they assumed should happen, and a more thoughtful approach to exploring possibilities with Giuseppe, indicative of a critically reflective stance. This is reflected in the following quotes:

- 'Don't make assumptions about him. Talk to him.'
- 'I would leave when he asked me to because he had not asked me to come.'
- 'I would ask if I could do anything for him or if I could drop by again.'
- 'I would like to firstly ask him if he wants involvement from a social worker and if he would like to know more about the help that is available to him.'
- 'I'd ask Giuseppe to tell me his own story – my assumptions may be wrong.'

The reasons that students articulated during Stage 2 of the research as to why they would prioritise the above issues also reflected a significant shift in their thinking towards a more critical approach to thinking and practice. See, for example, the following statements:

- 'I would like to make sure he is aware of his options.'
- 'Because I could make assumptions about what should happen but if we haven't communicated with him, how do we know what he wants and whether we're just going off on a tangent?'
- 'Because understanding the situation from Guiseppe's perspective is something I now regard as an imperative first step.'
- 'Because the most obvious thing is to develop a positive client–worker relationship.'
- 'Because we need to interact. There's no point in making assumptions without taking to him.'
- 'Need more information so need to communicate. Need communication to build rapport and trust.'
- 'You need to ask Giuseppe what is happening because he is the expert on his own life.'
- 'Talk to Guiseppe and ask him if there is anything he needs.'
- 'I would leave when asked because he did not ask for help and by pushing him it could alienate him more. I would try to establish a relationship by asking if I could call by again so maybe eventually I could get to know him.'
- 'Because it's up to Giuseppe.'

Overall, the Stage 2 data indicated a move away from the paternalism of the establishment theories to a more critical approach that respects and facilitates the autonomy of others.

These critical theory/practice themes were even more developed in the responses to the questionnaire from final-year students who had completed their social work program (Stage 3). For example, a majority of students (78%) made reference to 'power', Giuseppe's level of 'powerlessness', or his need to be 'empowered' in identifying the main issues in the case study. They also used both structural and poststructural concepts – talking about both 'class' and 'socioeconomic' disadvantage and disempowering 'discourses' – in reflecting on the issues. Closely associated with power was addressing language/communication barriers (76%), which was expressed in terms of consulting with Giuseppe about whether he would like to work with an 'interpreter' or 'translator'. Final-year students also identified Giuseppe's 'culture' or 'ethnicity' (62%) or his 'gender' and 'masculinity' issues (53%) and some referred to these as a potential basis for disadvantage or 'human rights' issues as one would expect from structural, feminist or anti-oppressive practitioners.

A number of final-year students identified that grief would be a significant issue for Giuseppe (37%). For some students there was an explicitly critical understanding of grief as a social issue. One student stated:

> Grief may well be a significant social issue, impacting on everything in Giuseppe's world, including his health, motivation to keep the house going or self care, and social connection. Even though his wife died years ago, grief has no time limit. It's a unique experience for every person and there may be a cultural dimension here as well. I wonder if he has ever had an opportunity to talk with anyone about his grief – if that is what he wants, and how life was before his wife died. If people have to carry on and keep things bottled up, it can have profound consequences for their health and wellbeing . . .

Another student, who prioritised different issues, also exemplified a critical approach to practice:

> Firstly, I would be aware of not buying into medicalised discourses and risk management discourses by falling into the trap of seeing his health and safety as the only or main concerns. Whilst it is important to consider the immediate issues, I also had other questions coming to mind as I read the case study, such as: how are ageist discourses playing out here? How does Giuseppe's ethnicity as an Italian man impact on this experience and expectations of me as a worker? How does gender come into play here? How might hegemonic constructions of masculinity impact on Giuseppe's experience of grief and/or social isolation?

The use of critical theory was particularly evident in the reflections of these final-year students in both their political awareness of Giuseppe's context and their preparedness to act in collaborative ways that would be empowering for him and others in similar circumstances. A student, who identified herself as a 'socialist-feminist', wrote:

> Reading this made me angry at both the situation and what I imagine will be the typical social work response. I bet most social workers would only want to deal with the individual and not the broader issues of age, gender, class and power. Obviously, you need both! Giuseppe is not an idiot. He speaks four languages for goodness sake! He deserves dignity and must be listened to with great care and the worker must avoid psychobabble labels. If he [Giuseppe] needs help, I imagine the services available (if any exist in his area) will be inadequate. That is where we have a responsibility to advocate and lobby for change both for Giuseppe and others in similar circumstances. We also need to challenge the complacency that Australia doesn't have 'real' poverty or inequality.

■ Summary

Theory is a 'way of looking' at aspects of the world, enabling us to interpret our own and others' experiences. It is impossible to separate theory from practice. Theory is therefore a central component of social work practice. In this chapter, we have examined a range of formal social work theories in relation to a case study concerning Giuseppe. As examples of establishment social work theories we have explored psychodynamic and cognitive psychological theories – also known as individualistic theories; and systems theory – a conservative social theory. We have contrasted these with a number of critical social work theories, including radical, Marxist, structural, feminist, anti-oppressive and poststructural theories.

Establishment social work theories tend to focus on the private problems of the person, who is seen as the problem, and it is the role of the practitioner to 'fix' or find solutions for them. This can have the effect of positioning the worker as the expert and holding service users responsible for the unjust situations in which they find themselves. Because establishment theories focus our attention on reforming or changing the individual, they can draw us, as workers, into complicity with dominant institutions and discourses that turn our gaze away from social factors and our role in social change. Establishment theories both reflect and reinforce the dominant discourses that maintain current power relations and inequalities in society. Many social work students often begin their studies with beliefs and values that are easily captured by establishment theories because dominant discourses and ideology reinforce conservative thinking within our media, education system, socialisation processes, and institutions as 'common sense'. Hence, many of us accept these beliefs as if they are our own, until they are challenged by another standpoint and we have a chance to critically reflect on them.

Adopting establishment social work theories in practice has displaced, deskilled and devalued many practitioners (Harris & White 2009; Lavalette 2011). This has resulted in reports of experienced practitioners feeling demoralised, alienated and angry about the gap between their aspirations for entering a career in social work and human services and the sort of work roles that they are currently undertaking (Baines 2010; Jones 2005). It is thus imperative that social work students, graduates and practitioners are connected with critical social work theories so that we can begin to resist and question dominant discourses and reclaim the meaning of our practice. A critical analysis and appreciation of the social and political context of people's lived experiences has clear implications for orientating social work practice towards progressive social change. This will be explored in more depth in the following chapter as we examine the ways theories guide our practice methods and processes in greater detail.

■ Review questions

- How do you feel about the various theoretical perspectives we have covered in this chapter?
- What do you consider to be the strengths and limitations of each of the perspectives?
- What do you consider to be the strengths and limitations of each of the perspectives?
- Which theories fit most comfortably with your own values, and why?
- Which theories do you feel most challenged by, and why?

■ Further reading

Agger, B., 2013, *Critical Social Theories: An Introduction*, 3rd edn, Oxford University Press, Oxford.

Allan, J., Briskman, L. and Pease, B., 2009, *Critical Social Work: Theories and Practices for a Socially Just World*, 2nd edn, Allen & Unwin, Crows Nest, NSW.

Garret, P., 2013, *Social Work and Social Theory: Making Connections*, Policy Press, Bristol, pp. 1–20.

Healy, K., 2005, 'Three waves of systems theories' in *Social Work Theories in Context: Creating Frameworks for Practice*, Palgrave Macmillan, Basingstoke, pp. 132–50.

Mullaly, B., 2007, 'The social work vision: A progressive view' in *The New Structural Social Work*, Oxford University Press, Ontario.

Payne, M., 2005, 'Psychodynamic perspectives' in *Modern Social Work Theory*, 3rd edn, Palgrave Macmillan, Basingstoke, pp. 73–96.

Webb, S. and Gray, M., 2013, *Social Work Theories and Methods*, 2nd edn, Sage, London.

7

Social work practice

■ Introduction

SOCIAL WORK PRACTICE may be conceptualised in a variety of ways. Sometimes practice is referred to as 'methods'. Establishment social work has tended to refer to different levels of practice: *micro methods*, including methods for working with individuals, such as casework, counselling and case management; and methods for working with couples and small groups, such as family group conferencing, mediation and group work; and *macro methods*, which are more collective methods of practice, such as advocacy, community development, policy development and analysis, research and social action (Allan 2009). Practice is also sometimes referred to in terms of the processes that characterise it from beginning to end; for example, engagement, assessment, intervention, termination and evaluation (Chenoweth & McAuliffe 2012).

While talking about the processes, methods and skills of practice can be useful for practitioners, social work practice involves more than these things. It does not always occur in a neat, straightforward, linear manner. The situations that social workers engage with are often messy, complex and dynamic. Moreover, some thinkers have raised concerns about the implications of the language that is used to describe practice methods, skills and processes (Dean 2011). For example, if you accessed a service for support, would you like to be 'assessed' and have a worker 'intervene' in your life, before 'terminating' you? If we subscribe to the *poststructural* view that 'words create worlds' (Hartman 1991, p. 275), or that the language we use can construct our view of reality, then as critical practitioners we need to be attentive to the terminology we use and the power relations it invokes.

Dean (1993, p. 60) points out that:

> The expressions 'diagnosis', 'assessment', 'therapy', and 'treatment' derive from the medical and research models and suggest that the client is sick and needs to recover. In addition, these terms turn the client or problem into a finite entity to be studied and diagnosed. Similarly problematic, the term 'interventions' defines a process in which the clinician does something to the client (or situation).

Obviously, we need to use some terms in order to describe what we mean, yet it is not possible to do this without invoking theory. Let's look at this now in relation to practice processes.

■ Practice processes

Engagement is often regarded as the first stage of a practice process. In simple terms, engagement may involve establishing rapport and a relationship with the person, group or community with whom we work (Chenoweth & McAuliffe 2012). While this may sound like an objective, factual description, there are different ways to 'engage' and these variations reflect our theoretical and cultural assumptions. For example, from an *establishment individualistic* perspective, engagement may be an opportunity to establish the practitioner's control and authority over the relationship with the service user by demonstrating expertise and determining the parameters of the work, explaining the nature of the problem or dysfunction (Perlman 1957). By contrast, from a *critical* perspective, engagement is an opportunity to reduce power differentials between the practitioner and service user by facilitating the service user's control over the process, and demystifying the practice, the organisation and the services offered through sharing information. This would be a two-way process in which the practitioner positions themselves as a resource to explore with the service user their perception of their needs, and how they want to use the time together. In this way we demonstrate that we 'cannot be experts at "knowing" another's meaning but only increasingly skilled at facilitating a conversation in which it will emerge' (Dean 2011, p. 79).

Assessment is often seen as the second stage of a practice process when practice is described in this linear fashion. At its most basic, assessment is often thought of as the process of defining the problem and identifying what needs to happen to respond to the problem (Chenoweth & McAuliffe 2012). This process typically consists of the worker asking the questions and the service user providing the information, with the worker then deciding on the best course of action, based on their assessment of the situation. Some assessments are conducted for specific purposes: for example, *psychosocial assessments* determine the nature of the person's situation and issues in their social environment (Healy 2005), while *risk assessments* determine safety and potential harm (Healy 2005). From an establishment social work perspective, assessments are often assumed to be objective processes that rely on various tools and **classificatory schemas** to remove what is regarded as the bias of the

Classificatory schemas are frameworks based on scientific theoretical understandings of human behaviour used to organise and interpret information or 'facts' collected about the service user, which classifies them into diagnostic categories (Greene 2008, p. 18).

practitioner from the knowledge that is believed to be uncovered or *found* by the assessment process (Greene 2008). However, from a critical perspective, the practitioner's values and interpretations cannot and should not be removed from the assessment process, as this may provide valuable insights into the situation. Such assessment from a critical perspective assumes that knowledge is *produced* (through the discussion that happens between practitioner and the service user), rather than found (see, for example, Fook 2012). Similarly, practitioners informed by critical perspectives do not seek to create a particular agenda by relying on predetermined questions, but rather to explore the insights and wisdom of the people with whom they work in order to construct a shared understanding of the issues and possible practice responses (see Greene 2008, p. 19 for comparative examples). As such, some critical practitioners have rejected the mainstream language of assessment to instead embrace the notion of developing a '**professional narrative**' to describe this practice process (Fook 2012). We will explore the ways in which theories impact on how practitioners produce professional narratives later in this chapter.

> A **professional narrative** is a term used to describe a critical approach to assessments in which the worker recognises that they are creating meanings of the service user's world and needs (Fook 2012, p. 135).

Intervention is often seen as the next part of the practice process after assessment. The term 'intervention' is used in establishment social work discourses to describe the practical elements of what practitioners do. Part of the difficulty that critical practitioners have with the term 'intervention' is that it positions the service user as the passive recipient and locates power with the expert practitioner who saves or changes the situation with their intervention. From a critical perspective, the professional narrative (or assessment) we create about a service user's story and needs will influence the type of intervention (or methods of practice) that we deem appropriate. However, as we discuss below, the ways that we perform practice methods is also informed by theory. Some critical practitioners may prefer the term 'involvement' as it suggests a quite different approach (Fook 2012).

Termination is a term used by mainstream social work to mark the end of a working relationship or formal disengagement of the service user from the service (Chenoweth & McAuliffe 2012).

Evaluation involves making a judgement about the adequacy of the practice (Chenoweth & McAuliffe 2012). Logically, the ways in which we define what is good, and who it is good for, will be contextual and contested, and as critical theories highlight, implicated in power relations. Critical practitioners often use critical reflection to evaluate and research their practice (Fook 2012).

■ Practice methods

In addition to processes, practice is also described in terms of the *methods* applied (or *interventions* applied if we use the establishment/mainstream term). As we have stated, practice is often categorised in terms of micro and macro methods. Micro methods refer to direct service components of social work practice. These include methods for working with individuals, such as casework, counselling, case management and advocacy. It also includes methods for working with couples, families and small groups, such as mediation and group work. The more collective methods of practice are often characterised as macro interventions and include community development, policy development and analysis, research and social action. Micro methods aim to respond directly to the needs of individuals and groups who we are working with. Macro interventions are potentially more focused on creating large-scale change within social and political systems (for further information see Healy 2012).

This is not to suggest that practitioners only use micro methods or macro methods. Indeed, as Allan (2009, p. 77) explains, critical practitioners use a combination of both for they 'see the need for multiple ways of working because individuals' experiences are shaped by and shape their broader world'. However, a common misconception is that we must use *individualistic* (conservative) theory if we are working with individuals – for instance, using counselling, casework or case management – or if the nature of the issues have been historically dominated by individualised (psychological) approaches, such as in the areas of mental health, grief and loss. Indeed, working with individuals can be conducted using establishment theories or critical theories. (See, for example, Fook 1993 for a discussion on how case work can be radical.) Similarly, some practitioners assume that because systems theory concerns the functioning of systems, all work with families, for instance, must be informed by systems theory. The same logic applies in that we assume that all community development must be innately progressive, or informed by structural theories, because it works at a macro level, but community development can, like any method, be practised conservatively or critically (Ife 2013). Ultimately, the theories we use to inform our understandings of methods, and inform the professional narratives we create (assessments), are more determining in this regard than the practice method itself.

It is therefore not meaningful to talk about practice methods or processes without an integrated discussion of how *theory* informs these concepts. Let's now explore this in relation to a number of practice methods.

Counselling is defined by the Psychotherapy and Counselling Federation of Australia (PACFA) as a 'professional activit[y] that utilise[s] an interpersonal relationship to enable people to develop self understanding and to make changes in their lives' (http://www.pacfa.org.au). From a critical perspective, however, this is problematic because it assumes there is a singular, universal way to define counselling as a practice. While all approaches to counselling involve relationship, and working in a one-on-one capacity, the PACFA definition reflects a conservative (establishment) position because it assumes that the problem, and therefore the target of intervention, is the service user, who is assumed to have not developed appropriate 'self understanding'. Change from this establishment view of counselling should be personal change – that is, change should occur in the life of the service user (individualised adjustment), rather than occurring in social structures (social change). However, from a critical perspective, counselling seeks to be both supportive and educational by working in partnership with individuals to explore the ways in which they are disadvantaged by social and political structures and working with them to find ways of resisting injustices in the system, both for personal liberation and for social change.

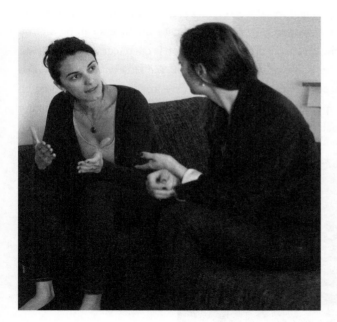

Figure 7.1

Similarly, *casework* has traditionally been defined as a process used by certain human welfare agencies to help individuals to 'cope more effectively with their problems in social functioning' (Perlman 1957, p. 4). Again, this definition reflects a conservative position because the problem is assumed to be the inadequate 'social functioning' of the service user that needs to be remedied by practice methods aimed at bolstering their capacity to 'cope' (even if their situation is unjust). Critical perspectives reject that anyone should have to cope with injustice and question how we can transform society to be more accommodating and responsive to people's needs. Referring to the same aspect of practice, taking a *modernist, critical perspective*, Fook (1993, p. 7) later defined *radical casework* as a practice that:

> first and foremost assumes an analysis which constantly links the causes of personal and social problems to problems in the socioeconomic structure, rather than to inadequacies inherent in individual people or in socially disadvantaged minority groups.

This definition more closely aligns with the intentions of critical social work, which seeks to examine and challenge the injustices that society creates for individuals, rather than helping people to adapt to them.

Case management is arguably the prevailing method in contemporary human service delivery and is required by some funding arrangements. The primary function of the case manager is to coordinate services for clients with multiple needs. The role of case manager is often filled by a qualified social worker; however, organisations may increasingly argue that the competencies typically required of case managers can be met by personnel from other disciplines. This deprofessionalisation is of concern from a critical perspective. Donna Dustin, in her evocatively titled book *The McDonaldization of Social Work* (2007, p. 52), suggests 'social workers working as care [case] managers should be under no illusion that they are working toward a more just society'; they're protecting resources and containing costs rather than engaging in preventative community work.

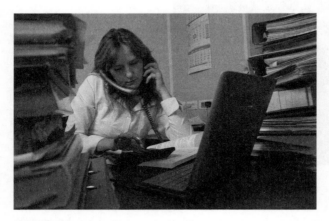

Figure 7.2

In a neoliberal climate, practitioners need to be cautious about case management being used to serve the interests of management rather than those of service users. As a technocratic practice that aims to simply manage issues rather than respond to the complexity of a situation in a holistic or sustainable way, case management may be less responsive to personalised needs of service users. From a critical perspective, the practice of case management may decrease the likelihood that existing systems will be criticised, meaning that newer and more responsive systems might not be developed. Case management does not create processes for service users to question the relevance of services and/or become empowered in the process of being case-managed. There are also increased possibilities that individual professional workers or case managers, whatever their occupational background, will bear the brunt of the blame/responsibility for the effectiveness of the case management process, regardless of the level of appropriateness of the resourcing available or authority they hold (Fook 2012, p. 170).

Another practice method, *group work*, can be most simply understood as work with groups. This type of work can vary from being educationally orientated, thera-peutic, activist in nature, or simply take the form of meeting around a particular cause. Social work with groups represents a broad domain of direct social work practice. (For further information see Healy 2012; Garvin, Gutierrez & Galinskey 2004.) As with the other methods, there is no guarantee that group work will necessarily be critical or emancipatory. The following definition of structured group work provides an example that is captured by dominant (establishment) thinking, rather than critical thinking. This definition states that 'the worker is the expert until her knowledge has been imparted to the group' (Middleman & Wood 1990, pp. 11–12).

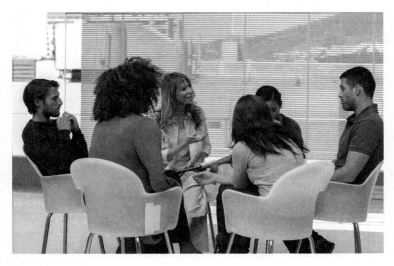

Figure 7.3

The theoretical perspective that informs the way we understand the practice method thus has a greater influence over how the method is practised than the method itself. And as we shall see in the following discussion, not all theoretical perspectives utilise all methods of practice. If we adopt an establishment social work approach, for example, and we assume that the individual with whom we work is our target for change, then we will only use individualistic methods, such as counselling, casework and case management (and we will do so using conservative theories).

Conservative (establishment) practitioners do not use more collective practices aimed at systemic change because these methods are seen as irrelevant given that they do not contribute to the goal of transforming the individual. Therefore, some methods of practice (those that focus more on societal/systemic reform rather than individual change, such as community development, policy development, social action, and advocacy) are only used by practitioners who subscribe to the more progressive (critical) theories that advocate social change (Allan 2009).

Community development (also sometimes referred to as community work or community capacity building) has been defined as a collective approach to achieving progressive social change that uses a structural analysis of the causes of issues impacting on people's daily lives, moving these seemingly private concerns into public action. It is considered 'bottom-up' work, where community members set the agenda for how the work will be undertaken and any other decision-making processes that affect them (Ife 2013; Kenny 2010). This approach 'builds social capital and enables groups of individuals to collectively create the kind of communities in which they wish to live, work and play' (Lathouras 2010, p. 21). This is not to suggest that community development is innately critical and emancipatory, or cannot be co-opted by establishment approaches. Indeed, like any practice method, community development can be practised in top-down ways and driven by expert practitioners who control the agenda and marginalise the community workers they purport to empower (Ife 2013). This is where critical reflection can be a useful tool to enable us to avoid causing harm to the people and communities we work with, despite our best intentions (Fook 2012).

Closely related to the practice of community development is *social activism* (sometimes also referred to as social action). Social activism may be defined as the intention to work with collective consciousness to promote, block or influence social, political, economic and/or environmental change or maintenance of the status quo. Activism can take a wide range of forms, such as participating in political demonstrations/campaigning, lobbying government, signing petitions, writing letters to newspapers or politicians, engaging in terrorism, imposing boycotts on buying certain products or alternatively preferencing some businesses, and holding rallies, street marches, strikes and sit-ins (Baines 2007; Ife 2013).

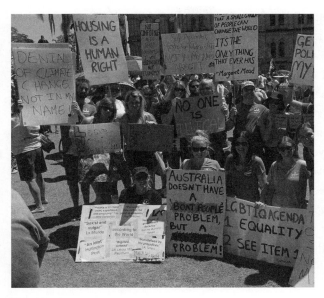

Figure 7.4

Policy development and *policy analysis* are related to activism because they seek to scrutinise and challenge oppressive policies and propose alternatives. A policy is a principle or rule to guide actions towards those that are most likely to achieve a desired outcome (for further information see Jamrozik 2009). Grants to encourage people to buy or build new homes are designed to provide an incentive to stimulate the economy. Baby bonus cash payments were designed to encourage people to have babies. Policies that apply a tax levy for Medicare are designed to encourage people to purchase private health insurance. Policies that penalise working parents in two-parent households by reducing their welfare benefits when they work are designed to keep one parent (typically the mother) at home. Social policies can create social advantage and disadvantage, social justice and injustice and promote social equality and inequality. Therefore, policy analysis and development are not inherently critical practices, but they can be if informed by a critical perspective (Bacchi 2009).

Research is another method of practice that may be more or less critical in its approach. Research sets out to explore the questions that beset social work practice. Sometimes our questions are quite specific to our daily practice: How should I approach this team meeting today? What is missing from my assessment of this family? How can I best advocate for the rights of my client in relation to her housing needs? Often our questions must be 'answered' on the spot, as we are called upon to (re)act quickly. However, sometimes questions persist over time and, as critical practitioners, we become passionate in our desire to explore them more fully and share our findings with others. This is where research is born.

As with all practice methods, research is inherently political and embedded in particular theoretical and ideological perspectives (Coppock & Dunn 2010; Healy 2000). As critical social workers our research should reflect our commitment to anti-oppressive practice and an orientation to emancipatory change and social justice agendas. As an example, one of us (Selma), in her PhD research, explored how living in a residential psychiatric disability support service, based on therapeutic community principles, affected people's lives (Macfarlane 2006). An establishment approach to this research question might have directed Selma to a systematic analysis of professional journals, such as the *Archives of General Psychiatry*, for scientific or medical-model analyses of outcomes for people with specific psychiatric diagnoses. Or perhaps the establishment researcher would have developed a questionnaire for mental health practitioners to elicit their views of effective service provision. Neither of these approaches is inherently bad, but both are limited.

REFLECTIVE EXERCISE 7.1

- Can you see some of the limitations, from a critical perspective, of the research methods described above?
- Whose voices are privileged, and whose are silenced?
- What might be an alternative approach?

Selma's research explored her question through in-depth, relatively unstructured interviews with current service users, past service users and program staff, in order to gather narratives that are often neglected or minimised: stories of lived experience. These stories were then positioned alongside mental health theories from the literature in order to share the power associated with being a legitimate producer of valuable knowledge (Macfarlane 2006). This approach is at odds with the more *positivist* research traditions, which are based on a hierarchy of what 'counts' as knowledge that positions hard scientific research (**randomised control trials** and experimental studies) at the pinnacle, and more qualitative research, such as narratives of lived experience of oppression and marginalisation and service users' perspectives at the bottom (if not totally absent). From a critical perspective, research in mental health should challenge ways in which scientific discourses have been privileged over those of lived experience. And, in retrospect, Selma realised that a truly critical approach would have actively involved service users in both the generation of the research project and the analysis of the findings (Macfarlane 2006).

Randomised control trials are studies in which people are allocated at random to receive one of several clinical interventions (Jadad 1998).

A critical approach to research, as a method of practice, draws our attention to the ethics of research conduct. A tragic example, in the Australian context, is that while Aboriginal people are one of the most researched groups in society, they remain among the most marginalised. Only in recent years have Aboriginal scholars, workers and community members begun to turn the tide by developing and implementing their own research and arguing for the legitimacy of Indigenous knowledge systems alongside often unquestioned Western approaches. (See, for example, Baskin 2006; Herbert 2003; Martin & Mirraboopa 2007; Smith 2005; Wilson 2003.)

■ Practice skills

In addition to methods and processes, practice is sometimes conceptualised in terms of skills and techniques. Establishment social work often conceptualises skills in two broad categories: skills necessary for *assessment*, and skills necessary for *intervention* (Compton & Galaway 1999, p. 9). Skills can be further categorised as generalist skills and specialist skills: generalist skills underpin all social work practice (such as inter-personal communication skills and writing skills), while specialist skills are related to expertise in particular fields of practice (such as counselling skills in working with bereaved persons, or skills in a particular approach to harm minimisation in drug and alcohol services) (Compton & Galaway 1999; Trevithick 2005). The general skill-set required for social workers is set out in the AASW Code of Ethics (2010). Go to https://www.aasw.asn.au/practitioner-resources/code-of-ethics.

REFLECTIVE EXERCISE 7.2

Go to the library and examine some introductory social work and/or human services texts.

- What do you notice about the ways that they discuss practice processes, methods and skills?
- What do these books tell you about how theory and context inform practice?

Some texts present information on practice methods and processes as if they are merely providing an objective description in technical terms, which is untainted by theory. They may also present theory in a separate discussion as if it is something we can graft onto practice as an afterthought.

- What do you think might happen if we fall into the trap of thinking that our practice can be separate from theory?
- List some of the consequences for your practice.

These *technicist* (skills- and competency-based) approaches focus on how to do practice as if it is a purely technical exercise. Students are often keen to learn the 'tools' of practice, and report feeling short-changed if we talk about theory instead of teaching the 'recipes' of how to do practice. Indeed, much of the way social work is taught inadvertently assumes that there is a separation between theory and practice. But technicist approaches that assume that practice can be adequate without theory have been criticised for perpetuating an artificial division between practice and context, thereby creating the view that practice is somehow unaffected by the dominance of *neoliberal, capitalist, colonialist, patriarchal* and *medicalised* influences (see, for example, Dominelli 2009). The inescapability of this means that simply focusing on skills or techniques tends to lead to individualistic and politically conservative practice that reinforces the status quo and may lead (uncritical) practitioners to inappropriately blame people for the social problems that have impacted their lives (i.e. victim blaming) (Mullaly 2010; Waldegrave 1990). Therefore, if we understand practice merely as a set of skills or competencies, the person or issue we work with is artificially separated from the political, social and historical context (Mullaly 2010; Waldegrave 1990). In addition, the focus on specific skills detracts practitioners from a broader vision of emancipatory change. As such, it is contended that social workers should seek to challenge the assumptions underpinning technicist approaches to practice, and instead promote critical analysis and critical reflection (Ife 2013).

Although practice is an activity that necessarily involves *doing*, it is not just a practical endeavour. In order to do practice, we need to first *think* about what it is that we will do. Hence, practice is also a moral, social, political and intellectual exercise. From a critical perspective, social work practice is an opportunity to create social change towards a more socially just world. Given that critical practice requires social and political analysis of society, power relations, dominant discourses, and so on, it cannot be reduced to a set of skills (Ife 2013; Moreau 1979; Mullaly 2010).

While it is important that practitioners have excellent skills, we also need to understand that the particular skill we choose in any given situation, and the ways in which we choose to use it, will be informed by theory. Theory, whether we are conscious of it or not, actually informs how we interpret a situation, how we understand the issues involved in that situation, how we view our role and, ultimately, how we will engage in practice. Social work practice is, therefore, not simply a collection of techniques, competencies or skills or tools that we *do* to people, but the thoughtful and intentional application of theory to action (Fook 2012).

Regrettably, the influence of neoliberalism on higher education has in many cases reduced social work education to competency-based skills acquisition aimed at accepting the status quo, rather than critically reflective, transformative learning. This encourages the promotion of conservative approaches, which are supported by a focus on techniques and competencies, rather than a critical analysis of social structures and power relations embedded in our current social arrangements. The omission of the latter results in the reshaping of education towards conservative, market-led demands that aim to produce technically proficient practitioners who unthinkingly conform to existing inequities in the system and are unable to see the broader implications of their work (Wehbi & Turcotte 2007).

Rather than facilitating an acceptance of the status quo by replacing the learning and teaching of social work and human services practices with a set of skills or competencies that are separated from theory, context and critical analysis, a critical approach provides a critique of technicist approaches and aims to raise awareness about the possibilities to challenge social injustices so that we do not unconsciously fall into the trap of becoming functionaries of the state who uncritically enforce oppressive social systems. This is vital to the continuation of social work in current contexts, where dangers exist for social work to be co-opted into neoliberal practices that work against the very core of social work's value base (Holscher & Sewpaul 2006; Madhu 2011).

While it is necessary to explore definitions of specific practice processes, methods and skills enable us to develop an initial understanding of some of the terms and concepts associated with practice (as is demonstrated above), the theoretical framework that the practitioner uses is more important in influencing whether and how a particular method, skill or process is practised. In the remainder of this chapter we will use the following case study about a young woman named Sarah to demonstrate how theory is directly linked to practice, particularly in relation to how our professional narrative (or assessment, if we are using establishment social work language) influences our use of practice methods (or interventions, in the words of establishment social work).

CASE STUDY
Sarah
You are working in a community-based residential program for people who have been diagnosed with a mental illness. In your geographical area (a rural town), the program offers a medium-term stay (12–24 months) for persons aged between 21 and 40 who have a psychiatric diagnosis and wish to work on getting their life back on track. The program offers one-to-one counselling support and group-work activities, and is aimed at developing skills that will allow participants to live more independently in the wider community and achieve greater wellbeing.

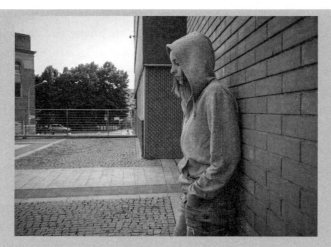

Figure 7.5

You are the 'keyworker' (designated support worker) for five of the 15 residents on the program. Sarah, one of the clients with whom you work, is aged 26, and has been a resident in the program for about six months. She was referred to the program by her doctor. Her parents also encouraged her to access the program as they felt she needed to move out of the family home. Sarah was diagnosed with a mood disorder approximately three years ago and has been hospitalised several times since then. A few months prior to her first hospitalisation, Sarah was sexually assaulted by a friend's cousin at a party she went to one night. Sarah tells you that you are the only person that she has told about this experience of sexual assault.

Sarah has never lived away from home. Her father (Peter, aged 52) is a real estate agent and her mother (Kath, aged 50) a nurse; her older brother, Geoff, is a physiotherapist. Sarah's parents have told you that they need to live their own lives and, despite their love for Sarah, feel it is not doing her any good to remain in the family home where she is either idle most of the time or madly engaged in vigorous activity.

Although the program is voluntary, Sarah has continually expressed to you that she does not want to be there, that it is not doing her any good, that she doesn't have problems like the other residents and that all she wants is for her parents to let her move back home. Sarah's parents ring you on a fairly regular basis, particularly when Sarah has appeared on their doorstep in the evening saying she wants to sleep there. Occasionally, her parents allow this, but other times they tell her she has to go back to the program. Sarah feels hurt. She expresses to you that she is angry with her parents and cannot understand why they will not let her move back home.

Sarah's evening visits to her parents' home (which is within walking distance of the facility) have escalated recently, and her parents have requested a meeting with you 'to sort things out'. Sarah is looking forward to the meeting and hopes it will result in her being allowed to move home. Her parents, on the other hand, seem to be expecting you to support them in their refusal to let Sarah sleep over or return home to live. You are concerned about how you will balance your roles as advocate/support worker for Sarah, and mediator of the discussion, while also feeling empathy with Sarah's parents.

- What are the major elements of this situation? Which stand out for you? (For example, what do you see are the main issues and difficulties? Who are the key players? What are the main problems?)
- Can you prioritise these?
- What does your prioritising indicate about which issues you regard as more important than others? (You might like to compare your priority list with those of other students.)
- What do the assumptions you have made indicate about the theories that are underpinning your thinking? For example, have you tended to focus on individual (conservative) or social (critical) explanations?
- Can you identify the theories you have used? Does it surprise you that you have drawn on these and not others? Why or why not?
- It might help when doing this exercise to make a long list of all the different theories that could be used to understand the situation. How do the different theories view the issues differently? And what implications might the theories have for your practice?

■ Constructing a professional narrative (assessment)

By answering the questions from this brainstorming exercise, you have taken the first steps in constructing your professional narrative (assessment) about Sarah's situation.

The professional narrative that we construct has been defined as the cornerstone of social work practice. Our professional narrative determines everything: how we see the person; how we make sense of, and work with, the issues that the people with whom we work present (Fook 2012). As with other practice processes, assessment has traditionally been presented as if it can happen without reference to theory. The implicit *objectivist* assumptions that underpin this construction means that the 'findings' of assessments often uncritically mirror *dominant* (neoliberal, positivist, colonialist, biomedical) concepts.

Hence the assumption that we can undertake assessments from a neutral and objective position is flawed. The notion that we can conduct assessments in an ordered, linear, 'one size fits all' approach has also been criticised, along with the assumptions of expertise and control that underlie establishment views of assessment. The construction of your professional narrative should be a co-construction of the story between you and the people with whom you work. It should be seen as a *process* that happens over time, rather than an event. It should be seen as potentially multiple, contradictory and changing, as different elements of the narrative are emphasised and excluded (Fook 2012). And, most importantly, it should involve turning the '**deconstructive gaze**' onto your own assumptions, values and interpretations of the narrative (Fook 1996, p. 198), as this will tell you much about the theories implicit in your practice. Such a *reflexive* stance will enable you to examine the social and political implications of your professional narrative, rather than just focusing on 'how to' do it. The major elements that stand out for you or the key issues or difficulties you identified when reading Sarah's story indicate a lot about the theories that you are using to guide your practice.

■ Individualist theories

If we were examining Sarah's story through the lens of an establishment individualistic theory, the most significant aspect we would privilege is the fact that Sarah has been diagnosed with a mental illness (a mood disorder that has resulted in her hospitalisation several times in the past three years).

Adopting a conservative approach that accepts the status quo, using an establishment individualistic theory, we would accept the power and authority invested in psychiatry and would defer to the assessment and diagnosis of the treating physician. This would lead us to understand that Sarah's behaviour is a result of her illness. The fact that she is either idle most of the time or madly engaged in vigorous activity would be seen as a symptom of her mood disorder; related to bipolar disorders in which 'patients' are seen as suffering from extreme highs and lows in mood, energy levels and behaviour. The fact that Sarah has continually expressed that she does not want to be in the residential facility would likely result in her being assessed as 'non-compliant' and 'resistant' to 'treatment'. (Note the use of medicalised language that characterises these perspectives.) Sarah's perception that the program is not doing her any good would be regarded as evidence that she is 'lacking insight' into her 'condition'. Her perception that she doesn't have problems like the other residents would be interpreted as Sarah being in 'denial' of her illness – a defence mechanism identified by psychodynamic approaches; other psychological approaches construct this as '**cognitive dissonance**' (Festinger 1957). That all Sarah wants is for her parents to let her move back home, and that she has never lived independently previously would be judged as 'pathological' and 'not normal', and therefore targeted as a site for change. The practitioner may be able to help Sarah by working with her to resolve unconscious issues that are assumed to have emerged from her childhood (Howe 2009). Hence, Sarah is viewed as the problem in need of intervention from the practitioner who tries to fix her issues with their expertise by 'helping' her 'accept treatment' that will enable her to 'manage' her 'illness'.

This establishment individualistic analysis fits comfortably with neoliberalism as this medicalised course of action is seen as the responsible thing to do. Given that individualist theories view the issues in Sarah's situation as her individual problem, counselling (working one-on-one with a practitioner in a therapeutic relationship) would be seen as an appropriate method of practice to work with Sarah. Counselling informed by cognitive behavioural and psychological techniques would be well suited to this purpose as it would aim to correct Sarah's 'faulty' belief system (Howe 2009). If Sarah raised her experience of sexual assault with a practitioner, informed by a medicalised perspective, it is likely that the practitioner may not see this as particularly relevant. At worst, it could be dismissed as a delusion arising from her mental illness, or seen as 'destabilising' and distracting from working on the main problem: the treatment and management of her mental illness (Morley 2005). In any case, from an individualist perspective, the goals of counselling would be to help Sarah accept and adjust to her illness, talking to her about changing her thinking and managing her behaviour (individual change). This, combined with medical treatment of her mood disorder, is assumed to enable Sarah to develop a more stable personality and the skills to live more independently in the wider community and achieve greater wellbeing. Macro practice methods (such as community development, advocacy, policy development and social action) that target society as the site of intervention would not be used while working with Sarah by establishment practitioners who use individualist theories, as macro practices are seen as irrelevant to the purpose and goals of their work, which is to fix/reform the individual.

■ Systems theory

Moving away from a strict focus on the individual, systems theory and other conservative social theories examine some contextual and environmental factors, such as Sarah's family. However, like the individualist theories that retain the goals of establishment social work (that is, to work towards maintaining the status quo and existing power relations), practitioners using conservative social theories take on the role of social control and social regulation. Hence, the ultimate aim would be to keep things as they are; Sarah should remain in the residential facility and her parents should be enabled to move on with their lives. The fact that Sarah is still living at home at age 26 and not working would be regarded as **deviant behaviour** that requires intervention by the practitioner. Sarah's behaviour would be viewed as disrupting others (her parents who have to take care of her) and having the potential to threaten the smooth functioning of society more broadly. If equilibrium is to be restored (which is the purpose of systems theory), Sarah needs to accept treatment for her illness so that she can manage it and then be able to live independently and make a contribution to

> **Deviant behaviour** refers to behaviour that does not confirm to socially constructed cultural norms (Howe 2009).

Mediation is an informal (not legally binding) process whereby participants engage in open discussions to resolve a dispute. (Roach Anleu 2010).

Differentiation relates to the family unit and how each member develops their sense of 'self' as an interdependent actor. From a systems perspective, those who are highly differentiated are believed to function at a higher level (Bowen 1978).

Family therapy refers to a set of practice approaches that view problems facing a family member as produced by family dynamics that are troubling for that individual, and therefore seek to transform unhelpful family dynamics (Healy 2012, p. 116).

A **family group meeting** is organised by the social worker to develop a shared understanding within the family and between the family and worker(s) about the family's concerns, and a plan of action to address these concerns (Healy 2012, p. 116).

Conflict resolution is the process of bringing together people who have seemingly incompatible needs, to reach a consensual outcome. There is an assumption that all parties are able to participate in the process equally (Roach Anleu 2010).

society by gaining employment. This will improve her functioning so that she can participate in society in a manner consistent with a normative consensus (social norms).

A systems theory approach that is uninformed by critical analysis would thus welcome the opportunity to meet with the family system (Sarah and her parents). Systems theory does not look at power or gender so the **mediation** role taken on by the worker facilitating the conversation would treat all participants as equal players (Healy 2005). From this perspective, there is no need for advocacy. The role of the mediator is, therefore, to be neutral and facilitate communication (healthy, functioning, open systems) (Payne 2005).

The practitioner would point out that Sarah is threatening the functioning of the healthy family system by leaving the facility and turning up at her parents' house. This is moving her away from her goal of 'normal', independent living. The worker would also point out that the parents need to be consistent in their refusal to allow Sarah to stay, as the failure to do so would be confusing for Sarah and indicate 'unhealthy boundary functioning' or problems with **differentiation**.

Hence, the practitioner aims to work with the family system in order to support the healthy functioning of the whole system. This work may take the form of **family therapy** or a **family group meeting** and involve skills including mediation and **conflict resolution**. If Sarah raised the issue of her sexual assault, as with her mental illness, this could be perceived as another threat to her functioning, and fulfilment of her expected roles – both in the family and in society. The neglect of gender and power in systems theory analysis does little to provide insight into the impact of the violence on Sarah (Mullaly 2010). A healthy functioning family system, in which each person knows and performs their appropriate role, from a systems perspective, is seen as a key component of a functional social order from a systems perspective. As with the establishment individualistic perspectives, macro methods (such as community development, policy development and social action that target society as a key site for intervention) are not seen as relevant by practitioners informed by establishment social theories. They are, however, less therapeutic than the individualist perspectives because the family unit is seen as the target of the intervention to ensure conformity towards the needs of the system, which is assumed to operate for the greater good (Howe 2009).

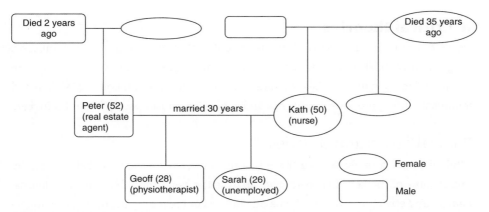

Figure 7.6 Genogram of Sarah's family: a diagram of the family's generation configuration (Compton & Galaway 1999, p. 69)

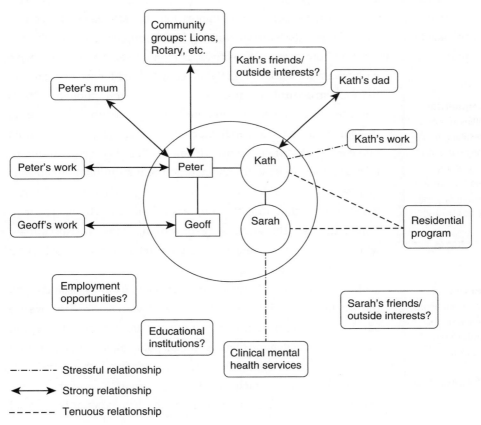

Figure 7.7 Eco-map of Sarah and her family: 'a diagram of the family within its social context' (Compton & Galaway 1999, pp. 69–70)

■ Critical theories

As we have previously discussed, the term 'critical theories' is used to encompass a range of theoretical perspectives, which highlight inequality and oppression and are change-oriented in intent. These include radical and structural theories, Marxism and feminism, anti-oppressive approaches and some elements of poststructural thinking.

Radical/structural theories

While we have already defined these theoretical perspectives, it is useful to briefly revisit some of the key ideas before we analyse the case study through these lenses. Radical and structural theories focus on patterns of inequality in society: the underlying social structures of class, race, ethnicity, age, gender, (dis)ability, sexual orientation, and so on (Fook 1993; Mullaly 2007). Marxist theories focus particularly on economic relations and class struggle, while feminist theories focus specifically on women's experiences and gender inequalities (Seidman 2013). Anti-oppressive approaches focus on unequal experiences of oppression and privilege and highlight the need for social workers to desist from creating further oppression through their practice (Mullaly 2010). From these perspectives, personal liberation of the people with whom we work is directly linked with broader social change to redress **structural inequalities**. Poststructural thought draws our attention to diversity and a multiplicity of truths, the power of discourse to construct individual and social life, and the fluid and complex nature of identity (Fook 2012). Hence, structural/feminist analyses assist us to understand the institutional dimensions of power (Fook 1993; Mullaly 2010), and poststructural theories assist us by highlighting that oppressive power relations are maintained through the acceptance of various dominant discourses, which we have the agency to **deconstruct** and resist (Fook 2012; Fook & Morley 2005).

So, how might these critical theories inform our assessment and the practice methods we would use to work with Sarah? First, we see Sarah not only within her family and community context, but within the context of wider and divisive (social, political, historical, cultural and gendered) structures. Our attention is drawn to her experience of sexual assault, which is all too common. For example, we know that one in five Australian women has experienced sexual

Structural inequalities refer to inequalities in power and resources resulting from people's positioning in social structures (class, gender, ethnicity, age, and so on) and not their personal or physical abilities (Fook & Morley 2005; Davis 2007).

Deconstruction involves questioning our assumptions, values and common sense notions that may be linked with dominant discourses (Fook 2012).

violence after the age of 15 years (Australian Bureau of Statistics 2006, cited by Victorian Centres Against Sexual Assault (CASA) Forum 2013). We also know that the links between being sexually assaulted and being *diagnosed* with a mental illness are well documented in the research literature (see, for example, Morley 2005). While critical workers might use some of the same individual practice methods as establishment workers, the ways in which they would use these methods is quite different. In addition, critical workers will also use macro-level practice methods since their focus is on the individual as well as society, and the ultimate goal is to address the fundamental causes of sexual assault.

In contrast to the establishment individualistic theories and systems theories, critical theories provide an alternative set of assumptions on which to base our practice when we work with victims/survivors of sexual assault who have been diagnosed with a mental illness. These include:

- that sexual assault is a fundamental violation of human rights and unacceptable in any form
- that all emotional and behavioural responses to sexual assault (regardless of the forms these take) are understandable, and that applying a psychiatric diagnosis to these responses is pathologising and stigmatising (Fook & Morley 2005)
- that diagnosing emotional responses to sexual assault and/or institutionalising the victim/survivor individualises the social problem of sexual assault, by depoliticising its patriarchal causes (Fook & Morley 2005) (see Chapter 2 for a more detailed discussion of how patriarchy contributes to violence against women)
- that this process blames the victim/survivor by shifting attention to her responses, while simultaneously covering up the need for changes to our society, which has historically sanctioned the patriarchal conditions that enable sexual violence against women and children to occur (Fook & Morley 2005)
- that preventing family violence is the responsibility of the whole community.

In addition to these concerns with individualistic approaches, a critical perspective rejects a systems response that overlooks power divisions (i.e. patriarchy) and simply seeks to activate or augment the existing system through, for example, employing more police, law reform or other social control measures that reinforce the existing social order.

As the worker, you may be aware that other service users have disclosed similar experiences to Sarah's, and voiced their concerns that they will be blamed or not

Universalising refers to the feminist / anti-oppressive counselling skill that encourages the service user to see their experience in light of structural inequalities that are shared by others (Scott, Walker & Gilmore 1995).

Contextualising is exploring with the victim/ survivor possible alternative contexts in which a situation, thought, feeling or behaviour considered unacceptable would be acceptable (Scott, Walker & Gilmore 1995).

'Reclaim the Night' (or in some countries 'Take Back the Night') rallies 'draw together women from diverse backgrounds and experiences to work together in addressing issues of men's sexual violence against women and children' (Reclaim the Night Australia 2013).

Consciousness raising relates to raising the awareness of those who are experiencing social and political oppression as to the structural conditions that cause personal problems (Fook 1993).

believed. This mirrors the research that tells us that the reasons most frequently cited by victims for not reporting an assault include fears of being disbelieved, and being made to feel that they contributed to the sexual assault in some way (see, for example, Brown 2007; Jordan 2012). Micro (individual level) methods of practice, such as counselling and/or group work (both educational and therapeutic), may be used to support Sarah, hear her story and affirm her blamelessness. These practice methods may enable Sarah to share (**universalise**) her experiences, thereby 'breaking the silence' that surrounds sexual assault, while **contextualising** her experiences. This would provide her with information about her rights, and a safe space to explore decisions that emerge from the sexual assault, including her right to make a complaint to police, recognising that sexual assault is a serious crime for which she is not to blame (a process known as deguilting) (Scott, Walker & Gilmore 1995).

We may also encourage Sarah to engage in social action aimed at preventing violence against women, such as '**Reclaim the Night**'. This would occur alongside utilising feminist practice skills of **consciousness raising** to debunk social myths that operate to deny the incidence and prevalence of sexual assault in our community (Scott, Walker & Gilmore 1995). Social myths about sexual assault are false beliefs that blame the victim/survivor and deflect attention from the perpetrator. (For example, she was raped because she was asking for it given what she was wearing, how she was behaving and her previous sexual history – factors that have nothing to do with the perpetrator's decision to harm her.) Such myths may take other forms. (For example, rape is about sex, which again transfers the responsibility to the victim for her sexual attractiveness, while denying that rape is about power – the intention to degrade, control, humiliate and disempower another person.) Other myths, such as the belief that women and children lie and fantasise about sexual assault, function to increase the likelihood that victims/survivors will remain silent about their experience (thereby protecting the perpetrator) and operate to discourage victims/survivors from accessing necessary supports (Morley 2014).

The robbery

POLICE OFFICER: Mr Smith, I understand that you were held up at gunpoint on the corner of Drummond and Mair Streets, Ballarat. Did you struggle with the robber?

MR SMITH: No, I did not.

POLICE OFFICER: Why not?

MR SMITH: The man had a gun.

POLICE OFFICER: Then you made a conscious decision to go along with the robbery, rather than fight back?

MR SMITH: Yes.

POLICE OFFICER: Did you scream or cry out?

MR SMITH: No, I was scared he would shoot me.

POLICE OFFICER: I see. Have you ever been held up before?

MR SMITH: No, never.

POLICE OFFICER: Have you ever given money away?

MR SMITH: Yes, of course.

POLICE OFFICER: Willingly?

MR SMITH: Yes – look Officer, what exactly are you getting at?

POLICE OFFICER: Well, let's put it this way. You have given money away in the past. In fact, you have quite a reputation for being free with your money. How can we be sure that you weren't contriving to have your money taken by force, then cry 'robbery'?

MR SMITH: That is not true!

POLICE OFFICER: What time did this robbery occur?

MR SMITH: About 11.00 pm.

POLICE OFFICER: You were on the street at 11.00 pm! Doing what?

MR SMITH: Just walking.

POLICE OFFICER: Just walking? You know that it is dangerous being out on the street that late at night. Weren't you aware you could have been held up?

MR SMITH: I hadn't thought about it.

POLICE OFFICER: What were you wearing?

MR SMITH: Let me see – I remember now. I was wearing a business suit.

POLICE OFFICER: An expensive suit?

MR SMITH: Well, yes – I am a successful businessman.

POLICE OFFICER: In other words, you were walking around the streets, late at night, in a suit that practically advertises the fact that you might be a good target for some easy money. Isn't that so? I mean, if we didn't know you better, Mr Smith, we might even think that you were asking for this to happen, mightn't we?

Reproduced from Claire Vernon, *Good Practices and London Rape Crisis Centre*, King George V Sexual Assault Service, 1994. Used with kind permission of Yvonne Traynor, CEO, Rape and Sexual Abuse Support Centre, Croydon, United Kingdom.

- What are your responses to this exchange between Mr Smith and the police officer?
- It may seem ludicrous to subject Mr Smith to this line of questioning. However, if we change the context of this interaction and consider the discussion in light of a sexual assault, this may be a fairly standard and acceptable line of questioning. Why do you think this is the case?
- What social myths were you able to identify in the police officer's questions and assumptions? How might these same myths impact on dominant understandings of sexual assault. How might a feminist analysis of sexual assault assist us to debunk these myths?

Normalisation refers to assessing feelings and emotional responses as common and legitimate by validating and reassuring the service user that their feelings, thoughts and behaviours are entirely justified given the outside pressures of their experiences (Scott, Walker & Gilmore 1995).

Validation refers to the skill of affirming the 'truth' of a person's subjective experience, affirming their telling of their story and what has occurred (Harms 2007; Scott, Walker & Gilmore 1995).

Counselling and group work could also be used to explore, **normalise** and **validate** the emotional responses to a sexual assault and honour the coping mechanisms Sarah has employed to survive her experience, while advocacy might be used to represent Sarah's interests vis-à-vis outside systems, such as police and/or medical and mental health professionals, and Sarah's family (Scott, Walker & Gilmore 1995). This stands in contrast to individualistic perspectives that do not see the need for advocacy and pathologise her emotional responses to the assault, thus justifying the medicalised, objectifying and potentially oppressive nature of involvement with the mental health systems (see, for example, Anthony 1993 and Deegan 1996). In challenging, rather than affirming, the status quo, once Sarah develops an understanding that the sexual assault was not her fault, and that her responses are 'normal', she may make the courageous decision to tell one or both of her parents about the assault; knowledge that would increase their potential capacity to support her. For example, this would provide Sarah's parents with an alternative understanding about Sarah's need to feel safe, and why this draws her back to her parent's house, thus invoking a different role for Sarah's parents in her recovery and a strengthening of their relationships with each other. In contrast to the establishment individualistic theories, applying a social and political analysis of Sarah's experiences of sexual assault and mental health/illness is the most important component of practice from a critical perspective while the other methods or skills are simply tools that enable us to put the emancipatory potential of critical theories into practice.

Critical approaches work at both micro (personal) and macro (political) levels to achieve emancipatory ideals. Given that critical perspectives view sexual assault as a community responsibility, rather than an individual problem (albeit while acknowledging and working with the personal impact of sexual violence on the victim/survivor), *social structures* are targeted as a site for social change. Therefore, community development and education are relevant practice methods aimed at combating widespread community ignorance of the social myths surrounding sexual assault (Australian Law Reform Commission (ALRC) 2010). The following 'tips to end rape' provide an example of this type of education. Often, education strategies locate responsibility for preventing sexual assault with potential victims through promoting messages such as 'don't walk home by yourself at night', 'don't leave your drink unattended in a nightclub' or 'don't talk to strangers', which is part of the process of ascribing blame to victims. A critical approach, however, more appropriately locates responsibility for preventing sexual violence with potential perpetrators.

---

10 top tips to end rape

1 Don't put drugs in women's drinks.
2 When you see a woman walking by herself, leave her alone.
3 If you pull over to help a woman whose car has broken down, remember not to rape her.
4 If you are in a lift and a woman gets in, don't rape her.
5 Never creep into a woman's home through an unlocked door or window, or spring out at her from between parked cars, or rape her.
6 USE THE BUDDY SYSTEM! If you are not able to stop yourself from assaulting people, ask a friend to stay with you while you are in public.
7 Don't forget: it's not sex with someone who's asleep or unconscious – it's RAPE!
8 Carry a whistle! If you are worried you might assault someone 'by accident' you can hand it to the person you are with, so they can call for help.
9 Don't forget: honesty is the best policy. If you have every intention of having sex later on with the woman you're dating regardless of how she feels about it, tell her directly that there is every chance you will rape her. If you don't communicate your intentions, she may take it as a sign that you do not plan to rape her and inadvertently feel safe.
10 Don't rape.

Reproduced with the kind permission of Eileen Maitland, Information and Resource Worker, Rape Crisis Scotland.

> **Social or public advocacy**
> is thinking of solutions and
> actions, big and small, needed
> for collective social change –
> to change the conditions that
> generate social problems
> (Baines 2007).

Social or public advocacy might be also used to raise awareness about sexual violence and lobby institutions, such as the legal system, to make legislative changes that are more responsive to victim/survivors' needs. Policy analysis and development is undertaken to expose and oppose the ways gendered inequalities that contribute to sexual violence are created at the political level, and research is undertaken as another practice method to provide evidence for these issues and push for structural change. As a practitioner, you would also *critically reflect* on your own level of expertise in working with women who have experienced sexual assault; you may determine that accessing specialist, feminist-based services would provide better support and assistance to Sarah, and you could support her in accessing such services (referral). Finally, using a feminist perspective you might also consider the expectations potentially being placed on Sarah's mother to provide care and nurturing for her adult daughter. Critical practitioners regard women's difficulties as inherently linked with the structures and institutions of a patriarchal society (see, for example, Dominelli 2002b; Orme 2013). This will assist you in recognising that women are often placed in positions where they are seen as being 'bad' or uncaring mothers, which generates enormous guilt and disempowerment. If it felt appropriate at the family meeting, along with acknowledging power imbalances that may exist within Sarah's family with reference to gender and age, you might also encourage a discussion around women's roles and how both Sarah and her mother may be striving to achieve a healthy balance of interdependence (Hurst 1995).

Acknowledging and exploring the potentially difficult aspects of living in a rural setting would also be part of a critical approach, in terms of access to education, meaningful employment and transition to independent living. Other questions to consider are what are Sarah's hopes and dreams and how does her social environment enable and/or entrap her? You could explore with Sarah how dominant discourses around young adulthood, femininity and productivity are shaping her personal experience and explore the possibility of more empowered alternative discourses, as well as the steps that might need to be taken to embrace this discourse. In acknowledging and validating Sarah's voice and lived experience, you could explore what it is about 'being home' that draws Sarah back to her parents' house. By valuing her story as a critical practitioner you would resist buying into the expert position, seeking to find answers with her, rather than for her, while always facilitating her control over the processes of your work together.

Furthermore, from a critical perspective, we might look at how class has shaped both Sarah and her family's notion of successful living. In particular, we might question how dominant notions of success have potentially positioned her as a 'failure', thus creating an experience of **internalised oppression** in which Sarah feels invisible and marginalised (Mullaly 2010). An exploration of this possibility could form part of our assessment as well as our 'intervention' with the family. This leads us to a brief discussion of the elements of postmodern thinking that would also inform and extend our critical approach.

> **Internalised oppression** refers to the 'incorporation and acceptance by individuals within an oppressed group of the prejudices against them within the dominant society' (Pheterson 1986, p. 148).

Poststructuralism

The key elements of poststructural thinking that are relevant to Sarah's story are around the concepts of fluidity of identity; resistance to binary thinking; **discourse analysis**; and the existence of multiple truths rather than singular grand narratives. To some extent all these concepts are interrelated, which will become apparent as this short section unfolds. Because we acknowledge that all individual identities are fluid and contextual, we would allow Sarah, and her parents, to be contradictory or ambivalent, and to fluctuate in their desires for change or maintenance of the status quo. Because we are attempting to resist binary thinking, we try not to be co-opted into 'either/or' constructs that suggest the following binaries: 'change versus maintaining the status quo'; 'Sarah's wishes versus her parents' wishes'; 'mental illness versus mental wellness'; 'micro or macro practices'; 'critical versus medical perspective'; and 'invalid knowledge versus valid knowledge'. (You might be able to think of more examples of binary thinking present in our analysis.) The result of this resistance means that we recognise that it is possible for some elements of Sarah and her family's position to change while others remain the same. So, for example, she might go home some nights but not others, but perhaps with an arrangement that she will ring before coming. We would question whether Sarah and her parents are totally at odds in their thinking, or if they have some elements in common while also acknowledging that total agreement is not necessary or perhaps even possible. We would also question how dominant discourses around mental illnesses have positioned both Sarah and her parents in particular ways and whether these positions are empowering or oppressive. In working with Sarah, we would consistently critically reflect on our own practice and the limitations and partiality of all theories we are drawing upon. For example, how might our own social location affect our 'take' on Sarah's situation? We need to be mindful of how this may both cloud and sharpen our vision.

> **Discourse analysis** refers to the language practices through which we construct our knowledge and understandings of 'reality' – what is true and what is false – which in turn determine our actions (Healy 2005).

'Critical poststructualism' is a term used to describe how modernist critical theories, such as feminism and Marxism (with their focus on universalised understandings of oppression and privilege – for example, 'all women's experience is the same' or 'all lower income earners are disempowered'), can combine with the emancipatory elements of poststructural thinking to extend critical practice. In many recent social work texts (see, for example, Allan, Briskman & Pease 2009; Fook 2012) the emancipatory forces of modernist and poststructural thinking have been combined within the term 'critical social work'. An important element of such a critical approach, as we have discussed in more detail in Chapter 6, is the practice of critical reflection, and it is on this note that this chapter concludes.

■ Summary

We began this chapter with a discussion of social work methods and processes, and how they are consciously or unconsciously formed and driven by theoretical and cultural assumptions. In the preceding section we teased apart the case study of Sarah in such a way that you will hopefully have been able to see how different theories lead to different ways of thinking and working. As social workers we will always be engaging in processes of some sort and our practice may be described in terms of method. However, it is our critical engagement with the strengths and limitations of these processes and methods, the assumptions and values that underlie them, and the effects they engender in local contexts of practice that are the key concerns of social work.

Critical reflection can, through the process of *deconstruction* and *reconstruction*, assist us in aligning the processes and methods we engage in with our critical, emancipatory and anti-oppressive ideals. Our critical practice, and the knowledge that informs it, develops as we subject our professional and organisational processes and methods to scrutiny in all their complexity, instability and contextual variability (Healy 2000). As Fook (2012, p. 179) reminds us, critical reflection can assist us to 'remake power relations in a contextually relevant way'. This requires a flexible approach to account for the subtle or not-so-subtle operation of power in diverse contexts. At the same time as we respond to the everyday concerns of the workplace and our potential for contextually relevant critical practice, we also acknowledge that our commitment is deeper and broader than our role as an employee; we are also committed to a broader vision of social justice in which our immediate struggles are part of a deeper, ongoing and multifaceted vision (Fook 2012, p. 182). As Pozzuto (2000) said nearly two decades ago, 'the task of critical social work is to lift the veil of the present to see the possibilities of the future'.

■ Review questions

- What questions has this chapter raised for you?
- Write a paragraph about how you understand the links between theory and practice.

Further reading

Allan, J., 2009, 'Doing critical social work' in J. Allan, L. Briskman and B. Pease, *Critical Social Work*, 2nd edn, Allen & Unwin, Crows Nest, NSW.

Fook, J., and Morley, C., 2005, 'Empowerment: A contextual perspective' in S. Hick, J. Fook and R. Pozzuto, eds, *Social Work: A Critical Turn*, Thompson, Toronto.

Rummery, F., 1996, 'Mad women or mad society: Towards a feminist practice with women survivors of child sexual assault' in R. Thorpe and J. Irwin, eds, *Women and Violence: Working for Change*, Hale & Iremonger, Sydney.

Scott, D., Walker, L. and Gilmore, K., 1995, 'Counselling support for adults who have been sexually assaulted' in *Breaking the Silence: A Guide to Supporting Adult Victim/ Survivors of Sexual Assault*, 2nd edn, CASA House, Melbourne.

8

Missing voices and working across difference

■ Introduction

THIS CHAPTER DRAWS attention to the often missing voices of the people whose needs we address in social work and human services delivery, variously labelled as 'service users', 'fellow citizens', 'consumers', 'customers' and 'clients'. In this light we explore the worker–client relationship and its inherent power dynamics, which relate not only to service delivery but also the control of research, participation in policy development, and the privileging of professional knowledge over client perspectives. Our main aim is to highlight the missing voices of marginalised discourses (such as feminism in a patriarchal society or consumer knowledge in a medicalised environment) and their capacity to illuminate and inform our work with others. We take this discussion further by exploring current concepts of working across difference and cultural background. Finally, we explore the **anthropocentric** limits of traditional conceptions of the client base of social work and suggest possibilities for extending this to include a more *eco-centric* (nature-centred) framework that values the integrity of nature and other beings. We hope this chapter encourages you to consider why and how some voices become dominant, while others are ignored or minimised, and the effects this has on our capacity for critical practice. To discuss how, why and what voices are missing from public and professional discourses, we need to identify how, why and what voices are most dominantly present. Therefore, we begin with an exploration of power and knowledge, and the complex ways they interact.

Anthropocentrism literally means human-centred and assumes humankind to be the final concern of the universe and views everything in terms of human experience.

In doing the exercise above, one of the authors (Selma) reflected on her experience in her family of origin where her father ruled the roost and had the most dominant voice in making decisions, while the voices of the women in the family were often unuttered or unheard. As social workers, we will often work with individuals, groups and communities whose voices have been silenced or marginalised: older people struggling on minimal fixed incomes, women suffering from domestic violence, troubled youth who have slipped through the cracks of education and employment, people living below the poverty line, and people who are homeless or experiencing mental illness. These voices are seldom heard or legitimised in public debate, and the knowledge they hold is rarely sought or validated. Their experiences of disempowerment are evident in the ways that they are defined by others more than they are able to define themselves. Foucault (1980) suggested that power and knowledge are inseparable: those whose views are dominant (whether this be men in a patriarchal society, psychiatrists in a medicalised model of mental illness or white people in a colonised country) are seen not only to hold the most valuable and legitimate knowledge, but also occupy positions of power to exert the 'rightness' of their perspective over other possible truths. As critical social workers, we are interested in how power, knowledge and 'help' are intertwined (Rossiter 1996): how do we use our knowledge and power in *emancipatory* ways and how can we best listen to, and advocate for, those voices that are marginalised to be heard? We will start by looking at power and knowledge in the worker–client relationship and the voice of the service user; then we will look at the often missing or marginalised voices of diverse knowledge systems and alternative discourses.

▪ The voice of the client/service user/consumer

It is unavoidable that we, as social workers, have and exercise a certain degree of power in our professional roles. After all, we are being paid to assess problems and situations, make decisions and devise appropriate interventions, and sometimes to act in ways that are mandated by law. We are accountable to the organisation we work for, to the wider community and society at large, and to our profession, as well as to the clients of our service. Our power, in some respects, also comes from the professional knowledge, expertise and skills we hold as the result of completing a university degree as well as experience gained in the field. Clients rightfully expect that we are able to assist them with difficulties they are experiencing. Someone – for example, a professional – who 'knows what others do not' may be precisely what *anyone* – including ourselves – might need when faced with oppressive circumstances or when life has 'fallen apart'.

REFLECTIVE EXERCISE 8.2

Think about your own practice if you are currently working in the field.

- What power do you hold and exercise? Examples might be the power to make assessments and determine the distribution of resources, and/or the power to define what is appropriate behaviour, and what is not.
- Is some of this power exercised because you have knowledge that the client does not? How might clients see you in relation to the power you hold and the value of your knowledge as compared to theirs?
- If you have been a client of welfare or human services, what power did you feel the worker held in relation to you and your life; how powerful did you feel? Did you feel that your own knowledge about yourself and your life was valued? Or, if you have had neither of these experiences, what do you think about the idea that social workers have power?

As critical practitioners, our aim is to try to unravel, in specific situations, how and for what reasons we exercise our professional power, how we enact our professional knowledge in more or less empowering ways, and how this fits with our critical intentions. At times, professional power can be seen – and experienced – as oppressive by service users, and as workers we are sometimes aware of this and become frustrated by the *social control* elements of our work. As *anti-oppressive*, *critical* social workers, our aim is to minimise power imbalances, not to further entrench them. At the same time, we acknowledge that power can be exercised in anti-oppressive ways for the benefit and empowerment of service users. Examples of this are when we engage in advocacy with clients to ensure their rights and needs are met, or in something as simple as using our position within an organisation to secure a room free of charge for a women's group to meet. So our professional power in the worker–client relationship is neither inherently good nor bad, but being the holder of professional knowledge is a powerful position.

Duncan (1998, p. 13) provides a powerful image when he suggests that 'dethroning' ourselves is one way to balance our professional knowledge with openness to the knowledge and power of the client. He suggests 'listening for change, and acknowledging that what clients "bring into the room" – their personal qualities, persistence, support, beliefs, life events – along with the creation of a supportive worker–client relationship, ha[s] as much to do with positive outcomes as anything else'. Rossiter (2011) draws our attention to a recognition that our professional knowledge and our professional narratives are always limited and fallible, and that we need to be open to the knowledge, wisdom and strength of others.

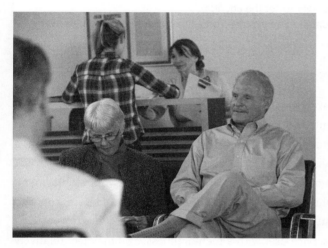

Figure 8.1

From a critical perspective it is important to be mindful of the power of 'service users' and to avoid a binary classification that sees them as powerless. Here, we have put 'service users' in quotation marks, because by acknowledging the power of a person who is labelled in this way, we are already undermining the discourse that suggests clients are passive, disempowered and unknowledgeable. Furthermore, service users are not necessarily fixed in their identity: we are all service users in different contexts and while this may be presented as a disempowering position to occupy, it is not the totality of a person's identity. In discussing and analysing her facilitation of a young mothers' group, Healy (2000) observed how the young women in the group had exercised power: their status as mothers meant they occupied a knowledgeable position that the facilitator – not a mother – did not. As the group was based upon a premise that lived experience created valuable knowledge, the group was able to question the overriding expertise of 'professional' knowledge. This points to a valuable implication of *poststructural thinking* for social work: that power can be shared and exercised in different ways by different people at different times. Our critical lens highlights the very real ways in which structural inequalities pose barriers to the exercise of power based on class, gender, ability, race, age, and so on, while also being mindful of the fluid nature of identity and how a person may be powerful in one context and less powerful in another.

REFLECTIVE EXERCISE 8.3

- Think of the various roles you occupy (e.g. student, friend, parent, sibling, worker).
- Do you feel you have more power in some of these roles or contexts than others (e. g decision making, or power to set the agenda)?
- Is your knowledge validated more in some contexts of your life than others? Why might this be so?

Social milieu was defined by Durkheim as the 'substratum of society' – the social environment that is composed of layers of interrelated and connected complex systems and communication mechanisms. (Sawyer 2002, p. 234).

Hegemony 'is the operation of one powerful group over others, such that the consensus of the subordinated groups is achieved by convincing people it is in their interests to agree with and follow the dominant group's ideas' (Germov & Poole 2011, p. 114).

Subject position refers to the social role constructed for an individual through a discourse; for example, the way in which people are turned into 'patients' by medical discourse (Gray 2007).

In the exercise above, you may have identified that, as a social work student, your knowledge, voice and power are more validated in your peer group than in the academic setting, and that in your role as a retail worker at a clothing outlet you have very little opportunity to set the agenda or make decisions about the terms of your employment. To add to this example, you may also be taking antidepressants and this element of your identity has the potential to construct you as a patient or service user with a mental illness. You may feel relatively powerless and hesitant to reveal this side of your experience to others. Your sense of validation and power in each of these aspects of your identity is, at least in part, due to social norms and expectations that result in certain social roles and institutions that uphold those norms. We have already discussed the way in which discourses become dominant in the **social milieu** of the time and place we occupy. In the example above, neoliberal discourses position workers as commodities and educational discourses position students as learners who must adapt and respond to the educational agenda that has been set. Psychiatric discourse positions a person experiencing psychological distress as the recipient of expert knowledge and treatment.

Dominant discourses become **hegemonic** when we internalise their norms and **subject positions** into our thinking and actions: often the subject positions created by the dominant discourse fix one person or group as inferior and the other as superior. The knowledge of the powerful group comes to maintain a certain legitimacy that excludes, negates or minimises the knowledge of the inferiorised group. We argue that the knowledge and voice of clients or service users is often minimised and excluded by practitioners and policymakers. Clearly, the knowledge of whole groups in Australia has been marginalised; nowhere is this more evident than in relation to Aboriginal and Torres Strait Islander knowledge systems. (We will discuss this further later in this chapter.) These voices are missing in myriad ways: from creating assessments and writing case notes, to decisions about how the organisation delivers services, to policy development and deciding what and how to conduct research into social problems.

REFLECTIVE EXERCISE 8.4

Pause for a moment and reflect on what you have read in the last few pages. Now that we have reached Chapter 8, you are hopefully finding that words and phrases such as 'hegemonic' and 'discourse' have become more familiar and understandable. You may even have found yourself thinking and speaking in this language. From a learning and teaching perspective, this is exactly what we would have hoped; however, as critical practitioners we also need to consider how to use our professional language anti-oppressively. After all, we want to demystify professional practice, not create another fence around expert knowledge!

In research conducted by one of us (Macfarlane 2014), the 'worker–client power divide' was pointed out by a participant who commented on how, in the time he spent as a resident in a psychiatric disability support service, the issue he never became accustomed to was the split between himself (an intelligent young man who had experienced psychosis and was currently identified as a service user) and his worker (an intelligent young man who occupied the role of support worker). Other participants commented on the power divide in a range of ways: the unnaturalness of a close supportive relationship that was curtailed by the worker 'clocking off' at 5 pm; how certain workers made them feel 'more sick'; the non-reciprocal nature of helping and advising; and the frustration of not being privy to the theory bases that were guiding the actions of workers. While some of these practices may not be amenable to change, they highlight the need for us to reflect critically on the way in which our power and role are experienced by those with whom we work and how we might change our practice to be more aligned with our anti-oppressive intent.

In the area of mental health, much has been written about and by the *consumer or recovery movement* – a movement that is characterised, like many social movements, by people coming together around a discourse of resistance to the dominant discourse that exercises power over their lives and identity (Coppock & Dunn 2010; Macfarlane 2009). Indeed, the discourse of recovery that has now found its way into policy and program initiatives was largely introduced by consumers of mental health services and has been embraced by the psychiatric disability support sector over the past three decades (Macfarlane 2009). The concept of recovery implies not so much a cure or denial of past events, but a 'mysterious and subjective process', as Anthony (1993, p. 17) puts it, encompassing the 'development of new meaning and purpose as one grown beyond the catastrophic effects of mental illness'. The recovery paradigm, as Anthony suggests, is a potentially 'unifying' one – in contrast to a more **'othering'** framework of medical model psychiatric discourse. Most of us can relate to experiences in our own lives that, while initially devastating and forever part of our story, we have more or less recovered from. Examples include the death of a loved one, divorce, severe or unexpected illness, or the loss of a dream that was core to our sense of self. Furthermore, the experience of mental illness or psychosis, subsequent hospitalisation, medication and/or treatment regimes, potential relapses and rehospitalisations often mean people have to recover not only from the illness experience but also from the trauma, stigma and loss associated with it (Anthony 1993).

> **Othering** refers to the way in which a dominant group classifies behaviour that is different from its own as 'other', enabling the othered group to be devalued and objectified (Mullaly 2010).

REFLECTIVE EXERCISE 8.5

During the course of Selma's research, when considering the meaning of 'othering', a service user once said: 'You [the workers] need to share the power to be the well ones.'

- What do you think he may have meant by this?
- What does this have to do with othering?

In a seminal text by Patricia Deegan (1988), she observed from her own experience that while recovery was vital to the rehabilitation process, it was overlooked in professional discourse because of its lack of fit with dominant scientific paradigms. She described three phases of recovery: denial, despair and then a mysterious transition to hope, which she compared to a tiny flame brought to life by two things – people who did not abandon her, and the 'possibility of being loved' (1988, p. 14). While recovery cannot be forced, Deegan (1988) said it could be nurtured in an environment that recognised the non-linear nature of the recovery process and the uniqueness of each person's journey. Some years later she wrote another inspiring article, 'Recovery as a journey of the heart' (1996), in which, again from her own experience, she cautions workers about misjudging their clients whose apparent apathy (giving up) and hardness of heart was actually a solution that protected them from wanting anything. 'If I didn't want anything then it couldn't be taken away; if I didn't try then I wouldn't have to undergo another failure; if I didn't care then nothing could hurt me again' (Deegan 1996, p. 95). Such insights, based on the knowledge and experience of the service user, are vital if we are to provide the professional narratives (assessments) and practice that may be helpful to each unique individual.

REFLECTIVE EXERCISE 8.6
- Do you think it is possible to learn just as much from an article written by a 'consumer' as an article written by a professional? Why, or why not? (And are 'professional' and consumer' necessarily fixed identities?)
- How might our reactions to this question be coloured by dominant discourses we are embedded within? (You might want to go the journal *Archives of General Psychiatry* and choose an article to read; then read Deegan's 1996 article referred to above.)
- What did you learn from each?
- How are they different?

◼ Our use of language

This is a good time to look critically at some of the words we have been using, including 'service user', 'consumer' and 'client', and consider whether, or how, these terms reflect elements of power and knowledge.

According to McLaughlin (2009, p. 1101) the labels we ascribe are very important, 'as they all conjure up differing identities identifying different relationships and differing power dynamics' – they actually tell us something about the nature of social work. In the 1970s, 'client' was the preferred term; this was later critiqued as objectifying – the client was constructed as a passive vessel in need of help, and the social worker as the powerful expert capable of providing this help. The terms 'customer' and 'consumer' emerged in the neoliberal 1980s and 1990s, turning the worker into more of a broker, and implying that the user of social services was able to rationally choose from various welfare commodities that were available. While these may be considered more empowering terms, the actual potential for clients to freely choose among a marketplace of services is questionable. 'Service user' was thought to be a more inclusive term; however, this term may also be critiqued as identifying the totality of the unique individual in terms of one aspect of their experience. Additionally, the division between service user and service provider is problematic as many of us may be both, and it also excludes people who may be in need of assistance but find the stigma of accessing services prohibitive (McLaughlin 2009). McLaughlin suggests that reclassifications of the worker–client relationship might include the term 'experts by experience', which makes a claim for the specialist knowledge life experience engenders; however, life experience does not make us experts in everything. Further suggestions include 'people', 'active consumers' and 'citizens' – each of which contains implications relating to power, voice and knowledge. Citizen, for example, implies equality within a democratic community. Barnes and Bowl (2001) remind us that language is a site of struggle while Pare (2004, p. 76) suggests that the terms that are used to describe people and situations locate us in relations of power.

REFLECTIVE EXERCISE 8.7
- What term would you like to be used to describe you if you were accessing a welfare or human services organisation?
- What term might clients choose if they exercised the power to label social workers in a way they felt encapsulated the worker–client relationship and involvement they experienced?
- Who has the right or the expertise to choose what language is appropriate to describe a person, group or experience at a given time in a given context? Why?

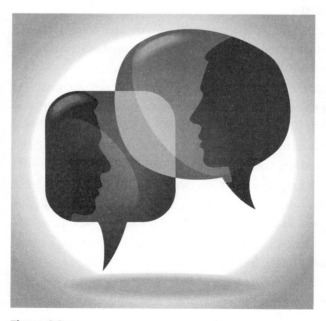

Figure 8.2

■ Including the voices that have been missing

Voices informing service development

The definitional problem leads us to consider what might be the role of consumers or active citizens in the development of services. Do service users have the knowledge, but not necessarily the power, to inform service delivery? Service user or consumer involvement in mental health-care delivery has been increasingly mandated as part of mental health policy and service development in Australia, Canada, the United Kingdom, the United States and other Western nations; however, the potential of this contribution is 'yet to be fully realised' (Healy & Renouf 2005, p. 45). Some service users have developed groundbreaking programs (such as local service user groups, consumer-led organisations, survivor websites and newsletters) and contribute to conventional mental health literature.

However, service user consultation or citizen participation can easily become tokenistic; consider what it would actually mean, in specific contexts, to include 'on equal terms, perspectives and knowledge sources which up until now may have been allowed a very restricted role in the construction of "mental health" ideas and praxis' (Beresford 2005, p. 109). Beresford suggests that key components would include services and support based on self-defined needs and rights; valuing holistic and complementary approaches to support, user-led training and education; encouragement of community development approaches; and developing new roles and approaches in mental health services and support. Some consumer/survivor groups prefer to work outside the conventional service system, arguing that as long as service user involvement is determined by the service provider it will simply reinforce the existing, undemocratic hierarchies of power and knowledge (Stickley 2006, p. 576). From a critical perspective, it is also important to question the assumption that simply 'speaking back to biomedicine' will necessarily be empowering; it can be costly, and some service users may not find telling their stories a rewarding experience; speaking out about one's own experience of depression, for example, when presenting a paper at a mental health conference can feel like a form of professional suicide. Similarly, sharing one's story of psychosis in a support group setting may reveal more than one wants others to know and make the development of ongoing relationships, in which one's personal story is revealed more gradually, difficult. In fact, silence can also be an effective means of agency for 'resisting "technologies of domination" that operate to compel confessions' (Foucault 1978, cited in Gray 2007, p. 427).

Voices informing research

Social work research could provide opportunities for consumers, clients or fellow citizens to move beyond mere participation to sharing leadership roles with practitioners. Turner and Beresford (2005) advocate user-controlled research in preference to other forms of research, including participatory research, because it involves consumers or community members (who are often the ones being researched) determining the aims, methods and uses of the research – not simply participating. We will further discuss missing voices in the development, ownership and implementation of research later in this chapter in relation to cultural imperialism and epistemological racism.

Voices informing education

Related debates take place about the need for service users to be involved in social work education. Some argue that as social work emphasises collaboration, empowerment and the sharing and valuing of diverse knowledge, the inclusion of consumers/clients/citizens in educating social work students is not only desirable, but essential (Pack 2013; Scheyett & Diehl 2004). Scheyett and Diehl describe a one-day workshop in which final-year students and consumers of mental health services engage in structured dialogue aimed at broadening students' awareness of the social work actions that were considered positive and empowering and those that were not.

Voices of carers

While the voice and role of carers is increasingly acknowledged as a vital part of the service system, particularly in relation to mental health, caring continues to be a challenging and often isolating experience for families and other non-professional support people. Shankar and Muthuswamy (2007) found that up to 75 per cent of individuals return home after discharge from Australian psychiatric facilities to families that are poorly equipped and not supported to provide care. This occurs in a context of reduced community services, brief inpatient treatment and poor community follow-up. Disturbingly, all the families they interviewed had experienced powerlessness and invalidation in their interactions with mental health services and workers, who they felt did not listen to them or ask for their opinions. While individuals may not, for varying reasons, want their family members involved, we make the point, from a critical social work perspective, that non-professional insights may be important sources of knowledge and not necessarily inferior to professional viewpoints.

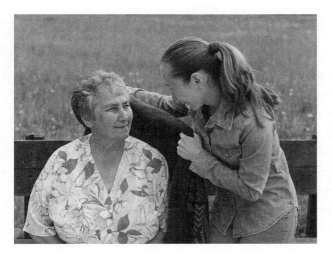

Figure 8.3

■ Diverse knowledge systems and alternative discourses

From a critical perspective we try to resist thinking in *binary* (either/or) terms that position professional knowledge and non-professional knowledge at opposite ends of a continuum, in which one end is valued and the other not. By positioning different forms of knowledge in opposition to one another, productive dialogue is curtailed and some forms of knowledge are potentially marginalised. One of the key tenets of a critical social work approach is the valuing of diverse forms and sources of knowledge and the acknowledgement that there are many truths. In this sense, *poststructural thinking* prioritises local contexts and acknowledges that social practices are complex and multifaceted, as well as shaped by history and culture (Healy 2000, p. 51). Poststructural thinking also draws our attention to ways in which some forms of knowledge, such as bodily and emotional, have been devalued as they do not fit with modernist notions of rationality and scientific fact (Healy 2000, p. 52). Local organisations and community members may have a wealth of knowledge to share, if only we listen and create opportunities for non-hierarchal dialogue and genuine consultation. We have met many people who, while not qualified social workers, work tirelessly to promote wellbeing and social change in their communities, drawing on knowledge and skills they have developed outside the parameters of a university degree. This is particularly true for people who have historically and politically been denied access to obtaining the qualifications that give professional status in Western society, such as indigenous people.

Cultural imperialism
refers to 'the dominance and control of one society's or group's culture by another' (Beilharz & Hogan 2012, pp. 542).

Cognitive imperialism
occurs when a particular way of thinking and expressing knowledge (cognition in the broad sense) is valued, while other ways are belittled or inferiorised.

You may have noticed that this chapter began with the 'inner circle' of the worker and client and has gradually been expanding outward, as we look at power and knowledge and the ways in which our social world and our own practice might exclude or devalue diverse truths and voices. We are now moving on to consider some 'big ideas' in terms of postcolonialism, epistemological racism, **cultural imperialism** and **cognitive imperialism**. While these may seem like abstract or grandiose concepts with little to do with the world of social work practice, as you develop your understanding of their meaning, you may see they have powerful implications for critical social work.

Postcolonialism

Postcolonialism (literally 'after' colonialism) is a contested concept, in that there is no general consensus on exactly what it means. For some, it is an aspiration, not yet achieved, in which the oppressive impact of colonialism would be fully challenged, removed and replaced with a more socially just paradigm; for others, it refers to an historical period that followed the colonial periods of the past; for others still, it is a description of anti-oppressive social attitudes to difference. One way of defining postcolonialism is as the social, political, economic and cultural practices which rise in response and resistance to colonialism (Gandhi 1998). The concept of postcolonialism is particularly relevant to critical social work in Western nation states (such as Australia, Canada and the Americas) and also to other parts of the world where colonisation occurred and where its impacts are still being felt.

In order to understand postcolonialism we need to look first at colonialism and what characterises the relations between colonised peoples and colonisers. Primary among these characteristics is unequal power and the construction of the colonised group in relation to the coloniser's supposed superior knowledge and belief system. Knowledge about the colonised group is produced from the dominant perspective of the coloniser, as if it were the only real knowledge; the coloniser group employs a normalising gaze that assesses the colonised group as its object – according to a hierarchical standard often characterised by the creation of *binary* opposites, in which one side of the binary is considered better than the other. Power is evident in this relationship between the binaries as the less valued side is often defined by virtue of its difference to the dominant side. Examples of this would be culture/nature, civilised/primitive, literate/illiterate, landowners/nomads, rational/irrational and normal/abnormal. Thinking about colonised people as objects creates a social and emotional distance between the coloniser and colonised that enables inhuman and inhumane actions, such as genocide

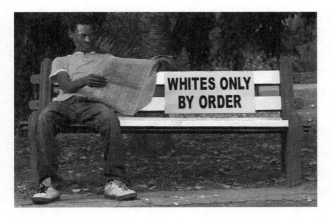

Figure 8.4

of indigenous peoples, to occur. Having control of the political system, education system, language, literature, religion and media ensures for the coloniser power to transmit ideology, values and attitudes, while at the same time destroying and forbidding the continuance of existing systems of local economy, political and spiritual beliefs, institutes, modes of governance and social and familial ties and roles.

> **REFLECTIVE EXERCISE 8.8**
> Read back through the previous paragraph.
> • Can you see how this process has played out in your own country?
> • What is your response to the suggestion that a postcolonialist stance and practice is vital for critical anti-oppressive social work?

Social work, historically, has sadly been implicated in colonialist practices, involving the removal of Aboriginal and Torres Strait Islander children from their families for no other reason than their 'racial identity' (see Haebich 2000 for an in-depth account of Indigenous Australian welfare policies) and the imposition of narrow cultural norms on groups that diverged from white Western practices. Gray (2008) suggests that establishment social work as a profession often exhibits a 'West is best' and 'West to the rest' orientation. This is often done unknowingly, from a position of assumed **normalcy** in which one's own cultural location is invisible. While social work claims to embrace a respect for diversity, without adequate interrogation of one's own cultural location, Gray (2008, p. 1)

Normalcy as used here relates to the way in which the dominant constructions of the 'family' (white, middle-class, heterosexual) are seen as 'normal' while all other family structures are seen as other or deviant (Mullaly 2010).

argues that social workers perpetrate '**professional imperialism**'. The transfer of knowledge from the 'top' (the West) to the 'bottom' (indigenous or developing countries' worldviews) is often one-way, meaning that the possibility of learning from indigenous or developing-world knowledge systems is rarely considered (Gray 2008).

Cognitive imperialism

A related concept is cognitive imperialism, whereby a particular way of thinking and expressing knowledge (cognition in the broad sense) is valued, while others are belittled or inferiorised (Wehbi 2013). An example of this is the notion of literacy – a much prized attainment in Western societies and arguably a necessary one. However, the predominant understanding of what comprises literacy is an example of cognitive imperialism by assuming that a particular means of expression – such as reading and writing (English) – is the sum total of what it means to be literate. Edwards (2010, p. 31) suggests a different definition of literacy, as 'the means with which to express, understand, provide for, and make sense of one's self and whole richness of one's self in its widest cultural, spiritual, intellectual and physical sense'. To be literate in one's environment, then, may mean having an understanding of the plants that provide nourishing food, locating water in dry environments, knowing when a storm is brewing, or empathically relating to people or other **sentient beings**. Literacy may also be described as 'the intelligence with which we meet life' (Olana Kaipo Ai, n.d., cited in Meyer 2003, p. ii).

REFLECTIVE EXERCISE 8.9

How does this different understanding of literacy cause us to question, for example, binary thinking around these concepts: civilised /primitive, literate/illiterate, intelligent/ ignorant and informed/uninformed?

Epistemological racism

Epistemological racism is probably a term most of us do not come across regularly, and on first glance is difficult to pronounce and to understand; you may even be thinking of skipping this paragraph! But we would encourage you to give us a go in explaining it. Basically, the word epistemology refers to how we know things: for example, through scientific experiments that discover universal truths (water always boils at 100°C at sea level); intuition and empathic connection; talking to other people; each person developing their own insights and truths over a lifetime; absorbing and learning from the culture around us; and internalising the dominant discourses we are embedded in. As a university student, you become aware of – and are asked to comply with – the dominant modes of academic learning that suggest, for example, that you learn things through reading what other people have said; and not just any people, but people who have had their work published and are thus considered credible. At times you may have rebelled against the idea that your own views and voice need to be filtered through, or backed up by, references to the literature. However, you are engaged in a process of epistemological learning that has continued over centuries.

Before putting the two words together, epistemological and racism, we should briefly remind ourselves of what we mean by racism and consider the various forms it takes. As we said in Chapter 2 *racism* refers to beliefs, statements or acts that render certain groups inferior on the basis that they do not belong to the culture of origin of the dominant ethnic group within a nation state (Hollinsworth 1997). Furthermore, *racial bias*, according to Scheurich and Young (1997, pp. 4–5) is 'typically understood ... in terms of individual acts of overt prejudice that are racially based' as well as other acts that are more covert; that is, hidden, subtle or not explicitly public. An example of overt racism might be a racist comment made by a lecturer in class against black people; covert racism may take the form of not promoting a minority group employee even though they have the same credentials and/or abilities, or higher, than a dominant group employee. *Institutional racism* exists when organisations, including educational institutions, have standard operating procedures that hurt or exclude members of one group: for example, testing what is congruent with white middle-class notions and values but not with the cultures of students of colour (Scheurich & Young 1997). *Societal racism* exists on a broad society-wide scale when social or cultural assumptions, norms and habits favour one racialised group over one or more other racialised groups; an example might be culturally based assumptions of the ideal family or 'normal' child-rearing. At the next level, *civilisational racism* concerns the way civilisation itself is defined by a dominant group, as to what is civilised and what is primitive, and how worldviews are constructed by dominant thinkers, generally of a particular race and culture (Scheurich & Young 1997). For some centuries, 'white' has implied a 'higher civilization based on superior inheritance' (Hacker 1992, cited in Scheurich & Young 1997, p. 7).

Epistemological racism is perhaps the most invisible form of racism; hence it may take us more time and thinking to understand it.

> We have used the term 'invisible' here and elsewhere for simplicity, but 'invisibilised' is another, perhaps more appropriate, term as it implies an active process, not just an outcome.

It is an important concept for us as critical social workers, as it may undermine our capacity to work and see the world in anti-oppressive ways. Epistemology – or how we know something – is culturally and historically produced according to the *worldviews* and *discourses* that are prominent in a particular time and place. Epistemologies arise 'out of the social history of a particular group' (Scheurich & Young 1997, p. 8) and are further legitimated by educational and other institutions as the 'right' way of producing knowledge and knowing things. In Western nations this means that the dominant race (whites) reflects and reinforces that social history and that racial group, while marginalising the epistemologies of other races and cultures. Often this is an unconscious process; most white researchers and academics do not consciously support racism. However, the uncritical acceptance of what are actually racially biased understandings in teaching, learning and ultimately practising as social workers is something for us to challenge. We can do this in the first instance by being aware of epistemological racism and how it affects our understanding of what is true and right, and supporting the work of diverse groups to develop and legitimise marginalised forms of knowing, researching and practising. In Australia, Indigenous social work is a developing field that will be built over time by Aboriginal and Torres Strait Islander people as a form of social work 'relevant to their communities' but also 'for non-Indigenous social workers as they develop respectful and emancipatory work with their Indigenous colleagues and clients' (Green & Baldry 2008, p. 390).

The exercise of power by dominant groups may range from coercive to persuasive in its methods; whether subtly or more overtly, a dominant group's knowledge system and status is imposed on others and is also accepted or consented to by less dominant groups. One voice becomes dominant; the other voice(s) become(s) **subjugated** as dominant views become 'common sense'. This consent is referred to as *hegemony*. As we stated earlier, hegemony is a term coined by the Italian Marxist Antonio Gramsci to explain the domination of one powerful group over others, where the consent of the subordinated groups is not achieved by physical force, but rather by convincing people it is in their interests to subscribe to the dominant group's ideas (Germov & Poole 2011, p. 114).

Subjugated views are those that differ from, or are alternative positions to, those of the dominant group and, as such, are often discounted and marginalised (Mullaly 2010).

The knowledge of the dominant group is further reflected through social institutions, such as the family, the education system and welfare services. Social work, as we have seen, is on many occasions co-opted into acceptance of dominant discourses – whether they be colonialist, patriarchal or neoliberal. Neoliberal norms are hegemonic today, as we have discussed earlier. These emphasise individualism (Deepak 2012; Gray 2008), competitive measures and consumerism as the best means to express oneself and be a productive member of society. As critical social workers, we propose a '**counter-hegemonic** vision ... of inclusion, community and valuing the contributions and health and well-being of ... marginalised populations' (Deepak 2012, p. 784).

> **Counter-hegemonic** refers to efforts opposing hegemonic power by organising to win a cultural consensus in favour of an alternative social ethic or program (e.g. the anti-apartheid movement, the civil rights movement).

REFLECTIVE EXERCISE 8.10
- How often, as a social work student or practitioner, do you read texts and journal articles from non-Western and non-indigenous authors?
- Have you observed, in your own or another's practice, times when as social workers we play the role of 'visiting expert', specifying the outcomes of practice before engaging in dialogue with the client or community?

■ Working across difference

Critical social workers have been considering the 'dilemma of difference' for decades. In 1985, Martha Minow observed that attempts at empowerment – one of the hallmarks of social work practice – may actually, at times, be disempowering; in other words, explicitly targeting groups in need of empowerment (e.g ethnic groups, people with disabilities, Aboriginal and Torres Strait Islander people) may unintentionally further stigmatise that group (Parker, Fook & Pease 1999). Rather than avoiding this dilemma, Minow (1985, cited in Parker, Fook & Pease 1999, p. 152) suggests we 'immerse ourselves' in it, not necessarily to achieve a resolution but to engage in a 'more productive struggle' for equitable processes and outcomes.

In the 1980s, in opposition to colonial and neo-colonial policies of assimilation, there emerged policies and discourses celebrating cultural diversity, such as **multiculturalism**, which was supposed to

> **Multiculturalism** refers to both the discourse and federal government policy from the 1980s to the early 2000s recognising and celebrating Australian cultural diversity and affirming that all cultural groups have equal rights to services and development.

Reconciliation is a contested concept; at its simplest, it refers to estranged parties becoming friendly, harmonious and compatible.

affirm that each cultural or ethnic group had the same rights to services and development as any other group in society. Policies of self-determination and **reconciliation** with Aboriginal and Torres Strait Islander people were likewise meant to recognise the unique history and situation of Australia's first inhabitants, with a view to redressing their particular needs and disadvantage. Sadly, however, and often with tragic results, 'stories of diversity are also stories of injustice, oppression and privilege' (Quinn 2009, p. 92). Although the terms 'race' and 'racism'[1] are contentious and rightly so, Quinn suggests that the language of race can be helpful in exposing the operation of power, privilege and oppression that still characterise nation states such as Australia. Citing Dominelli (2008), she identifies race and racism as 'the attitudes and processes involved in categorising, stereotyping, and assigning value and power to people on the basis of their differences, including physical attributes (particularly colour) and culture and language – processes of "racialisation" and "politicisation"' (Quinn 2008, p. 93). A key component of this discussion, from a critical perspective, is that racism is not simply an issue for the people who are marginalised and oppressed by racial constructions, but that everyone is involved in race relations. In the Australian context,

White privilege refers to superiority presumed by those with white skin as dominant members of society, thus affording benefits over those with non-white skin. This attitude contributes to racism (Hollinsworth 2006).

where the dominant racialised group consists of (largely white) descendants of the British colonisers, this turns the focus to those who benefit from **white privilege**, often in ways are that are invisible to that group but very visible to the groups who suffer and are silenced as a result (McIntosh 1998; Pease 2010). Privilege has also been described as a form of unearned advantage (Bailey 2004) that enables assets to accrue to members of dominant groups simply on the basis of being born into that group: for example, being white in a racially biased country, or male in a patriarchal society, or heterosexual in a homophobic society. Bailey (2004, p. 306) contrasts these unearned advantages or privileges with 'earned advantages' that accrue when a person works hard to buy a house or obtain a degree. However, even earned advantages may be easier to obtain for those who benefit from, for example, white privilege.

---

[1] While the language of 'white' and 'black' is useful in highlighting power and injustice, as well as difference, such language can also be dangerous as it categorises people in narrow, simplistic and fixed ways (Quinn 2009).

Concepts of oppression and privilege are crucial to the practice of critical social work, and to an understanding of how some voices are silenced, marginalised and not treated as legitimate, while others come to represent the 'norm' and a standard to which all are expected to ascribe. In an article entitled 'About being Mununga (white-fella): Making covert group racism visible', Kessaris (2006, p. 347) describes how racism in Australia 'commonly occurs as normal, shared, social activity amongst ordinary decent, Mununga [white/non-Aboriginal] folk, [covertly] linked to colonial beliefs and practices'. She goes on to describe how potentially well-meaning Mununga exhibit racism on a day-to-day basis without even knowing it, grouping these practices under five themes. In brief, the first theme is 'making, unmaking and remaking the Mununga self' – a practice in which dominant discourses co-opt Mununga individuals into oppression of blackfellas by accepting negative stereotypes, and remaining ignorant of the violent history of colonisation and its ongoing impacts. In other words, the marginalisation of Aboriginal people is accepted as normal. The second theme, which is closely related, is a 'deep shared understanding' that positions Aboriginal people as unworthy in Australian society. The third theme is that of 'violence, silence and benevolence' – often manifested in silence that tacitly condones ongoing threats and experiences of violence that have been perpetrated on Aboriginal people since colonisation. Kessaris takes the definition of violence further, by observing that benevolence and charity can be passive forms of violence as they set up uneven power dynamics and maintain power with Mununga.

Kessaris' fourth theme is that of racist practice, which she refers to as 'unconstrained Mununga talk' – 'talk that knows no courtesy boundaries, is passively or benevolently violent ... [is] characterised by a sense of entitlement and is legitimating of land theft as one of its primary purposes' (2006, p. 350). This includes white people speaking about Aboriginal people, often in their presence, as if they were not there; the example is given of black students in mainstream classrooms. The final theme is 'turning things around', which refers to how white people absolve themselves of responsibility for injustices experienced by black people, with blacks seen as the cause of the problems. For example, 'the White problem of indiscriminate prejudice and unearned privilege was inverted to be "the Black problem" of primitiveness, non-adaptability and poverty' (Kessaris 2006, p. 357). She concludes that until white people take responsibility for and work to eradicate racism, no real progress can be made. This needs more than cultural awareness training; it requires 'understanding the self in the midst of unbalanced power relationships', and working as allies with Aboriginal people to develop counternarratives that name and challenge colonial attitudes, talk and behaviour (Kessaris 2006, pp. 358–9).

REFLECTIVE EXERCISE 8.12

In relation to cultural awareness, Kessaris (2006, p. 358) poses several questions we might ask ourselves:

- Who have we been socialised to feel and behave superior or inferior to?
- How might we be colluding with the oppression of others or self-oppression?
- What can we do to work against the pressure of compliance in order to break the cycle of normalised racism?

The makeup of professional bodies often mirrors the power dynamics and cultural assumptions of the wider society in which they are situated. In an article outlining the findings of her research project, Bennett (2013) explores barriers to successful engagement between Aboriginal and Torres Strait Islander social workers and the Australian professional body, the AASW. Interviews with Aboriginal and Torres Strait Islander social workers across Australia raised issues such as cultural safety, tokenism and lack of connection with the individuals who led the organisation. Participants also felt that the AASW had not adequately recognised the ongoing impacts of colonialism, were pretending that racism was 'over and done with' and that 'the discussion of Whiteness is so dominant at the moment that to even suggest these things to people can make them feel insulted, challenged and uncomfortable' (Bennett 2013, p. 7). Genuine change was needed, participants suggested, to move beyond rhetoric and pose this challenge to social workers:

> If you say you are committed and you put these words in books and you don't have any actions that go with that – that is a form of theft. Because what you are doing is

stealing to bolster your own image by being associated with saying these things but if you never follow through … you are taking from Aboriginal and Torres Strait Islander people and giving nothing back (Bennett 2013, p. 9).

Participants provided a number of recommendations to address racism within the social work profession.

REFLECTIVE EXERCISE 8.13

Access and read this article: B. Bennett, 'Stop deploying your white privilege on me! Aboriginal and Torres Strait Islander engagement with the Australian Association of Social Workers', *Australian Social Work*, 2013, http://www.tandfonline.com/doi/abs/10.1080/0312407X.2013.840325#.U0TOFqLm7Sd.

What are the author's recommendations? What is your response to this reading?

Cultural awareness

This brings us to a discussion of culture and cultural awareness. As Quinn (2009, pp. 97–8) states, 'culture' is a frequently used term, which aims to describe the complex and 'distinctive ways of life and shared values, beliefs and meanings common to groups of people … the understandings and expectations which guide actions and interactions with others'. In our globalised world we need to have knowledge and awareness of our cultural location, as well as particular cultural knowledge of others with whom we work and live. To remain culturally ignorant is antithetical to critical social work practice: 'an informed and particular cultural knowledge is essential for "just" and healing practice' (Quinn 2009, p. 99). Uncritical acceptance of Western understandings and theories runs the risk of harming and oppressing those we claim to be helping; for example, when working with children and families it is important to listen to and learn from the cultural context of that family and the cultural nuances of identity, belonging and meaningfulness they find important.

You have probably heard of the phrase 'a little bit of knowledge is a dangerous thing': in the context of cultural practice this is particularly so. Waldegrave (1990, cited in Quinn 2009, p. 101) warns against the sort of 'cultural tourism' that dupes workers into 'moving around culture' in insensitive and ignorant ways. Operating from a position of inadequate knowledge can also lead workers to collude with stereotypes and retreat to a position of judgement based on uncritical assumptions.

In recent years, cultural awareness training has become popular across organisations, from commercial to non-profit to governmental. This training takes various approaches, and is no doubt well intended and beneficial to many. However, as Quinn points out, some of the theory underpinning cross-cultural practice fails to acknowledge that the issue is not simply diversity, but the historical legacy, social structures and processes of racism, oppression and privilege at personal and structural levels. Learning about cultural diversity, meaning and ways is a lifelong and ongoing process of negotiation and commitment that requires accepting the position of learner with respect and humility, and a willingness to give up the position of dominance. This may involve exposure to, and immersion in, particular cultural contexts and the ability to experience both discomfort and enlightenment.

■ The voice of the planet (through a human lens)

Finally, we turn to an aspect of social work ethics, vision and practice that draws our critical attention back to what is often called the cornerstone of social work: a focus on the person in environment. But how do we define 'environment'? Establishment social work has tended to focus on the individual's immediate social context, from the family to the immediate system of supports and resources available to the client. Structural approaches to social work broadened the environmental focus to include social inequalities and patterns of oppression that surround and shape the individual and their community. Social constructionist and poststructural perspectives have further extended the social work lens to consider the role of discourse in constructing our experience of the environment and that there is no direct access to the natural world except through our social constructions. This includes new conceptualisations of identity and power in acknowledging the complexity of one's environment. However, there is still an important voice that is missing in social work discourse: the voice of the planet, of the natural world and all living beings.

In recent years, social work academics and practitioners have drawn our attention to green social work (Dominelli 2012), ecosocial work (Norton 2012), the integration of nature into social work (Heinsch 2012), environmental justice (Miller, Hayward & Shaw 2012), environmental ethics in social work (Gray & Coates 2012) and the nexus between social work and the environment (McKinnon 2008). Although the focus of each is somewhat different, they are all suggesting that social work should be concerned about the natural environment, and that we have lagged behind others in acknowledging our responsibility. In terms of green social work, there are a variety of approaches to non-human nature and the environment, ranging from more conservative anthropocentric or human-centred approaches to radically eco-centric or nature-centred approaches. The former propose that nature should be protected as it provides health benefits for people: that humans have an innate need to be connected somehow to the natural world and that this connection promotes wellbeing (Heinsch 2012). The latter approaches, by contrast, suggest that the ecosystem and other living beings do not exist for human purposes but have their own integrity and purposes, in which human beings have only a minor (often destructive) role. Both perspectives have something to offer social work and it is important to avoid reinforcing destructive binaries between human beings and nature. After all, human beings are part of nature and we need to find ways to live in a sustainable harmony with our environment.

REFLECTIVE EXERCISE 8.14
- Should social workers be concerned about climate change, global warming, environmental degradation, pollution, chemical contamination, the wellbeing of non-human animals, sustainable agriculture and the protection of wilderness? (See Gray & Coates 2012, p. 239.)
- Why or why not?

In our industrialised Western world, where relatively few totally untouched environments remain, perhaps nature can be defined as:

> the spectrum of habitats from wilderness areas to farms and gardens ... [as well as] any single element of the natural environment (such as plants, animals, soil, water or air) and includes domestic and companion animals as well as cultivated pot plants (Maller et al., cited in Heinsch 2012, pp. 310–11).

Nature is thought to have soothing and calming effects that are experienced by living close to large green spaces; being in the outdoors, whether farming, gardening or trekking; or simply viewing images of the natural world. Living with companion animals, sharing outdoor adventures with others and working in community gardens have been further identified as sources of comfort and social connectedness (Heinsch 2012). These are elements we can incorporate into our social work practice in a range of settings.

From a critical perspective, it is essential to improve our awareness of the importance of the human–animal bond for many people with whom we work. This has important implications for service delivery and our practice (Morley & Fook 2005). We also need to expand the moral framework by seriously considering the plight of creatures besides human beings, and formulating practice responses to animal cruelty, exploitation and oppression, as well as championing the rights of animals as we do with human beings (Ryan, T. 2011).

We (the authors) have been variously involved in assisting the broadening of the traditional understandings of our practice with environment by developing shared

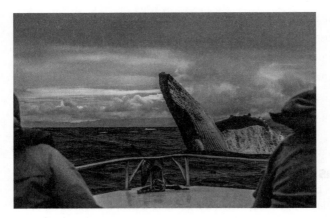

Figure 8.5

gardens in residential services, taking groups camping to relax in less urbanised areas, and supporting people who are grieving due to the loss of a companion animal. These are all simple ways of enabling the missing voice of the natural world to be heard in our lives.

In the Australian context, McKinnon (2008) describes some of the challenges involved in bringing environmental consciousness into the realm of social work practice: high levels of managerialism that question the value of work considered 'non-core', lack of evidence that environmental interests are important, and poor links in university curricula between social justice, environmental justice and sustainability. She draws attention to some key environmental issues facing Australia, which include an ever-decreasing number of bird and mammal species; the damming and regulation of waterways; rising salinity; deterioration in the health of water bodies; and habitat loss that has occurred since colonisation resulting from cropping, grazing, forestry, mining and human settlement. McKinnon (2008) points to expectations that environmental refugees will swell in numbers in coming years as sea levels and global temperatures rise, as environmental pollutants affect health, and as the environmental degradation of land, coastal ecosystems and fisheries result in loss of livelihood and displacement. She suggests that an awareness of the social consequences of environmental issues is vital for social workers.

The importance of human interconnection with nature has also been theorised in terms of alienation, suggesting that alienation from the natural world – the planet as a whole – is a key source not only of environmental but personal problems (Norton 2009, cited in Norton 2012, p. 299). Social workers such as Coates (2003, cited in Norton 2012, p. 301) have been critical of the ways in which traditional social work ('a domesticated profession') has focused on helping people adjust to the stresses of modern life, instead of promoting a new paradigm in which we connect with our ecological selves. Ecosocial work draws us to advocacy around policies that enhance rather than destroy the natural world, by partnering with environmental organisations, working to embed connectedness with nature in institutional settings where we work and supporting community actions promoting environmental sustainability, as well as understanding how the lives of those with whom we work may be impacted by connection or lack thereof with the natural world. Eco-spirituality has long been recognised by indigenous cultures, and in this aspect especially, social work theory and practice can be significantly enhanced by learning from indigenous knowledge systems.

Neoliberalism's uncritical focus on economic growth is antithetical to a principled critical social work approach that incorporates a sense of environmental ethics. Exploitation of the earth has resulted in social injustice and poverty for many who inhabit our planet, while providing riches for others (Gray & Coates 2012; McKinnon 2008; Miller, Hayward & Shaw 2012). It is argued that those most affected by degradation of the natural environment are the poor and marginalised people of the world. Miller, Hayward and Shaw (2012, p. 272, citing Claudio 2007) point out that a social work approach based on notions of environmental justice is attuned to how 'race, ethnicity, socioeconomic status, immigration status, lack of land ownership, geographic isolation, formal education, occupational characteristics, political power [and] gender' all put people at disproportionate risks of being exposed to environmental hazards. Social work's response, they suggest, should be aligned with principles of environmental justice that are cognisant of the impacts of resource depletion on local communities, promote community solidarity around environmental issues, draw attention to and protect people's rights to safe and healthy environments, and educate present and future generations on environmental issues. Gray and Coates (2012, p. 241) suggest that as a profession social work 'needs to walk a fine line between enlightened self-interest, which saves nature so humans can survive, and an ecocentric approach, which values nature for the sake of nature'.

REFLECTIVE EXERCISE 8.15
- Does social work have a responsibility to the natural world, and, if so, is this because of its impact on humans, or because the natural world is valuable in its own right?
- Going back to previous discussions about binary thinking, is constructing life in terms of human/non-human or man/nature an example of binary thinking. If so, what are the impacts of thinking in this way? Where does this discourse of separation come from?

The realm of eco-psychology suggests a link between our disconnection from nature, the destruction of the natural environment and an intensification of human problems; in other words, our *anthropocentric* focus has not only put at risk our survival but also our mental health and capacity to form nurturing and empathic relations (Norton 2011). In this sense, we play into the hands of individualising neoliberal ideology by rejecting our inherent interdependence as a species. Canadian professor of social work Cassandra Hanrahan (2011) has suggested social work should challenge anthropocentrism on the basis of our ethical and spiritual value base. Extending arguments that social work has neglected the role of nature generally in wellbeing, she turns the focus specifically on 'interspecies interactions to consider all the inhabitants of the Earth and their experiences of environments managed by humans' (Hanrahan 2011, p. 277). An holistic anti-oppressive approach, she contends, needs to acknowledge the significance of human–animal bonds, the welfare of non-human animals generally and ecological sustainability within nature. Human beings, she posits, compromise their own integrity by continually positioning themselves as the 'conceptual centre of the universe' (Hanrahan 2011, p. 278). The commodification of virtually everything in a capitalist society, coupled with neoliberalism's narrow focus on economic rationalism and 'survival of the fittest' in the marketplace, may mean that critical social workers, now more than ever, cannot continue to engage in the sort of *speciesism* that places a lesser value on non-human species in the web of life. Hudson (2011, p. 1675) puts it beautifully when she says:

> To become truly human requires a different kind of becoming animal, and a different mode of relating to animals and our own animality. We need not stand outside the

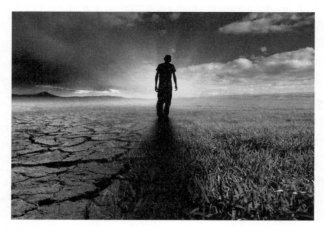

Figure 8.6

natural world as observers. We need to engage it as participants in a metabolism of the nature.

REFLECTIVE EXERCISE 8.16

What do you think? Should social workers be concerned with factory farming, cruelty to domesticated animals, animal experimentation, diminishing wilderness and species extinction? Why or why not?

REFLECTIVE EXERCISE 8.17

Refer back to the section in Chapter 1 where we outlined the key tenets of a critical approach.

• How does the material covered in this chapter 'fit' with that section?
• Has this material broadened your idea of whom we might work with as social workers, or the sort of practices in which we might be engaged? How?

■ Summary

Despite all we have said in this chapter, the task of the critical social worker is not necessarily to uncover hidden voices – this in itself implies the power to do things to others. The voices are already there: the voices of different truths, cultural wisdom, lived experiences, subjugated discourses, the voices of nature. Social workers can learn from these voices and advocate for them to be heard in their own right but only if we are first attentive enough to hear them and listen carefully. There are many other missing voices in social work, as in every discipline: novels, films, poems, music all have the potential to move us, inform us and present their own truths. One of us recently asked a group of students, in a class where they were discussing poststructural identities, to write a three-line description of themselves. Many wrote a description that described their social roles (mother, support worker, and so on), but one student wrote the most beautiful poem about his relationship with the ocean and with others he met on his life journey. The class then discussed how easy it would be, in the course of a potentially lengthy worker–client relationship, to never hear or know this aspect of the person's identity and what a loss that would be to understanding and working together.

■ Review questions

- Why is it important for social workers to understand power (both in relation to social structures and systems and our relationships with service users)?
- What voices or sources of knowledge are important to developing and practising critical social work?
- How might social workers encourage these voices to be heard?
- How has your understanding of racism, oppression and privilege expanded through engaging with this chapter?

■ Further reading

Fraser, H. and Briskman, L., 2013, 'Through the eye of a needle: The challenge of getting justice in Australia if you are indigenous or seeking asylum' in I. Ferguson, M. Lavalette and E. Whitmore, eds, *Globalisation, Global Justice and Social Work*, Taylor & Francis, Abingdon.

Hanrahan, C., 2011, 'Challenging anthropocentricism in social work through ethics and spirituality: Lessons from studies in human–animal bonds', *Journal of Religion and Spirituality in Social Work: Social Thought*, 30 (3): 272–93.

Kessaris, T. N., 2006, 'About being Mununga (whitefella): Making covert group racism visible', *Journal of Community & Applied Social Psychology*, 16: 347–62.

McIntosh, P., 1998, 'White privilege: Unpacking the invisible knapsack' in M. McGoldrick, ed, *Re-visioning Family Therapy: Race, Culture and Gender in Clinical Practice*, The Guildford Press, New York.

McKinnon, J., 2008, 'Exploring the nexus between social work and the environment', *Australian Social Work*, 61 (3): 256–68.

Quinn, M., 2009, 'Towards anti-racist and culturally affirming practices' in J. Allan, L. Briskman and B. Pease, eds, *Critical Social Work: Theories and Practices for a Socially Just World*, 2nd edn, Allen & Unwin, Crows Nest, NSW.

Volume 21, 2012, of the *International Journal of Social Welfare* (focuses on social work and the environment).

9

Fields of practice

■ Introduction

THIS CHAPTER DRAWS on our own and other authors' research and experience to introduce you to a range of social work practice fields and some of the current debates within those fields. We have already covered several fields of practice throughout this text, such as unemployment (and masculinity issues – see the case study of Peter in Chapter 3); working across difference, and with 'missing voices' (Chapter 8); health (and issues associated with masculinity, ageing, grief and loss, and working with migrants – see the case study of Giuseppe in Chapter 6); and sexual assault (see the case study of Sarah in Chapter 7), and touched on other fields, such as homelessness and substance abuse (both addressed in Chapter 2). In this chapter we focus on the fields of aged care, mental health and child protection. We have deliberately chosen these fields because historically, critical practice has only been considered possible in community-based organisations with an explicit mandate for social change. It has been, and still is, assumed that critical practice in mental health, child protection and aged care settings is extremely difficult (if not impossible). This chapter discusses the relevance of critical approaches and their potential to inform social work in all fields of practice, especially those fields in which critical practice is seen to be at odds with the dominant discourses and associated institutional structures and cultures.

Before exploring our three areas of focus, it must be said that fields of practice, although spoken of as discrete areas, often intersect and overlap. For example, if we are working in a sexual assault service, our work with people may cover grief and loss, substance abuse, disability issues, health and mental health, housing and homelessness, unemployment and poverty, cross-cultural issues, and so on. This reflects the complexity of human experience as well as the ripple effect that certain experiences can potentially have on all aspects of one's life. Another example of this crossover of issues may be seen if we take the example of working in the housing field. As you may know, homelessness occurs on a number of levels. Primary homelessness refers to people without conventional accommodation, living on the streets, under bridges, and so on. Secondary homelessness refers to people moving between various forms of temporary shelter – for example, friends, emergency accommodation and hostels. Finally, tertiary homelessness means people living permanently in single rooms in private boarding houses without security of tenure, nor a bathroom or kitchen to call their own (Kunnen & McKay 2009). While the 'presenting problem' (most obvious immediate concern) is the housing issue, unless other aspects of the person's experience are addressed – physical and mental health, safety, financial issues, poverty, past trauma, lack of support systems, institutionalisation, drug or alcohol issues, oppression in various forms – simply finding the person a place to live may not enable them to live well or to maintain their residency. From a critical perspective, services aim to respond to service users' immediate need for shelter, and additionally address and respond to a range of other related issues and needs, while simultaneously working towards broader structural changes to inhibit the social, political and economic inequalities that contribute to homelessness.

REFLECTIVE EXERCISE 9.1

Using a search engine, such as Google, try to find a homelessness program and see how the service describes its work. How does it acknowledge the complexity and multilayered experience and needs of service users?

The following sections will look at a number of fields of practice from a critical perspective. As you read, keep in mind that while we are constructing various fields of practice as separate spheres of activity, they will undoubtedly interact with other fields of practice and should not be considered in isolation.

■ Aged care

Because critical reflection on our own assumptions and beliefs is an important part of social work practice, we'll start this section with an exercise.

REFLECTIVE EXERCISE 9.2

What does the phrase 'aged care' conjure up for you? Does an image come to mind? Where does this image come from and how does it make you feel or think about being old? (What's the difference between ageing and being old?)

By engaging with reflective exercise 9,2, we have already begun to think critically about the field of practice often known as aged care. When we put on our professional hat, we do not leave our own views, values and biases behind: whatever stage of life we are currently at, we will have some understanding of what it means to be old, whether it is based on observations, experience, or dominant discourses and images that surround us. It is important to be aware of how these personal and social perspectives shape our work with others. Whether we work specifically in this field of practice or not, we may work with older people or their families. As the concept of 'aged care' may be laden with negative connotations for many of us, we might consider whether the phrase 'working with older people' enables us to refrain from 'othering' and engage more positively with people experiencing 'late adulthood' (Harms 2010).

REFLECTIVE EXERCISE 9.3

When is someone old? Is being old a generalisable category or is the experience different based on gender, race/culture, income, place of living, traumas experienced through life course, whether coupled or single, whether straight or gay?

Late adulthood is defined by Hutchinson (2003, cited in Harms 2010, pp. 359–60) as age 65 onwards, with 'young old age' ranging from 65 to 74 years, 'middle old age' from 75 to 84 years, and the 'oldest old' covering age 85 and over. In Australia, as in other Western countries, the population is ageing as people are living longer and birth rates are falling (Jamrozik 2009, p. 104). The ageing of the population is often constructed in economic and social terms as a problem and looming crisis: with relatively fewer taxpayers to fill government coffers, who will pay for the care and support of the growing aged population? One answer to this has been the policy development of superannuation as an enforced means of individuals saving money for their retirement. This fits with neo-liberal discourses of individual rather than state responsibility. However, from a critical perspective, reliance on superannuation demonstrates the lack of wealth and assets of much of the ageing population. While some may look forward to a comfortable, well-resourced and secure old age, others may worry about how they will cope, particularly if they do not own a home and have accumulated little superannuation.

Older adults may experience vulnerabilities not only in relation to income and housing, but also in relation to health. While many older adults do not fit the clichéd image of frailty, ineptitude and sexlessness (Macnab 1992 cited in Harms 2010, p. 360), health can be an issue. A significant proportion of government expenditure on health is for services to the aged population as older people experience more health problems, use medical

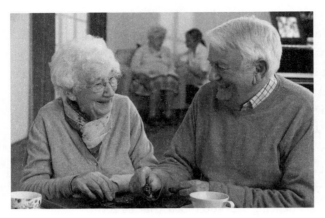

Figure 9.1

services more often and use more medications than younger people: most services for 'the aged' are health-related (Jamrozik 2009). Social policy directions in recent years have been aimed at developing programs and initiatives to support people as long as possible to remain at home; despite changing demographics and the rising participation of women in the paid workforce, women remain primary caregivers well into old age.

REFLECTIVE EXERCISE 9.4
- Why might we have put 'the aged' in quotation marks?
- What are we trying to draw attention to?

As previously mentioned, from a critical perspective we are mindful that categorising people into a universalised group, such as 'the aged' (or 'youth' or 'migrants'), can in some ways gloss over or negate the great diversity within that category and the unique needs and experiences of individuals. As well as this diversity, we know there may be shared experiences as well. For example, one common experience for older people may be described as *ageism*: that a person's age sets them apart or divides them from the rest of society in terms of power, resources and the way they are perceived by others, which they then may internalise.

REFLECTIVE EXERCISE 9.5
- Do we live in an ageist society – say, a society that glorifies youthfulness?
- (How) are older people oppressed?
- How might your response be different based on your own age and experiences?

Neil Thompson's (1998) work on oppression and discrimination remains seminal in teasing out what is meant by ageism and how this attitude generates oppression and discrimination for (at least some) older people. He uses the words **stereotyping**, **invisibilisation**, **marginalisation**, **infantilisation**, **medicalisation**, **dehumanisation** and **trivialisation** to help us understand what oppression and discrimination actually mean in daily experience. A crucial role for us, as critical social workers, is to be mindful of and challenge these forms of oppression in our day-to-day interactions with older people, as well as at the organisational or service delivery level, and in terms of policy advocacy and research.

From a critical perspective we acknowledge that various elements of oppression or privilege are likely to intersect in old age. For example, we would be mindful of gender and how ageing may in some ways be experienced differently by men and women. Grenier (2008) and other feminist writers (e.g. Estes 2005; Fausto-Sterling 1999) suggest that women, throughout their life course in a patriarchal society, are often judged by physical appearance; thus older women may come to define themselves negatively as their physical body matures and changes. Women may also take pride throughout their lives in their multitasking skills, as they care for and nurture others as well as lead active and fulfilling lives; their sense of self may be affected as becoming older impacts on these personally and socially desirable activities. As critical social workers, we need to be attentive to the narratives of complex and unique individual women, which may contain elements of loss and rupture (from a previous sense of self) as well as strength, empowerment and liberation (Grenier 2008; Maidment & Macfarlane 2011).

Negative social images of older age can be internalised as depression or anxiety. Older people may be experiencing grief or feelings of loss in relation to various aspects of their life, including loss of loved ones, degrees of loss of independence (for example, having to give up one's driver's licence, or even one's home) and loss of youth (Grenier 2008; Harms 2010). An overemphasis on risk and health care may mean that, as workers, we ignore or minimise emotional and other important elements of life experience. Sometimes we are able to work with an older person over a period of time, but often our work with older people will be at times of crisis, change and transition; our task

Stereotyping refers to an oversimplified, biased and inflexible conception of a social group (Thompson 1998).

Invisibilisation refers to the process of making a group invisible through under-representation in public discourse (Thompson 1998).

Marginalisation is the process of decentring and/or pushing someone or something else to the margins of society (excluding them from meaningful participation) (Thompson 1998).

Infantilisation involves treating individuals or a group of people like babies or children (Thompson 1998).

Medicalisation places people in the domain of the medical profession (so they are ascribed a sick or invalid status) (Thompson 1998).

Dehumanisation involves treating individuals or a group of people as objects (Thompson 1998).

Trivialisation entails not taking a group of people's views, issues and self-definitions seriously (Thompson 1998).

is to work positively with people who are potentially experiencing complex and frightening situations (Ray & Phillips 2002, p. 203). At the same time, our critical perspective directs our practice in terms of critical reflection and critical action (Ray & Phillips 2002).

Critical action is concerned with tackling inequalities and working towards empowerment of service users in the face of disempowering structural circumstances (Ray & Phillips 2002). This can be encapsulated in small yet important acts, such as exploring how service users see their problems and issues, or ensuring that the voice of the older person is heard in decision making about their lives. Our task is to challenge assumptions (our own included) that buy into ageist attitudes, such as a tendency to categorise all older people as the same. Black (2009, citing Victor 1991) suggests that this is one of the strongest stereotypes in relation to older people and minimises or ignores how health, culture, living arrangements, sexuality, mental health, and/or (dis)ability may create diverse experiences of older age. There are great differences, for example, in assets and income, with older women particularly susceptible to living on very limited incomes. As critical social workers we need to be mindful of, and challenge, the tendency for older people to be lumped into a 'problem' category that negates or minimises their diversity, complex life narratives and self-definition (Chambers 2004; Maidment & Macfarlane 2011).

Sexuality and aged care

In a *heterosexist* (or *homophobic*) society, gay and lesbian elders face discrimination in old age, as throughout their life course. In a research project exploring the experiences of lesbian, gay, bisexual, transgender and intersex (LGBTI) seniors in aged care services, Barrett (2008) identified a number of core issues, which in turn point to suggestions for critical practice. One key issue was the impact of historical experiences of discrimination – many LGBTI seniors had never experienced a time when they felt safe disclosing their sexual/gender identity because they feared disclosure would result in discrimination or a diminished standard of care. On the whole, they did not feel that aged care service providers understood what LGBTI culture means, or how to meet their needs. The impact of identity concealment further meant that some LGBTI seniors suffered from depression and other negative experiences. At the same time, some LGBTI seniors were unable to hide their sexual/gender identity and were thus exposed to discrimination. The impact of dementia may further complicate their needs to have their relationships recognised and be protected from discrimination by staff and other clients in aged care services (Barrett 2008).

Examples of heterosexist privilege

- I can talk about the romantic getaway my husband and I are planning for our anniversary and expect nods, winks and smiles. I have never been accused of being 'disgusting', of flaunting my sexuality, or of being obsessed with sex for sharing this.
- I never worry my children will be rejected at school because their mommy loves a man (or their daddy loves a woman).
- I have never been accused of hating women because I am married to a man.
- If my teenage daughter is having problems with her boyfriend, I can be sure that a school counsellor will be willing to talk to her and to assure her that she is normal.
- I have never feared my child would be taken away from me based solely on the gender of whom I loved.
- I've never been asked if I'm heterosexual because I have [had] a bad homosexual experience.
- I proudly display a picture of my family on my desk at work. I do not fear I will lose my job or the respect of my co-workers.
- When questioned about my family or relaying the events of the weekend, I do not have to think of creative ways to talk about my husband without ever referring to his gender.
- My romantic relationships have never been reduced to being based upon a preferred sex act.
- I can turn on the TV, go to a movie or flip through a magazine on a daily basis without ever seeing anything that testifies to the existence of any relationship that isn't heterosexual like my own.
- No one assumes my husband is just a good friend or my brother.
- When I mention I am married no one asks me why I have to tell them about my sex life.
- When my fiancée and I shopped for rings, we never feared ridicule from the salespeople.
- I have never had to leave my religious institution because condemnation of my relationship was preached from the pulpit.

As critical workers, we need to ensure that we do not contribute to discriminatory behaviours; indeed, our role is to skilfully challenge heterosexism and homophobia by making connections with the LGBTI community and creating a safe environment in which one's sexuality/gender can be expressed without fear of discrimination. Support for LGBTI-specific services and the need for education on the needs of LGBTI seniors in mainstream aged care services have been identified as key strategies to address the range of concerns expressed in research such as that conducted by Barrett (2008).

REFLECTIVE EXERCISE 9.7

- How might we embrace diversity in our work with older people? Using an internet search engine see if you can find aged care services that cater to the specific needs of various groups – for example, Indigenous aged care, Greek or Vietnamese aged care, or LGBTI aged care.
- What might dominant groups learn from diverse cultural approaches to aged care?

Before moving on to the next section on mental health as a field of practice, you might also want to think briefly about any implications from the previous section for understanding and working with Giuseppe (our case study from Chapter 6).

■ Mental health

The field of mental health is a huge area, permeating every other field of practice, and we will only scratch the surface in relation to critical approaches in mental health in this section. To start, you might wish to revisit some of the key concepts integral to a critical approach in social work, as outlined in Chapter 1.

In Australia and other Western countries, the biomedical or medical model is the approach to mental illness adopted by most doctors, psychiatrists and other mental health professionals, based on the idea that 'organic or biomedical causes will eventually be found for all forms of mental disorder' (Golightley 2008, p. 22). The 'psychiatric establishment', according to Fabrega (2008, p. 183), remains 'society's officially recognised organ [handling] a special class of behaviour conditions'. Doctors (psychiatrists or GPs) provide an assessment of the individual's disorder in the form of a diagnosis that acts as a pathway to specialised care and treatment, often in the form of prescribed medications (Golightley 2008, p. 25). The diagnosis is based on the *Diagnostic and Statistical Manual of Mental Disorders* of the American Psychiatric Association, often referred to as the DSM. Currently in its fifth version, it has grown from a 'small spiral-bound notebook of less than 150 pages' that clinicians could purchase for less than $5 in 1968 (Kutchins & Kirk 1997, p. 40) to the latest revision, DSM-V (2013), comprising 991 pages.

Areas of significant expansion in recent revisions have included mental and behavioural disorders of children, and sexual function disorders among women. Simultaneously, pharmaceutical companies, often the sponsors of mental health research, have continued to expand, heavily marketing their products among medical professionals; so much so that it has been argued that they now play a significant role in shaping the way we view the nature of psychiatric disorders and how they are best treated (Moncrieff 2006, p. 124; Timimi 2006). A diagnosis of mental illness may be experienced in different ways by different people at different times – sometimes as a relief to 'know what's wrong', sometimes as a useful gateway to psychiatric medication and counselling, sometimes as an oppressive and stigmatising label that does not take account of the wholeness of the person. You may have had your own experience of being diagnosed with a mental illness, or have seen this happen to someone in your family or friendship circle. Your own experience has likely created a particular view or bias about the oppressive or beneficial nature of diagnosis.

REFLECTIVE EXERCISE 9.8
Watch the first 10 minutes (or the whole clip if you have time) of this documentary: 'Diagnostic and Statistical Manual: Pyschiatry's Deadliest Scam', http://www.cchr.org/videos/diagnostic-statistical-manual.html.
    What are your personal and professional responses to this short video?

Mary Boyle (2007), Professor of Clinical Psychology at the University of East London, has suggested that psychiatric diagnosis should be abandoned entirely, not only because people's behaviour and emotions do not fit neatly into diagnostic categories, but also because diagnostic categories are poor predictors of outcomes, interventions or experiences. Dr Rufus May, a psychologist, highlights the importance of finding out how mental health service users experience being given a diagnosis. One of the criticisms made by consumers/survivors of the top-down medical model approach is that once a diagnosis is given, mental health professionals tend to focus on professional interventions and neglect the expertise of the consumer/survivor. May (2007, pp. 3–4) adopts what he calls a community psychology approach, which 'puts service users' views at the centre', helping people express their experience in their own terms and facilitating opportunities for self-help, recovery and peer mentoring groups. This approach resonates well with critical social work.

Service users/consumers themselves have been largely responsible for the introduction of a discourse that counters the medical model, often referred to as a *recovery discourse* (see, for example, Deegan 1988, 1996; Leibrich 1998; Lovejoy 1984). This discourse has been embraced by the psychiatric disability support sector over the past three decades. The concept of recovery implies not so much a cure or denial of past or current events, but a 'mysterious and subjective process [encompassing] the development of new meaning and purpose as one grown beyond the catastrophic effects of mental illness' (Anthony 1993, p. 17). The discourse of recovery, Anthony argues, is

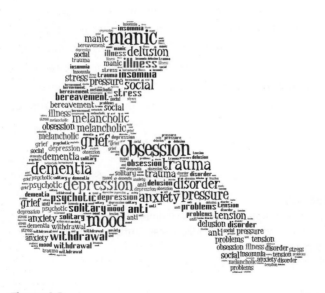

Figure 9.2

unifying rather than othering: we have all experienced loss and upheaval in some form and recovery journeys from that loss. Psychological recovery may not be dependent on whether or not the person continues to experience some symptoms or requires ongoing medication or support; it is more about an individual's sense of self-worth, meaning and purpose (Watkins 1996, p. 188).

A crucial role for social work in mental health is our capacity to question a medical construction of mental illness as the single legitimate voice in understanding and working with mental health issues; a sole reliance on this particular perspective – *the dominant narrative* – enables the silencing and undermining of other equally legitimate perspectives (Morley 2003b, p. 74). Our aim as practitioners is not to totally reject medical models but to think more critically about their effects – the costs, benefits and implications of the assignment of diagnostic labels and how they create identity and relations in more or less empowering ways (Cosgrove 2005). We also need to draw attention to how oppression and inequality shape mental and emotional wellbeing.

There is considerable evidence that some people's class, race, gender or sexual orientation (e.g. being poor, black, female or homosexual) makes them more likely to experience psychological problems than their supposed counterparts (Brown 2008; Coppock & Dunn 2010; Green 2007; Read 2004; Tew 2005). Brown (2003, 2008), for example, points to the consequences of racialised hopelessness among black men in the United States – manifested in suicide, substance abuse and criminality – and the 'anti-self issues' that occur as racial minorities try to maintain a positive identity in a society that consistently constructs 'the other' as defective (Brown 2003, p. 296). In Australia, the primary causes of poor social and emotional wellbeing for Aboriginal and Torres Strait Islander people has been identified as 'originating from the ongoing consequences of colonialism … [the] impact and effects [of which] have varied over time across Australia, but have resulted in trauma, grief and loss for successive generations' (Swan & Raphael 1995, cited in Garvey 2008, p. 7). Critical social workers need to understand that Indigenous definitions of health go beyond the limitations of the biomedical view of disease and take a holistic approach that includes 'the importance of land, culture, spirituality, ancestry, family – and acknowledge their inherent resilience' (Henderson et al. 2004, p. 142).

Understanding the implications of patriarchy and sexism is also crucial to critical mental health practice. Gender is particularly salient to personal psychological wellbeing. Williams (2005) focuses on the damage to women's mental health that arises from lack of access to resources that promote mental health (money, work status), from exposure to mental health risks (devalued or unpaid work, relations with men, abuse and violence) and from processes that maintain the status quo (being a 'good woman', devaluing emotionality). She suggests that workers cannot adequately support women unless they have an awareness of structural disadvantage and how psychiatric discourse masks social determinants of mental distress. A striking example, provided by Morley (2003b), is applying a medical label to the response of women who have been sexually assaulted, medicating their pain and outrage, and individualising the causes of, and solutions to, 'her problem'.

Hart's (2007) research into the construction of women's depression in Western mainstream magazines highlights the disciplinary mechanisms inherent in locating 'the problem' within the individual woman's body and mind while minimising the complexity of cultural, social and political factors surrounding her. Women are encouraged to engage in self-monitoring and disciplining and expected to pursue whatever self-improvement and self-transformation is necessary to control problematic experiences. This creates a reliable scapegoat for social inequalities while creating unattainable ideals of femininity and mental health. Existential questions 'about the meaningfulness of one's life and sociopolitical questions about happiness (e.g. should I stay married, have children and leave work, try to look younger, slimmer, etc.) [are transformed] into technical questions about the most effective ways of coping or managing one's emotional life and malfunction' (Rose 1996, cited in Fullagar & Gattuso 2002, p. 10).

> **Rurality** relates to non-urban communities whose economies are largely dependent on primary production such as agriculture (Alston 2012, p. 516).

Alston and Kent (2008) have written about the impact of **rurality** and patriarchy on the mental health of rural men, particularly farmers, and how dominant discourses of maleness and masculinity create an image of strength, stoicism and unemotionality that prevents men from acknowledging depression, anxiety and/or thoughts of suicide, and from seeking help. This has been exacerbated in Australia by recent years of drought and other threats to the viability of farmers and farming communities. Alston and Kent (2008, p. 144) suggest that social workers must recognise the significance of the context of **hegemonic masculinity** that surrounds men; workers need to not only pay attention to individual health outcomes but also to see dominant rural masculinities as a 'construction to be exposed as inherently unhealthy' and work with men to create discourses that are more health-inducing. The identity of rural men is often tied to their notion of self as farmer, with many men (and women) drawing a strong sense of identity and wellbeing from their work. When their work is threatened or unproductive, their wellbeing consequently suffers (Alston 2012, p. 518).

> **Hegemonic masculinity** refers to the dominant social form and expectations of masculinity within a patriarchal culture.

Work has been strongly linked to mental health in recent years, with employment serving as both a buffer from and a contributor to mental ill-health. It is easy to see how unemployment and poverty place severe stress on individuals, families and entire

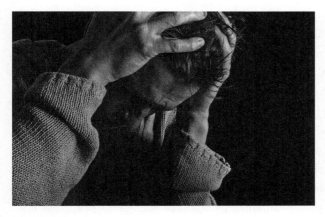

Figure 9.3

communities. Overemployment, underemployment and unhealthy jobs have also been identified as contributors to mental ill-health (Morrow, Verins & Willis 2002; Rogers & Pilgrim 2003) and exclusion from meaningful work is also recognised as a contributor to mental and psychological distress.

REFLECTIVE EXERCISE 9.9
Consider the implications of the preceding section for working with Peter (the case study presented in Chapter 3).

Migration and resettlement, homelessness, housing insecurity, being gay or lesbian in a heterosexist society, being or having been involved in the criminal justice system, living in poverty and being old in an ageist society are all factors that can have strikingly adverse affects on mental health. Working in any field of practice, social workers will be involved with people who may be experiencing psychological distress that is intertwined with structural disadvantage. Migrants and refugees may experience sadness, grief and isolation due to being in another society and/or past trauma, not to mention the devastating effects of being held in detention by a host country in conditions that exacerbate and engender psychological trauma, and racist exclusion from the wider community. In the prison system, the level of mental health problems and disorders is three to four times higher among inmates than in the general Australian population (Rogers 2008), resulting in jails and juvenile detention centres being referred to as 'de facto mental institutions' (Henderson 2008, p. 69). Some studies have suggested that mental illness within female prison populations – the majority of whom, if mothers, had sole care and responsibility for their children – may be as high as 100 per cent, with medication, rather than counselling or other support, being the primary response (Martin 2003, p. 167).

Homelessness clearly places the mental health and wellbeing of people at risk; it has been estimated that a third of people who are homeless in urban areas have a severe mental illness and when they are discharged from a psychiatric unit they often return to the unstable (or total lack of) accommodation they previously experienced (National Survey of Mental Health and Wellbeing 2007, cited in Commonwealth of Australia 2008, p. 9). In their research into housing insecurities, Hulse and Saugeres (2008) found that more than half the women and men they interviewed talked about having mental health problems. As is increasingly acknowledged in policy, many factors that influence the mental health of individuals 'lie outside the health system', with housing, employment, sport and recreation, education and income security all pivotal in effectively addressing mental ill-health and promoting social and emotional wellbeing (Victorian Health Promotion Foundation 2005, p. 3). Still, after nearly two decades of mental health reform in Australia, 'any person seeking mental health care runs the serious risk that his or her basic needs will be ignored, trivialised or neglected' (Mental Health Council of Australia 2005, p. 2). This is a sad indictment of our social and political priorities, and also a call to social workers to work from a holistic and critical perspective in addressing mental health needs.

Social workers have never been the dominant professionals in the field of mental health 'in terms of power, influence or legitimacy. For a century their involvement has been guided by medical authorities and their roles, while varied, have been viewed as supplementary' (Kirk 2005, p. 10). While this has changed somewhat as demand for outpatient, community-based support services has grown (as well as the capacity of mental health social workers in Australia to offer Medicare rebates for counselling), social workers still tend to adapt to the priorities and judgements of others in order to survive professionally (Kirk 2005; Morley 2003b; Morley & Macfarlane 2008). The radical potential for social work to act as a force for emancipatory social change has always sat uneasily beside expectations that social work should engage in practices of social control, resource rationing and surveillance (Ferguson 2008; Pozzuto, Brent Angell & Dezendorf 2005). Kirk (2005, p. 10) suggests that social work's 'failure to critically discuss the implications of the … biomedical paradigm of mental disorders is all the more surprising because the paradigm directly diminishes the importance of the social environment as both contributing cause and element of treatment'. He concludes that social workers need to 'be more sceptical of psychiatric claims and more critically minded about mental health practice' (Kirk 2005, p. 13). Furthermore, Kirk (2005, p. 17) proposes that workers are well placed to raise questions about established practices, examine fundamental beliefs and assumptions, and propose alternative views or interpretations. Morley (2003b) challenges social workers to consider that potentially emancipatory models of social work practice (such as strengths-based empowerment, advocacy and consumer participation models) do not go far enough in questioning the medical 'truth' on which they are based. She concludes that these models must be coupled with a critical analysis of the issues, which involves questioning oppressive social structures that shape individual wellbeing and the **reframing** and validating of individual experiences and responses that have been medically defined as pathological.

> **Reframing** refers to a process of re-examining negative and disempowering self-concepts, through drawing on the service user's strengths and offering another way a situation can be viewed (Lundy 2004).

■ Child protection

In this section we look at the emotionally and ethically charged area of child protection and explore how this field of practice might be informed by a critical social work approach, with particular attention to discourse and power. From the outset it must be stressed that approaching this field of practice critically in no way discounts or minimises the seriousness of harm to children and the need for vulnerable persons to be protected. Child protection work is an extremely difficult and important field of practice, with workers facing high caseloads in very pressurised settings while working in a bureaucratic 'system in meltdown' (Tucci & Goddard 2010, p. 9). The media reminds us that children continue to die and be seriously injured needlessly within the context of their families. There are far too few foster care or residential facilities available in which to place all children and the threshold of seriousness is set so high that many children in need fall through the net (Tucci & Goddard 2010, p. 9).

Mandell (2008) describes four key concerns among child welfare workers: struggle with the dual roles of authority and support; tendency to be judgemental about the parents; difficulty of witnessing the maltreatment of children on a regular basis; and angst over the difficult decisions that must be made in the context of the child protection mandate. She discusses the complexities of child protection and how work in this field draws out the individual worker's 'personhood, emotional history, values, commitment to social justice, biases, attitudes, anxieties, self concept, protective instincts, cultural backgrounds and social identity, and the same is so in the parent or child's experience of the worker' (Mandell 2008, p. 244). A critical perspective is thus necessary for this reason alone: critical reflection is crucial in order for workers to be mindful of how their own personhood and **social location** shapes their understanding of their role, the role of parents, the role of the state, and the strengths and limitations of interpretations and interventions in the lives of children, families and communities.

> **Social location** is how we would describe ourselves in such terms as gender, race, ethnicity, class, nationality, sexual orientation, age, disability and language as well as affiliations we may be involved in, such as religion and politics (Kirk & Okazawa-Rey 2004).

How does one make sense of such a complex, personally and professionally challenging and distressing issue as **child abuse**? Professionals in any field of practice need to identify (frame or assess) problems in order to 'solve' them; 'setting the problem' means that we select what are considered to be the crucial elements of a situation, 'the boundaries of our attention to it ... and impose upon it a coherence which allows us to say what is wrong and in what directions the situation needs to be changed' (Weick 1995, p. 9). Social policies and organisational mandates are powerful 'sensegivers' in that they provide such a framework for assessing and responding to a situation, creating order out of chaos and unpredictability and providing us with guidance as to how to approach what might be incomprehensible and uncontrollable scenarios (Weick 1995, p. 10).

> **Child abuse** can involve physical abuse, sexual abuse, emotional abuse and/or neglect (Queensland Government 2014).

Spratt and Houston (1999) put forward six *ideological* positions for making sense of the options available to child protection workers:

- *Penal:* the individual is seen as exercising free will in choosing to abuse a child; professional responses are punitive and based on 'dangerousness'.
- *Retributive/blame:* the worker must be seen to act in order to avoid possible error and blame for not having acted.
- *Medical:* the perpetration of child abuse is beyond the control of the individual and is seen as a disease.
- *Bureaucratic:* reliance on classification and processing – case management systems, registers and highly routinised procedures.
- *Technocratic:* the belief that there is a technical fix for the problem, via professional specialities, competency-based training and risk assessment of individual parents.
- *Humanistic:* focus on structural processes, such as inequalities; compassionate and rehabilitative leaning towards parents and families.

REFLECTIVE EXERCISE 9.10

- Which of the above positions resonates most strongly with your views and beliefs?
- Where has your view come from? For example, how has the media or lived experience impacted your assumptions?
- Can you imagine how each ideological position might lead to particular interventions?
- Which position do you think would most closely align with a critical approach and why?

Ideologies are expressed through the way we understand an issue such as child abuse and how we respond to the problem. Ideologies can be expressed in overt or more subtle ways: even the way a worker dresses can be an expression of ideology, as can the furnishings of an interview room, holding a case discussion in a family's home rather than an office, and the ideas that hold primary importance in a case conference (Pinkerton 2002, p. 98). Spratt and Houston (1999) suggest that workers will often be caught between ideologies, with some taking precedence over others. As social workers, we believe in children's rights to freedom from all forms of abuse, while at the same time we may believe that children are best brought up with their families and that parents are individuals who deserve respect for their rights, strengths and needs (Pinkerton 2002, p. 99). As previously mentioned, the organisation and its legal and social mandate exert a strong influence on the choices made by workers and constrains and directs actions according to particular ideological and theoretical constructions, which may or may not fit perfectly with the individual worker's values and views.

What might a critical approach to child protection work look like? You might remember that one of the features of critical social work is questioning taken-for-granted assumptions. In relation to child protection, Pinkerton (2002) foregrounds constant, critical questioning as a key element of practice. He suggests we engage in questioning not only our own and our colleagues' actions, but also the structural constraints and opportunities present for ourselves and the families we work with, at organisational and societal levels. This questioning is best addressed in the context of day-to-day practice and service delivery: 'how is practice measuring up to the worker's vision and values; what working hypotheses [theories or ideologies] are being tested in practice; and how is the balance of power being negotiated?' (Pinkerton 2002, p. 97). Power – no matter how kind, self-aware or careful the worker may be – cannot be removed from the encounter between worker and service user. Indeed, 'ensuring the safety of children can require the naked display of state power' (Pinkerton 2002, p. 103). While social workers exercise power over service users they are also subject to the power of the organisational and managerial mandate. Acknowledging this power is important not only when advocating for a client at a case conference but also when presenting staff interests to management (Pinkerton 2002).

Critical theories also provide us with an analysis of the structural dimensions of child abuse and neglect, such as the impact of patriarchy in creating male-dominated households where dominant hegemonic constructions of masculinity sanction men in exercising power and control over children. Critical analyses similarly provide us with insights into the social, political and economic factors that impact adversely on families, creating many strains and hardships, rather than supporting caring and nurturing environments in which children can flourish. Critical theories provide us with relevant information about the structural factors that potentially impact children's development. (For one concrete example of this, turn back to Chapter 2 and reread the section on social inequality in the education system on page 39.)

Critical theories also draw our attention to the importance of language. Todd and Wade (2004), for example, demonstrate how the language used in the dominant discourse surrounding violence operates in similar ways to social myths: to obscure the nature of the violence; to strategically diminish the perpetrator's responsibility; to hide the victim's resistance to abuse; and to blame and pathologise the victim of the abuse. It is crucial that workers in this field have the ability to recognise the ways that dominant discourses may infiltrate our thinking and practice so that we do not inadvertently cause harm to the people we aim to support.

Another element of a critical approach is attention to our potential to engage in binary thinking and how this is affecting our work. In highly regulated settings, the unique nature of each individual can – and perhaps must, in order to allow routinised practice – be overlooked. People become categorised or 'typified' in particular ways. Pinkerton (2002, p. 102) suggests that the critical practitioner will refuse to 'reduce people, workers and service users alike . . . to either the victims or villains of child abuse or the heroes of child protection'. Refusing to think in binary terms may be particularly challenging in child protection work as the rules and regulations of a bureaucratic system, while reducing professional autonomy, serve the function of guarding workers from some of the anxiety produced by their role. Collings and Davis (2008, p. 182) encapsulate this when they state 'workers may find comfort in institutional discourses premised on the rescue of children from inadequate or culpable parents because such a dichotomous view of children and their parents can . . . distance themselves from this pain that may accompany removing children'.

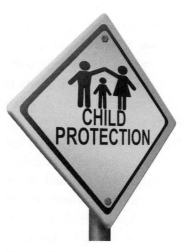

Figure 9.4

Working in partnership, a hallmark of social work practice, is certainly constrained by the involuntary nature of some worker–client relationships, particularly when the worker also carries a significant amount of power to intervene in the client's life. However, some of the basic requirements of a working relationship can still be met: providing information, making manageable practical arrangements, advising and providing emotional support. While goals may not be shared (that is, the worker may have different goals to the client), it is nonetheless important to make goals transparent. It has been suggested that in child protection perhaps the term 'negotiated agreement' rather than 'partnership' is more accurate (Pinkerton 2002). Negotiating an agreement means more than one person communicating the rules to another, although this may form part of the negotiations. While the power may remain primarily with the worker and the social mandate of the organisation, this is communication that more closely resembles the 'ideal speech situation' identified by Habermas (1990, p. 86) whereby all are allowed to speak and be listened to, as well as to question the views of others (Spratt & Houston 1999). Opening up communication in this way might be a more empowering approach to working with families. This ideal speech situation aimed at negotiating an agreement is in stark contrast to what Hennum (2012, p. 546) describes in relation to child protection in Norway: she asserts that 'the dialogues conducted by the child welfare services … are used more to confirm the cultural, moral, political and theoretical viewpoints of the participating professionals rather than to assist the parents in their struggle to create a life of dignity'.

In the Australian context, there is a heavy over-representation of Aboriginal and Torres Strait Islander families and children, who have come under the gaze and intervention of child welfare. At a recent summit, Indigenous child protection workers expressed the view that many of the interventions in Aboriginal and Torres Strait Islander communities lacked context-specific and culturally informed knowledge on the part of practitioners and that non-Indigenous workers rarely listened to what Indigenous staff and community members had to say about the protection of children (Ryan, F. 2011). From a critical perspective, listening deeply and respectfully to each other, caring for each other and taking the time to build relationships should not be seen as a waste of precious time, but rather the essential avenue for improving services and enhancing wellbeing. Awareness of the historical context is also a vital element in understanding the lives and experiences of Indigenous Australians: the traumatic and ongoing impact of colonisation, social and economic inequality and power imbalances have had ripple effects throughout Aboriginal and Torres Strait Islander communities. Despite dispossession and oppression, Aboriginal and Torres Strait Islander people have continued to struggle to create **nourishing terrains** for their children and families; these strengths should be highlighted and learned from.

> **Nourishing terrains** refers to an Indigenous Australian understanding of 'wilderness' that reflects a long history of human use and nourishment from the land (country), the concepts of 'country' and 'kinship' being inseparable to culture (Bird 1996).

In order to truly benefit and learn from Indigenous knowledge and experience, practitioners must be willing to examine their own social and cultural location and interrogate the theories and assumptions that inform their practice. Non-Indigenous Western models and theories may have limited relevance in Aboriginal and Torres Strait Islander contexts. Fiona Ryan (2011) provides a useful example in her deconstruction and reconstruction of the concept of attachment, a theory that under-pins much child protection practice. Attachment theory, as developed by John Bowlby in the 1950s, holds that the nature of the emotional bond between the child (from infancy) and primary caregiver (generally assumed to be the mother) is a significant contributor to the ongoing formation and healthy development of the adult. Certain forms of attachment are considered favourable and healthy, while others are consid-ered problematic (Freeman 2005). A critique of attachment theory has been that it ascribes 'normalcy' to Western constructs of the healthy relationship between mother and child, which are culturally biased and do not take into account other healthy ways of relating to children. Furthermore, an uncritical acceptance of attachment theory also neglects the contested nature of what actually constitutes optimum development for an individual (see, for example, Ryan, F. 2011).

Attachment theory is based on the assumption that secure attachment to a single primary caregiver is necessary for healthy ongoing development. However, Aboriginal and Torres Strait Islander and other non-Western worldviews and social patterns may be based on notions of multiple mothering and the involvement of siblings and other children in caring for the younger family members. While attachment theory suggests that competencies of the growing child revolve around the development of autonomy and individual resilience, Indigenous Australian perspectives may place more value on interdependence, group cohesion, and spiritual, community and land-based connec-tions. Based on this construction of healthy development, self-reliance and children's peer support of each other may not mean that caregivers are negligent or unaware of their children's actions; indeed such practice may be a result of 'ancient and deeply nurturing values' (Ryan, F. 2011, p. 189). From a critical perspective, our focus should be on supporting local community initiatives developed and owned by local people, hum-bly and respectfully learning from Aboriginal and Torres Strait Islander practitioners about their people and communities and encouraging the employment of more Indigenous workers in professional positions (Bessarab & Crawford 2010).

■ Summary

This chapter has explored the possibilities for critical practice in the fields of aged care, mental health and child protection. These fields of practice do not exist in isolation and will necessarily intersect and overlap with other fields and issues. For example, we could not discuss aged care without also referring to the challenges for the LGBTI populations in this setting. While we have covered a number of different fields of practice throughout the text, we intentionally chose to focus on these three fields here because they are not often associated with critical practice. It is often assumed, for example, that practitioners cannot work in critical ways in the child protection system due to the statutory nature of much child protection practice. Similarly, many practitioners assume that the medically dominated nature of most mental health and aged care settings will prevent the goals and values of critical practice from being relevant in these fields. Our purpose in this chapter, however, has been to provide you with some examples of the ways in which we may bring the values, analysis and experiences of critical approaches to all fields of practice, regardless of the other frameworks that inform them.

■ Review questions

- What are your responses to our overview of each of these fields of practice?
- Are you drawn to working in any of these fields? Or are you passionate about working in other fields of practice, and why?
- What do you think are some of the main challenges of working in the fields of aged care, mental health and child protection?
- Make some notes about how you imagine you would work to resolve these challenges. How might a critical analysis assist you in this process?
- Write a brief paragraph summarising the key ideas about how critical perspectives might inform your practice in each of the three fields of practice covered in this chapter.

■ Further reading

Barrett, C., 2008, *My People: A Project Exploring the Experiences of Gay, Lesbian, Bisexual, Transgender and Intersex Seniors in Aged-Care Services*, Matrix Guild, Victoria.

Black, B., 2009, 'Empowering and rights-based approaches to working with older people' in J. Allan, L. Briskman and B. Pease, eds, *Critical Social Work: Theories and Practices for a Socially Just World*, 2nd edn, Allen & Unwin, Crows Nest, NSW.

Grenier, A., 2008, 'Recognising and responding to loss and "rupture" in older women's accounts', *Journal of Social Work Practice*, 22 (2): 195–209.

Healy, K, 2012, 'Working with mandated individuals' in *Social Work Methods and Skills*, Palgrave Macmillan, Basingstoke, pp. 84–108.

Macfarlane, S, 2009, 'Opening spaces for alternative understandings in mental health practice' in J. Allan, B. Pease and L. Briskman, eds, *Critical Social Work, Theories and Practices for a Socially Just World*, 2nd edn, Allen & Unwin, Crows Nest.

Morley, C, 2003, 'Towards critical social work practice in mental health', *Journal for Progressive Human Services*, 14 (1), pp. 61–84.

Ryan, F, 2011, 'Kanyininpa (holding): A way of nurturing children in Aboriginal Australia', *Australian Social Work*, 64 (2), pp. 183–97.

Todd, N and Wade, A, (with Renoux, M), 2004, 'Coming to terms with violence and resistance' in T. Strong and D. Pare, eds, *Furthering Talk: Advances in Discursive Therapies*, Springer, New York.

10

Challenges and opportunities for critical social work

■ Introduction

I N CHAPTER 1 we invited you to consider the critical potential of social work: the potential for us as individual workers, and collectively as a profession, to question the social conditions and discourses that give rise to human suffering and what we might do about these. The critical standpoint is one that sensitises us to social injustice and the need for transformation. Being a critical practitioner is challenging: while we may decide this is the path we wish to take, it is an ongoing process, borne out in day-to-day and week-to-week activities. Becoming a critical practitioner is not a single act of commitment but an often arduous journey of revelation and struggle. There are many potential setbacks along this journey. As the words of a great 20th-century social reformer, Martin Luther King, remind us: 'Human progress is neither automatic nor inevitable ... Every step towards the goal of justice requires sacrifice, suffering and struggle; the tireless exertions and passionate concerns of dedicated individuals.' Critical social workers are among those dedicated individuals with passionate concerns. However, we need to be mindful of both the obstacles and strategies of renewal if our concerns and passions are to be sustained. In this concluding chapter we elaborate on common challenges experienced by social workers and suggest ways in which these may be turned into learning opportunities and possibly even liberating experiences.

Social work, as we have shown, addresses itself to the problems of our power-divided world, characterised by *gendered*, *racialised* and *class* oppressions, for example, caused by the interconnections of *global capitalism*, *neoliberalism*, *managerialism*, *patriarchy*, *biomedical dominance*, *government* and the *law*. Social workers are generally engaged in assisting individuals, groups or communities to overcome life issues and crises that stem from these various forms of oppression. However, social workers in daily practice often meet people at a low ebb: people in need of resources, experiencing oppression and/or emotional vulnerabilty due to crises or ongoing challenges. This means that social work can and often does create stress or fatigue for its practitioners (Figley 2002; Lloyd, King &

Chenoweth 2002). At times we can absorb the suffering of service users in ways that are painful to ourselves (Zellmer 2004–05). Some service users are involuntary and do not want to interact with us; and most would prefer to be in better circumstances. Social workers are dedicated to creating a more *socially just* world, and we necessarily feel a strong pull to assist the people with whom we work, but we are accountable not only to them, but also to our organisation and its funding bodies, and the general public, to achieve externally determined outcomes. Meeting these multiple accountabilities can be a testing balancing act for even the most experienced practitioner.

It is important to remember, as we have said throughout this book, that being a critical practitioner means more than making a critical analysis of society. It also means having the capacity to turn the critical lens back on ourselves. This entails questioning ourselves, where we stand and what role we play in maintaining or countering oppressive practices and conditions. In claiming to be critical we aim to oppose oppression, but are our words and deeds as social workers always consistent with this intent? We have described this self-questioning – and the changes in practice it may engender – as *critical reflection*. The point of such questioning is not to wallow in our shortcomings but, on the contrary, to remove barriers to our work. We believe this is an essential prerequisite for critical practitioners to sustain their practice and not despair in the face of the organisational pressures and the conundrums of institutional practice that often seem far removed or at odds with our values and visions.

The obstacles to *emancipatory* practice are real but they can be unintentionally amplified by our own constructions of the situation, which may uncritically reproduce the dominant discourses of our workplaces and political contexts. This can result in us blaming ourselves for the gap between our critical intent and what we feel we actually achieve in practice, leaving us feeling stuck and frustrated. Such constructions require careful, yet hopeful interrogation.

There are many challenges to critical practice, but some of the important ones can be summarised under the following four headings: (1) the challenge of the 'failed activist', (2) the challenge of the 'lone crusader', (3) the challenge of embracing discomfort and uncertainty and (4) the challenge of believing that 'there is no alternative'. We now discuss these interconnected dilemmas, looking at how critical reflection may assist us in challenging and working through their problematic constructions.

■ The challenge of the 'failed activist'

The challenge of the failed activist refers to the perceived gap between our desire to contribute to *progressive* social change ideals (as highlighted by *critical theories*) and what we feel we actually achieve in practice, particularly within highly *bureaucratic* and *managerialist* environments. It is tempting to feel that this gap – between our critical aspirations and our actual practice within organisational contexts that are dominated by neoliberal discourses – represents our own personal and professional failure, and it is easy to feel like a failed activist (Rossiter 2005). An example of this might include having to terminate our work with a service user after four weeks, as required by the organisation's funding agreement, when we think we have only just started to establish a working relationship. Another example might be that a young women's support group is axed because its success cannot be measured in economic terms. Or, as an educator, being told by the administrators who control the deadlines that students will no longer be able to receive extensions of more than one week, regardless of their circumstances. It is easy to become disheartened and jaded when power is imposed in an arbitrary fashion 'from above' according to criteria that seem to work against the goal of the practice or the program one is engaged in.

However, the use of critical reflection can be a means of enabling us to step back from practice, and see some of the historical, social and political complexities that may constrain our commitment to social justice (Rossiter 2005). Social workers, according to Rossiter (2005), are 'often placed within forcefields of contradictions' that shape our practice just as significantly as our theoretical frameworks and social justice goals. Social justice is a process for which we are continually developing our understanding in each context of practice (Rossiter 2005).

Van Soest's (2012, pp. 104–5) words also encourage a counter-discourse to that of the failed activist:

> Taking even one small step on the journey changes one's perspective on the landscape. Action, either practical or symbolic, overcomes ... inertia ... you don't have to do everything, be everything ... this is a trap. It keeps us from taking action. No matter how small each individual effort might seem, know that every single one of us can make a difference because it is our combined efforts that produce change.

In the examples of potential practice challenges outlined above, the worker who needs to terminate their practice may choose to advocate by representing the service user's needs to management to argue for more sessions with that service user, or advise the service user regarding ways to work around the policy, or provide information about how to raise complaints to challenge policies that are operating contrary to their needs. The worker facilitating the young women's group might suggest to the young women that they continue their support group without the worker's formal facilitation and outside of the office hours of the organisation. The worker could continue to support the group by obtaining permission from the organisation for the women to use one of the rooms. The educator might negotiate with her faculty that if a student has produced a draft of their assignment, a more flexible arrangement in terms of extensions can be implemented.

In all of these examples, to order to overcome the challenge of becoming a 'failed activist', critical practitioners need to do two things: (1) abandon the idea that the whole system needs to change in order for our work to be worthwhile and effective and (2) let go of the view that there is only one, correct way to achieve emancipatory outcomes or to do critical practice. Healy (2000, p. 145) describes what she calls *pragmatic activist* social work, which, in place of grand plans, or all-or-nothing ideals, frees workers to focus on 'local, contextual and modest proposals for change'. This was a major theme to emerge from research that one of us (Christine) undertook that examined the ways in which practitioners who worked in the field of sexual assault could set about challenging oppressive aspects of the legal process. Interestingly, most of the research participants were so unhappy with the legal response to victims/ survivors of sexual assault that they felt the whole judicial system needed to be dismantled, changed and replaced with a more effective and compassionate process before victims/survivors would have a real opportunity to obtain justice from the legal system. However, one of the key consequences of this belief is that it resulted in practitioners feeling powerless to effectively advocate and support victims/survivors. At the same time, this belief resulted in practitioners devaluing the casework and counselling they were engaged in with victims/survivors by comparing it (dichoto- mously) to social change – something from which they felt too removed to be able to contribute (Morley 2014).

Christine's research used critical reflection as a method of inquiry to generate different ways to think about the problems with the legal system (*deconstruction*) and to *reconstruct* new ways to think about practice. Significantly, the practitioners who participated in the research developed a range of alterative strategies to challenge oppressive legal processes without changing the whole system. The new thinking and practices they developed were not of a structural nature – that is, none of the proposed changed practices formally altered key problems they identified, such as the traditional professional hierarchies between sexual assault practitioners and legal or medical professionals; or legislation concerning the formal operations of systems. However, all of the new practices have the potential to deliver better processes and outcomes for victims/survivors. To provide a brief example, one participant watched in horror as the child victim/survivor she had been supporting through the legal process was savagely discredited by a defence lawyer. This participant reimagined her practice to include possibilities for her to influence the ways that the judiciary responds to child witnesses. This took the form of arranging for the prosecution to subpoena her as an expert witness so that she could provide information about the social myths that surround sexual assault, children's developmental stages and the ways that these affect how children give evidence. While this practice does not structurally change

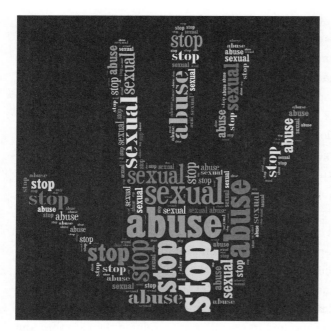

Figure 10.1

the legal system, it does facilitate the conditions for transformation by creating possibilities for sexual assault practitioners to influence the way the legal system understands and responds to victims/survivors in ways that might result in their experiences being validated (Morley 2014).

Therefore, pragmatic activism celebrates the smaller, local acts of resistance that contribute to and create the conditions for emancipatory changes. At the same time, it sacrifices the notion that there is only one, right way to achieve critical outcomes. This latter belief is one to which many critical social workers can succumb, particularly if they are not able to integrate *poststructural theory*, which examines multiple constructions of situations and subsequently creates multiple practice options. Paralleling this, Healy (2000) suggests that resisting oppressive practices needs to be relevant to the specific context and anchored in the community's experience; a 'one-size-fits-all' or an 'all-or-nothing' approach will not necessarily be useful, especially if it ignores local conditions and needs.

Consider the practitioner who judges and labels another worker's practice or another organisation as 'unethical' because they take a different approach to practice. Consider the student who berates and ridicules another student for not being 'critical' or 'anti-oppressive' enough, while executing a traditional top-down of model of expertise. Consider the social work educator who claims to be teaching a critical approach to practice, yet intimidates and silences students with an authoritarian style of facilitation by not allowing alternative viewpoints and positions to be heard. In all of these examples, the assumption of having the single, 'right' approach can lead to an arrogance or form of intellectual elitism that is anything but critical or emancipatory! In fact, an unreflective 'critical' approach, even with the best intentions, can result in oppressive practices that can be harmful for those with whom we work.

> Consider the history of Marxism. The communist parties that waged successful revolutions (for example, in Russia, China and Korea) emphasised the scientific objectivist side of Marx's work as a universal guide to revolution – codifying it as a rigid orthodoxy to justify their own domination. This should warn critical social workers that even the most radical theory can be abused by power to serve the opposite of its intent. Paradoxically, in the capitalist West, Marxist perspectives retained their critical spirit.

Fook (2012) reminds us of the gap that may occur between theory and practice. The goal of the practice should be clearly evident in the means employed to achieve the goal. Therefore, we are not just focused on the outcome; the process is equally important. The language of critical social work is meaningless unless we can integrate our values and theories into our practice. We also need to consider the ways in which language can be co-opted by dominant discourses. For example, the term 'empowerment' has been used to justify a range of theoretical perspectives, including establishment ones, in which empowerment has been seen as an opportunity to shift responsibility on to the individual (Fook & Morley 2005). Similarly, the term 'participation' has been used by the Australian Government Department of Human Services to require mothers with children over the age of seven to compulsorily work in order to receive financial entitlements.

SERVICE USER'S PERSPECTIVE

My children are aged six and seven. I receive the single-parent pension and have just completed a Bachelor of Education degree. I currently work 23 hours per fortnight at a primary school as a teacher's aide. Since completing my degree, I have now accepted a position as a full-time teacher with the same school. My contract for this position begins in five weeks; the day after my existing contract expires at the beginning of the school year. However, now that my youngest child has turned six I am required to participate in job seeking for an additional three-hour position per week, by demonstrating that I have applied for a minimum of four positions per fortnight, because recipients of the single-parent pension are required to work a minimum number of hours per fortnight or study full-time (whilst also parenting our children on our own) to be exempt from job seeker participation. *(Trinity, personal communication, January 2014)*

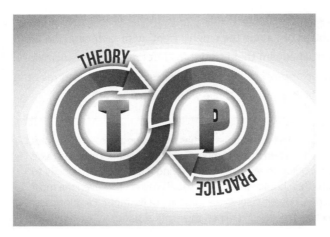

Figure 10.2

Transparency too has been valued as a goal of critical practice, yet transparency in situations of unequal power can put at risk those who are vulnerable. While a blanket reading of transparency can sound good in principle for open and democratic processes, it can be used as a tool by managers – for example, to discipline and extract more labour/value from employees (that is, for exploitation) (Garrett 2013). As Bakhtin (cited in Garrett 2013, p. 165) points out, 'In practical terms transparency is most closely associated with tyranny' rather than autonomy. Consider the plight of people who are reluctant to make information about their lives transparent to the state. In such situations the language of critical theory and practice can simply become empty rhetoric. Critical reflection can improve our practice by assisting us to identify gaps between the theories that we imagine we are using and the ways in which our actual practices are experienced by others (Fook 2012).

REFLECTIVE EXERCISE 10.1
Think about the practice of advocacy: a social work method and skill that is clearly relevant to critical anti-oppressive practice. Can you imagine a practice situation in which it might be inappropriate or not in the 'best interests' of a service user to advocate with them, or on their behalf?

Case example

Here we will focus on a specific incident, within the context of social work education, to critically examine the use of *advocacy* as a tool of empowerment. The scenario is one where a student has been withdrawn from her **fieldwork placement** on the grounds of lack of attendance and complaints by workers in the agency that she had engaged in inappropriate behaviour. After some negotiation, and advocacy for the student on the part of the **liaison officer**, it was agreed that the student would terminate the placement. The student did not accept that there was anything wrong with her behaviour on the placement and maintained that the agency personnel were unsupportive. Some weeks later the student suggested another placement option that she was keen to pursue. Although the liaison officer was unsure, as a result of the previous placement experience and other factors, about regrading the student's readiness to successfully complete the placement, she was convinced by the student that this new placement opportunity would be more conducive to success than the previous one and advocated on behalf of the student to commence the new placement.

> **Fieldwork placement** is an educative process whereby students develop a range of professional skills under supervision in a variety of workplace settings (AASW 2012).

> The **liaison officer** is a university representative who maintains regular contact with students on fieldwork placement to clarify educational issues, monitor progress of the placement, mediate any difficulties and assess student progress (AASW 2012).

Several weeks into the placement, problems began to emerge again in relation to attendance and unprofessional behaviour. Once again the student was withdrawn from placement at the request of the agency. While being informed by a critical perspective, the liaison officer would routinely seek to support and advocate for the needs of students. However, on this occasion the liaison officer questioned whether the use of advocacy had been the most beneficial practice for the student, given that the student had now been withdrawn from two placements and accrued a fail.

When we deconstruct this incident, through critical reflection, we focus on the specific context in which the events unfolded: the worker was operating from a value and theory base that suggested advocacy on behalf of the student was appropriate and necessary for critical practice aimed at student empowerment; she also supported the potentially marginalised voice of the student in terms of her readiness for placement. The liaison officer felt she was using her considerable power to pave the way for the student to successfully complete her placement. While these intentions clearly fall within a critical approach to practice, in this instance they may have contributed to the student feeling disempowered due to the termination of two placements and a fail result, and the liaison officer feeling guilty and somewhat incompetent, also potentially having jeopardised the relationship with the organisation in terms of future placements. When reconstructing the incident, the liaison officer acknowledged that the power to determine outcomes was potentially shared between herself, the university, the student (who was not totally powerless) and the placement organisation, all of whom had input into the scenario. The liaison officer also realised that discourses of advocacy, while often crucial to anti-oppressive process and outcomes, may, in some specific contexts, not have desired results. Further, by engaging in binary thinking – seeing her options as advocacy versus abandoning the student – the liaison officer had engaged in somewhat simplistic thinking around what might produce the most empowering outcome.

Before discounting oneself or one's theory as a 'failure' in practice, we need to recall that critical theory is not a total account of reality; nor is it a dogmatic or prescriptive guide to activism regardless of context. Rather, it provides moments of clarity for how we might realise our values in action, but those actions (and the theory behind it) will always have to be reassessed in the light of our current and changing circumstances. What is constant is the basic intent or value base of the theory; to enable all people to lead meaningful and dignified lives in a just, participatory and sustainable community. There is no one-size-fits-all model or program that we can simply copy to achieve this. Rather, the challenge is to be constantly alert to emancipatory possibilities and ways we might bring them about anew in each different context.

■ The challenge of the 'lone crusader'

The next (and related) dilemma is that of the 'lone crusader'; another potentially disempowering position that we may occupy as critical social workers. Fook (2000) describes how constructing oneself as the only one with the 'right' (socially just) attitude and analysis means that we generally construct others as enemies, with the resultant effect of leaving us stuck and alienated from taking responsibility to create even minimal change. The lone crusader often subscribes, like the failed activist, to the belief that the only good change is total change, which for one person acting alone is probably always going to be unattainable. Fook (2000) suggests that we rethink our notions of change, away from all-or-nothing conceptions towards the notion of 'unfinished change', which, although incomplete, is nevertheless valuable.

REFLECTIVE EXERCISE 10.2
- How do you feel about the notion of unfinished change?
- How does it compare to the feeling of failure?
- Can you think of a situation from your practice or in your life, where this reconstruction from 'failure' to 'unfinished change' may be a useful concept to apply?

Another consequence of adopting the 'lone crusader' outlook is that it can leave social workers (both individually and collectively) feeling that they are indispensable to meaningful social change; that social change rests primarily on their shoulders and that without their expertise it will not happen. Bertha Reynolds (1963, p. 184) referred to this belief as the profession's 'God Complex' and thought that Marxism relieved the social worker of this construction by emphasising the agency and self-organising capacity of the impoverished and oppressed. In other words, it is not social workers but the oppressed themselves who will ultimately liberate the oppressed. Nevertheless, Reynolds (1963, p. 184) believed social work could help with this process in its own 'particularly useful way'. Impoverished and destitute people may not have the energy, time or skills to organise themselves collectively. However, social workers may have the critical analysis, skills and institutional resources that can assist in such organising while also providing immediate relief. If institutional barriers impede this, then it may also mean that critical social workers will, as the need arises, help form or join organisations outside the workplace to bring about change. One of the most disempowering aspects with the 'lone crusader' construction is precisely the attempt to act *alone*, when in fact collective strength, and the diversity it brings to a situation, can achieve much more in terms of emancipatory change.

Social workers will often work in multidisciplinary teams (sometimes referred to as interprofessional or interdisciplinary teams) in which the team members represent various disciplines and professions, each with a range of aims, theories, processes and desired outcomes. In these contexts, the tendency to feel like a 'lone crusader' may be further exacerbated. Some tensions between team members can stem from a lack of understanding of what each professional can bring to the problem or issue at hand, as well as anxiety that one's specific role and unique contribution will be over-taken or co-opted by others (Coppock & Dunn 2010). Social workers in mental health settings, for example, may find it particularly difficult to espouse and enact a critical perspective in a context heavily dominated by medical model professionals and discourses. In such a scenario we may find ourselves constructing others who do not share our orientation as enemies, rather than allies, in trying to achieve wellbeing for our clients. One way to counter this binary tendency is to consider our professional practice as working both with, and within, whole contexts. Fook (2012) suggests that the true service user of the social worker is the context; thus the whole organisation – and the political culture of service delivery, and the social structures that make up our society – may be perceived as our client.

Framing dilemmas in oppositional ways, such as ally and enemy, creates a sense in workers that they are 'caught in impossible binds with dichotomous and mutually exclusive choices about whether to meet the needs of powerless clients or subjugate

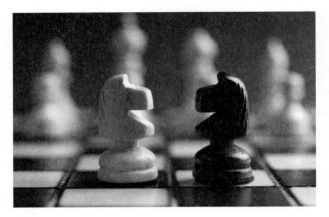

Figure 10.3

themselves to the demands of organisations and managers' (Fook 2012, p. 167). This construction leaves little room to see where opportunities for creative choices may exist and can also imprison us in a self-protective cocoon of blaming others rather than seeing where possibilities to create change might exist. Fook (2012, p. 173) suggests that we try to 're-theorise' the enemy by coming up with new ways of seeing colleagues and situations that might enable us to change the situation. There will, of course, always be some people who decide to make us their 'enemy'; people who oppose entire programs in which we and our service users are invested, but a critical practitioner will always persist in building the widest possible base of allies, win over the middle ground and minimise the number of outright opponents.

The leadership of the revolutionary and peace activist Nelson Mandela (1918–2013) is instructive here. As he stated:

For to be free is not merely to cast off one's chains, but to live in a way that respects and enhances the freedom of others (Mandela 1995, p. 755).
If you want to make peace with your enemy, you have to work with your enemy (Mandela 2013, p. 50).

PRACTITIONER'S PERSPECTIVE

Selma was working as a support worker in a residential psychiatric disability support service. This is not a title that gives one much status in the mental health hierarchy, which is fine from a critical point of view because critical practitioners derive their value and worth from their connection and usefulness to services users, rather than dominant discourses about professionalism. However, when working in this role, tensions between those members of the hierarchy with more status and those with lower status can come to the fore. In this scenario, tensions had developed between the clinical workers at the mental health clinic and the support workers at the residence, with the professionalism and insight of the former seeming to take precedence over that of the latter. It was easy for the support workers to feel like misunderstood lone crusaders who were on the side of clients made powerless by the mental health system. This, however, created something of a stalemate between people who needed to work together if the best interests of the client were to be achieved. As Selma explains:

> While we were not totally aware of what we were doing, we engaged in a process of reconstruction of our 'enemies': we invited them to come to monthly educational exchanges in which they taught us, the support workers, more about the different medications and treatments clients were receiving, and we shared some of the theory and underpinnings of our approach to support within a community setting. Thus we came closer, in an unfinished process of change, to constructing each other as potential allies on some issues despite our differences, and engendering greater mutual respect that ultimately served the clients with whom we worked.

■ The challenge of embracing uncertainty and discomfort

REFLECTIVE EXERCISE 10.3

We now turn our attention to the experience of uncertainty and discomfort.
- What do you immediately feel or think when you read the words 'uncertainty' and 'discomfort'?
- What impact or connotation do these feelings generally have, in your experience?

When doing reflective exercise 10.3, you may have thought about times in your life when you felt confused, unsettled or unhappy. On further consideration, however, you might begin to contemplate that, at times, feelings of discomfort and uncertainty were ultimately important and useful in making changes in your interpretations and practices. They may have led you to make changes, great or small, that expanded your horizons and created a greater sense of wellbeing, movement or achievement. Times of discomfort or uncertainty can actually provide us with 'messages' that we need to be attentive to, and encourage us to consider that change may be required.

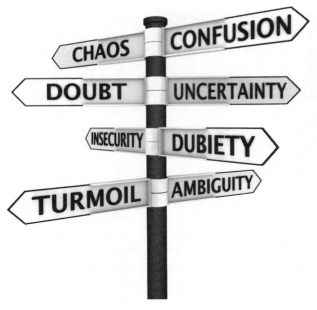

Figure 10.4

However, these experiences are not particularly valued in current contexts that tend towards the management and elimination of risk and uncertainty over the prioritising of needs and rights. Increasingly technicised practices, intent on creating predictability and uniformity, quantitative economic measures based on supposedly 'objective' notions of efficiency, and narrowly defined parameters of 'evidence' can feel like rigid constraints for critical practitioners. Indeed, there is little space within the current dominant discourses permeating our contemporary practice contexts to discuss feelings of discomfort or uncertainty. This would seem to be at odds with critical reflective practice that relishes the inevitable complexities and uncertainties of professional practice and the many moments of 'not knowing' by regarding these as opportunities to generate new learning and knowledge (Napier & Fook 2000, p. 10).

Even in organisations that pride themselves on being 'learning organisations' that are supposedly devoted to professional development of staff, the rhetoric of learning is often hollow, and opportunities to honestly reveal worker discontent and uncertainty about practice and service delivery are limited and feared (Beddoe 2009). Beddoe's research with human services workers in New Zealand revealed that workers often found it very difficult to give honest feedback to their organisation as they felt it was a 'low trust environment'; that learning from mistakes was not valued, so discussing uncertainties was taboo; that most professional development was 'top-down' (initiated by management rather than lower-level workers); and that 'continuous improvement' often meant change for no real benefit. Beddoe proposed that critical questions to be posed around professional development included: Learning for whom? Who benefits? What learning is valued? Does the organisation learn from us (social workers)?

Rather than avoid or minimise the uncertainty we experience sometimes as workers attempting to create change in complex circumstances with people, a critical approach calls us to embrace uncertainty as one of the hallmarks of professional practice. We are not talking about uncertainty that is paralysing (although pausing to breathe, be still and looking around might sometimes be beneficial), but uncertainty that engenders the critical questions that are the trademark of our profession. Rossiter (2011, p. 12) suggests that uncertainty or unsettledness in practice is ethical practice: 'an orientation ... that allows us to suspend assumptions, place what we think we know at risk and leave ourselves open to the revelation of the other'. This means active listening, respect, and a fluid orientation to possibilities: 'there is no professional story that adequately represents the singularity of a person' (Rossiter 2011, p. 15).

Furthermore, there is a misconception in our culture that the more experienced and knowledgeable we become (especially as leaders), the more certain we must be in having the correct answers or solutions to practical problems. In this, we mistake certainty for truth. In fact, humility may be a far better guide than certainty for decision making in the human services. As Napier and Fook (2000, p. 214) remind us:

> We are never too experienced to learn from the newest graduate or the most 'down and out' service user. We are never too inexperienced to create insights into the most enduring professional dilemmas. We are never too practised to revisit our successes or failures, our certainties or uncertainties to recreate new theories for new situations. Professional social work practice must be critically reflective to stay alive.

Ultimately, we suggest that this constant reflective capacity is the source of wiser decisions more than heedless certainty. You must be able to say confidently, I *think* that I am right, but *know* that I could be wrong; and so remain open to changing circumstances.

Discomfort, like uncertainty, can be a less-than-desirable state or experience. Discomfort, which is often equated with unhappiness, is something that our consumerist, acquisitive culture encourages us to avoid by quickly achieving a more comfortable position. However, as critical social workers we need to be constantly able to step out of our comfort zones, not only for personal and professional growth, but also to take steps along various roads towards social transformation. Invitations to leave our comfort zones can occur when old beliefs are challenged, when things don't go to plan, when we feel incompetent, when confronted with difference, or when painfully confronted with our own privilege or power (Wong 2004). Wong (2004) suggests we open ourselves to the

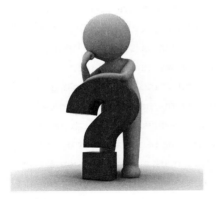

Figure 10.5

feeling of discomfort as a teacher and friend, providing opportunity for growth, suggesting we take time to listen non-judgementally to what this feeling is telling us instead of being busy reacting and defending, and being open to the possibility that a place of discomfort is a place where change can begin. Critical, anti-oppressive practice may be especially uncomfortable at times, because we may be challenging existing modes of thinking and working, not only in others, but equally importantly, within ourselves.

■ The challenge of believing that 'there is no alternative'

Conservative British Prime Minister and proponent of neoliberal policy Margaret Thatcher was noted for her frequent use of the phrase 'there is no alternative', by which she meant that there was in her view no alternative to global capitalism, with its assumption of free markets and trade (Berlinski 2008). In neoliberal times, we all face the challenge of becoming complicit in this widespread, dominant belief. According to Stewart-Harawira (2005, p. 160), one of the most dangerously incorrect constructions of neoliberal discourse is its sense of inevitability – that there simply is no other way, that alternatives do not exist. Creating *counter-hegemonic* visions, we have argued, is a key role for critical social work. A precondition for such visions lies in our capacity for hope, not just any wishful thinking but an 'educated hope' or 'critical hope' (Amsler 2011; Giroux 2001 2004; Webb 2013). Such hope begins with a thorough critique of what is flawed or ruptured in the current societal situation in the light of how it might look if the situation were unflawed and made whole. It then attempts to discern possibilities in the current situation that might lead in the direction of the desired outcome if sufficient effort were made to realise it. 'Hope' may sound like a pie in the sky or fluffy notion; however, even the dry, rationalist discourse of neoliberalism contains a parti-cular version of hope and hopefulness. It is a self-focused hope, 'a notion of hope that is utterly personal, displacing social and collective hopes with the narrow convictions of the entrepreneurial self . . . [without] social responsibility and public accountability': a neoliberal utopia (Giroux 2001, p. 228). However, this version of utopia can be, and is, challenged by an inclusive social utopianism that is an optimistic construction of society 'animated by a determined effort . . . to address pressing social problems and realizable tasks' (Giroux 2001, p. 236). Educated hope fits well with a critical and reflective approach to social work practice. We cannot begin to change or even criticise present conditions if we do not have a view of what to hope for in their place. Only in the light of a possible future can we see how far the present situation falls short of a worthy and dignified human existence.

The role of social work educators, students and practitioners in exploring ways to resist neoliberalism and other oppressive discourses is first to 'to dream differently' (Friere 2001, cited in Amsler 2011, p. 49) and this can start in your social work education. Again, this is not an easy task. Current educational discourses demand learning to be 'fun'. However, acquiring critical knowledge about the social world and changing it may not always make you feel good. As you will now know from reading this book, it may be challenging, confronting, potentially painful, yet entirely worth the effort. Learning about social justice and change is not necessarily therapeutic for the learner; it is not about acquiring the quick 'fix', or the recipe with step-by-step instructions. While it may be that we all learn better when we are enjoying the experience, this need not preclude other emotions from being part of our learning. Amsler (2011, p. 55) evocatively suggests, from a critical perspective, that the obligatory demand for an always 'happy consciousness' is cause for alarm, not celebration. This does not mean that the opposite is true either. Critical learning can be exhilarating and a passionate joy but this may not happen unless we are also willing to experience the discomfort involved in challenging deeply rooted assumptions and dominant discourses, and to be willing to be transformed by what we learn (Amsler 2011, p. 58). Developing a critical consciousness involves discomfort with the status quo and a desire to challenge the horizons of possibility inherent in our situation. For example, higher education, though currently dominated by neoliberal discourse, has historically been a site for both questioning and transforming society, providing a conduit to challenge discourses whose dominance often leads us to believe there are no alternatives (Stewart-Harawira 2005). Hope, as a source of critique and social transformation, is an integral part of the critical social work agenda that allows us to generate the vision and energy we need to engage for change in our local contexts of practice.

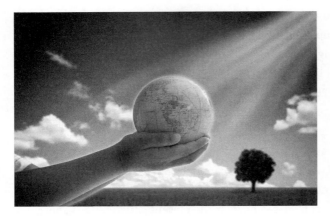

Figure 10.6

■ Summary

This book is an invitation to participate in social work as a critical and hopeful practice of social change for social justice. We believe that despite all the obstacles outlined here, and many others you will encounter in the field, that this practice is not only possible but is actually happening in many places and in many forms, providing robust resistance to dominant social forces, and making a difference in the lives and experiences of the people affected by them. We do not have to accept the prevailing conceptions of the world as one of inevitable inequality and suffering, nor do we have to accept the establishment version of social work as a disciplining device or pain-killing therapy for disadvantaged individuals. As Iain Ferguson (2009) has argued, not only is another world possible, as the anti-capitalist movement loudly proclaims, but so, too, 'another social work is possible'. This is a social work that values human dignity, is prepared to struggle in the discretionary spaces of institutional practice for just outcomes, to accompany our service users as fellow citizens in collective action and not to impose if they do not want our help (2009, pp. 94–6). This is the challenge of critical social work and we believe it is a worthy one.

■ Further reading

Ferguson, I. and Lavalette, M., 2013, '"Another world is possible": Social work and the struggle for social justice' in I. Ferguson, M. Lavallete and E. Whitmore, eds, *Globalisation, Global Justice and Social Work*, Taylor & Francis, Abingdon.

Fook, J., 2000, 'The lone crusader: Constructing enemies and allies in the workplace' in L. Napier and J. Fook, eds, *Breakthroughs in Practice: Theorising Critical Moments in Social Work*, Whiting and Birch, London.

Ife, J., 2012, 'Achieving human rights through social work practice' in *Human Rights and Social Work: Towards Rights-Based Practice*, 3rd edn, Cambridge University Press, Port Melbourne.

Morley, C., 2009, 'Using critical reflection to improve feminist practice' in J. Allan, L. Briskman and B. Pease, eds, *Critical Social Work: Theories and Practices for a Socially Just World*, 2nd edn, Allen & Unwin, Crows Nest, NSW.

Reynolds, V., 2011, 'Resisting burnout with justice-doing', *The International Journal of Narrative Therapy and Community Work*, 4: 27–45.

Glossary

Ableism refers to the personal prejudices, cultural expressions and social forces that marginalise people with disabilities and portrays them in a negative light based on their failure to conform to the prevailing cultural definition of normality (Mullaly 2010, p. 215).

Absolute confidentiality is 'when information revealed to a professional is never passed on to anyone in any form. Such information would never be shared with agency staff, fed into a computer or written in a case record. In reality, absolute confidentiality is rarely achieved' (Zastrow 2010, p. 99).

Activism can take a wide range of forms from participating in political demonstrations/ campaigning, lobbying government, signing petitions, writing letters to newspapers or politicians, terrorism, imposing boycotts on buying certain products or alternatively preferencing some businesses, rallies, street marches, strikes and sit-ins (Baines 2007; Ife 2013).

Activists are people who engage in activism.

Advocacy involves an attempt to influence the behaviour of decision-makers and is something that social workers practise on a regular basis. It aims to improve the responsiveness of social arrangements to people's needs out of a basic respect for an individual's human rights (O'Connor et al. 2008, p. 83).

Ageism refers to negative attitudes towards elderly individuals, which associates them with degeneracy, senility and frailty, and a drain on resources as they make no contribution to a capitalist society (Mullaly 2010).

Agency is the 'ability of people, individually and collectively, to influence their own lives and the society in which we live' (Germov & Poole 2011).

Agrarian refers to an economy based on the farming of land in small communities using human and/or animal labour.

Almoners were chaplains or church officers in charge of distributing money (alms) to the 'deserving poor'; their positions were later filled by hospital social workers (Gleeson 2006).

Anthropocentrism means human-centred and assumes humankind to be the final concern of the universe and views everything in terms of human experience (see Ryan, T. 2011).

Anti-imperialist is one who is opposed to the ideas and beliefs of imperial (territorial) expansion of a country beyond its established borders, including wars to conquer and subjugate people of different cultures (Ife 2013).

Anti-oppressive social work 'is a form of social work practice which addresses social divisions and structural inequalities in the work that is done with "clients" (users) or workers. Anti-oppressive practice aims to provide more appropriate and sensitive services by responding to people's needs regardless of their social status' (Dominelli 1998, p. 24).

Anti-racist theories refer to a range of theories that expose and oppose the use of race, ethnicity and culture as a basis of oppression, discrimination or exploitation (see, for example, Hollinsworth 2006).

Anti-socialist means being opposed to the theoretical and political positions within socialism, which include communism, Marxism and social democracy (Mullaly 2007). The COSs believed that their role was to 'prevent people from becoming hungry' by addressing undesirable social traits and attributed failings to moral relapses. However, by the 1890s some COS workers were aware of the causes of distress (Bremner 1988, p. 98).

Assessment involves 'making a professional judgment about the problematic aspects of a situation' (Fook 2012, p. 132).

Assimilation is the 'Acceptance of a minority group by a majority population, in which the group takes on the values and norms of the dominant culture (Giddens & Sutton 2013).

Attachment theory, as developed by John Bowlby in the 1950s, holds that the nature of the emotional bond between the child (from infancy) and primary caregiver (generally assumed to be the mother) is a significant contributor to the ongoing formation and healthy development of the adult (Freeman 2005).

Bias is a partial and subjective view that is often seen as a negative or undesirable. However, from a critical perspective all information (including scientific evidence) is connected with values, assumptions and constructions, and is therefore biased (see, for example, Morley 2013).

Binary thinking (or dichotomous thinking) sees the world in terms of two mutually exclusive, often opposing, categories (Fook 2012) – for example, black or white; establishment or critical; male or female; able-bodied or disabled.

Biography refers to our social, economic, political, cultural, gendered and historical positioning and experiences, which shape our interpretive lens of the world (Fook 1999).

Biomedical discourses refer to the ideas, languages and practices used to justify the medical model (which is based on the biological sciences) as the dominant approach to health and illness (Healy 2005).

Biomedical model refers to the current, dominant approach to health and illness that is based on the biological sciences (Healy 2005).

Birth of civilisation refers to the period around 6000 BCE when towns and urban centres emerged alongside villages in what is now the Middle East. Specialised food crop cultivation allowed surplus food production to sustain urbanisation, new technologies for the manufacture of metal tools and weapons were developed, commodities such as pottery and textiles were mass produced, social classes began to develop as those who controlled resources or had political power grew personal wealth, and writing became the dominant means of communication and record keeping (Nagle 2010).

Bureaucracy rests on the idea that citizens need to be ruled efficiently by experts (Giddens & Sutton 2013).

Capitalism is the current dominant socioeconomic system throughout the world, and is based on the private ownership of productive resources. Economically it turns all things into marketable commodities. Socially, it produces fundamental and inequitable class divisions between owners and non-owners of capital (Giddens & Sutton 2013; Marx & Engels [1848] 1969).

Care-based ethics is an action-oriented approach that focuses on nurturing, patience, relationship and connection (Bowles et al. 2006).

Case management is arguably the prevailing method in contemporary human service delivery and is required by some funding arrangements. Critical practitioners have critiqued case management as a technocratic practice that aims to simply manage issues rather than respond to the complexity of a situation in a holistic or sustainable way (Dustin 2007).

Casework has traditionally been defined as a process used by certain human welfare agencies to help individuals to 'cope more effectively with their problems in social functioning' (Perlman 1957, p. 4).

Charitable Organisation Societies (COSs), which began in England in the 1840s, were funded by philanthropists and run by volunteers to provide direct service to people in need. COSs used scientific means to assess, measure and administer relief to those who were the deserving poor. Data was collected and used to analyse social problems (Chenoweth & McAuliffe 2012, p. 35).

Child abuse can involve physical abuse, sexual abuse, emotional abuse and/or neglect (Queensland Government 2014).

Civilisational racism concerns the way civilisation itself is defined by a dominant group, as to what is civilised and what is primitive, and how worldviews are constructed by dominant thinkers, generally of a particular race and culture (Scheurich & Young 1997).

Class is a term used to refer to major social divisions that arise from the unequal distribution of economic resources in society (Van Krieken et al. 2012).

Classificatory schemas are frameworks used by establishment social workers that are based on scientific theoretical understandings of human behaviour used to organise and interpret information or 'facts' collected about the service user, which classifies them into diagnostic categories in order to direct a future course of action (Greene 2008, p. 18).

Climate change 'is the by-product of industrialization models promoted by Western entrepreneurs [and the excesses of our unsustainable Western lifestyles, including consumerism] exploiting natural resources to produce goods that make a profit, while discharging greenhouse gases and other pollutants into the atmosphere and water because this was the cheapest method of waste disposal. These activities subsequently caused air temperatures to rise to levels that threaten all forms of life on Earth' (Dominelli 2012, p. 12).

Cognitive behavioural theories are a category of individualist approaches to social work practice, aimed at changing the behaviour of people by changing their thinking (see, for example, Payne 2005).

Cognitive dissonance is the psychological discomfort experienced when holding two or more conflicting beliefs or when there are discrepancies between our behaviour and our beliefs (Festinger 1957).

Cognitive imperialism occurs when a particular way of thinking and expressing knowledge (cognition in the broad sense) is valued, while other ways are belittled or inferiorised (see, for example, Wehbi 2013).

Colonial settler invasion, or **settler colonialism**, is a pattern of one people invading and occupying the territory of another people in order to establish a lasting, highly populated society based on primary production or mining (e.g. Australia, the United States and New Zealand). It differs from 'absentee' colonialism, where the occupying elite is small relative to the indigenous population and only pursues the extraction of goods or profits rather than social development (e.g. the Spanish in the Philippines, the Dutch in Indonesia and the French in Indo-China) (Beilharz & Hogan 2012, p. 558).

Colonialism 'involves the act of colonising, invading, conquering, moving in and then taking over another people's land, resources, wealth, culture and identity' (Ife 2013, p. 198).

Commodities are anything sold on a market for profit (Giddens & Sutton 2013).

Communism is a form of socialism that aims to build a classless society, without private property, money or a state. The dominant communist movement of the 20th century was the revolutionary Marxism–Leninism of the Bolshevik Party led by Lenin, which seized power in Russia in 1917. It advocated a planned economy focused on human need over a free market geared towards profits for a few; public ownership of productive property for the benefit of all; and reduction of social inequalities (Mullaly 2007, p. 115).

Community development (also sometimes referred to as community work, or community capacity building) seeks to re-establish the community as the location of significant human experience and for the meeting of human need, rather than relying on larger, more impersonal and less accessible structures, such as the welfare state, the economy and professional elites (see Ife 2013).

Competitive tendering emerged as one of the processes governments developed as they changed their role from providing to managing welfare service provision. Non-government organisations (NGOs) would compete with each other to be providers of services that are deemed appropriate in the 'market' created by the state (McDonald et al 2011, p. 52).

Conflict resolution is the process of bringing together people who have seemingly incompatible needs, to reach a consensual outcome. There is an assumption that all parties are able to participate in the process equally (Roach Anleu 2010).

Consciousness raising relates to raising the awareness of those who are experiencing social and political oppression as to the structural conditions that cause personal problems (Fook 1993).

Consequentialist (or 'teleological') **ethics** emphasise the consequences of decisions or actions, suggesting that the greatest good for the greatest number of people should be pursued (also sometimes called 'utilitarianism') (Bowles et al. 2006).

Conservative refers to a political stance that preserves the existing social order (including its inequities and injustices) (Mullaly 2007).

Constructions are products of human organisation or creation (Parton & O'Byrne 2000).

Consumer or recovery movement is a movement that is characterised by people coming together around the aim of resistance to the dominant discourse that exercises power over their lives and identity. Indeed, the discourse of recovery that has now found its way into policy and programme initiatives was largely introduced by consumers of mental health services and embraced by the psychiatric disability support sector over the past three decades (Coppock & Dunn 2010; Macfarlane 2009).

Consumerism refers to the increasing affluence in Western countries, which has resulted in a greater emphasis on consumption and leisure. Opportunities to consume have massively increased and are promoted extensively through the media and the internet (Giddens & Sutton 2013).

Context refers to the complex layers that surround, impact upon and shape our understandings and actions.

Contextualising is exploring with the victim/survivor possible alternative contexts in which a situation, thought, feeling or behaviour considered unacceptable would be acceptable (Scott, Walker & Gilmore 1995).

Contracting out involves the government buying the services of a non-state provider. The relationship is managed by a legally binding contract between the purchaser (government) and provider (private provider) (McDonald et al. 2011, p. 52).

Contradictory consciousness refers to the situation whereby subordinated groups and individuals recognise their oppression from practical experience but simultaneously express dominant ideas about the reasonableness and fairness of the system producing their oppression (see Gramsci 1971).

Counselling is a professional practice that can be defined in various ways. From a critical perspective, counselling seeks to be both supportive and educational by working in partnership with individuals to explore the ways in which they are disadvantaged by social and political structures and working with them to find ways of resisting injustices in the system, both for personal liberation and for social change (Fook & Morley 2005; Morley 2014).

Counter-hegemonic refers to efforts opposing hegemonic power by organising to win a cultural consensus in favour of an alternative social ethic or program (the apartheid movement, the civil rights movement) (see, for example, Pratt 2004; Mullaly 2010).

Critical action is concerned with tackling inequalities and working towards empowerment of service users in the face of disempowering structural circumstances (Ray & Phillips 2002).

Critical postmodernism is a term used to describe how modernist critical theories, such as feminism and structural theory (with their focus on universalised understandings of oppression and privilege), can combine with the emancipatory elements of poststructural thinking to extend critical practice (Allan, Briskman & Pease 2009; Fook 2012).

Critical reflection is the process involved in understanding the ways our own values, beliefs and assumptions influence and shape our view of the world (Fook 2012).

Critical social work is a progressive view of social work that questions and challenges the harmful divisions, unequal power relations, injustices and social disadvantages that characterise our society (see, for example, Allan, Briskman & Pease 2009).

Critical theories 'are concerned with possibilities for liberatory, social transformation ... a key point is not just to understand the world but to change it' (Healy 2000, p. 13).

Cultural imperialism refers to 'the dominance and control of one society's or group's culture by another' (Beilharz & Hogan 2012, p. 542).

Cultural models of ethical decision-making prioritise the cultural context, suggest consultation with cultural experts and favour consensus (McAuliffe & Chenoweth 2008).

Culture is a term that aims to describe the complex and 'distinctive ways of life and shared values, beliefs and meanings common to groups of people ... the understandings and expectations which guide actions and interactions with others' (Quinn 2009, pp. 97–8).

Deconstruction involves questioning our assumptions, values and common sense notions that may be linked with dominant discourses (Fook 2012).

Deconstructive gaze is the process of recognising that we ourselves have constructed our understandings of the world and thus we have the ability to change them by challenging the ways in which we have constructed and continue to construct our ideas (Fook 1996, p. 198).

Decontextualisation refers to a process whereby problems are examined at the individual or group level while ignoring the social structural context. In this way, 'differences' between marginalised and dominant groups are identified as the problem, and strategies to 'correct' the differences in the marginal group so that they can be more like the dominant group are employed (Mullaly 2010).

Defence mechanisms are those unconscious strategies that serve to protect the individual from emotions such as pain, anxiety and guilt. Defences arise as a reasonable response to unreasonable circumstances; however, they mask the true nature of the anxiety (Howe 2009).

Deguilting is a critical practice that involves removing blame (Scott, Walker & Gilmore 1995).

Dehumanisation involves treating individuals or a group of people as objects (Thompson 1998).

Democracy is the idea that we govern ourselves as citizens and have a role in shaping the development of laws (Giddens & Sutton 2013).

Demystifying is a critical practice concerned with sharing power that involves taking the mystery out of social work practices. It involves explaining the organisation and the services offered through sharing information. (For further information see Moreau 1979.)

Denial means negating or refusing to accept as real something that is real (e.g. the death of a loved one) (Longres 1995, p. 422).

Deontological (or duty-based) **ethics** infers that some acts are obligatory regardless of their consequences; that because some principles sit above others (that is, we have a duty to follow them), choices are clear and absolute. They are either right (consistent with rules) or wrong (against the rules) and the law must be followed to the letter (Bowles et al. 2006).

Deterritorialisation refers to processes whereby social space becomes more global and not located in a particular place (Scholte 2000, cited in Dower 2003, pp. 42–3).

Deviant behaviour refers to behaviour that does not confirm to socially constructed cultural norms (Howe 2009).

Dialogical processes or relationships are mutual and two-way, with the participants in the dialogue each learning from and teaching each other. 'Both work together so that they can ask the questions as well as think about the answers' (Mullaly 2010, p. 240), which then will inform their actions.

Differentiation relates to the family unit and how each member develops their sense of 'self' as an interdependent actor. From a systems perspective, the degree of differentiation determines the capacity of each to manage their emotions and connections to others. Those who are highly differentiated are believed to function at a higher level by managing their emotional responses compared to those with the greatest fusion, particularly in times of stress (Bowen 1978).

Discourse is a poststructuralist term referring to a set of ideas or language about a particular topic with shared meanings and assumptions that reflect and reinforce particular power relations (Fook 2012). There will always be range of discourses contesting the construction of a human problem or social situation and one or more of these may be dominant at any given time.

Discourse analysis refers to the language practices through which we construct our knowledge and understandings of 'reality' – what is true and what is false – which in turn determines our actions (Healy 2005).

Discrimination refers to the way marginalised groups are excluded, harassed, ridiculed, intimidated and sometimes attacked by dominant groups because of their physical, behavioural or cultural differences (McDonald et al. 2011).

Dispossession refers to the denial of citizenship of Aboriginal people by colonising Europeans, resulting in their separation from land, physical ill-treatment, social disruption, population decline, economic exploitation, discrimination and cultural devastation (Gardiner-Garden 1999).

Dominant discourse is the term given to whichever discourse is dominant in the social construction of a particular human problem or social situation at any particular point in time. The term is similar to **dominant ideology** (but a dominant discourse need not be class-based and may reflect other power relations; see, for example, Fook 2012).

Dominant ideology is a term used by Marxists to describe the ideology of the ruling/ capitalist class, which misrepresents its interests as if these were in the interests of society as a whole. It is therefore a political tool used by the ruling class to reinforce the subordination of workers by masking exploitation and promoting capitalism as natural and beneficial (Van Krieken et al. 2012). (See also **hegemony**.)

Duty of care is defined by the AASW as 'The obligation to take reasonable care to avoid acts or omissions which one can reasonably foresee would be likely to injure another; also, the duty of people in particular circumstances and occupations to protect and control others (AASW 2002, p. 26).

Duty to disclose refers to the release of confidential information in particular situations if, for example, a client may be at risk of harm (Swain & Rice 2009).

Eclecticism refers to mixing theories uncritically, even if the assumptions underpinning the theories contradict each other (Plionis 2004).

Eco-centric means nature-centred.

Ecological perspectives/theories are those that encompass interactions with both human and non-human environments (Healy 2005).

Economic rationalism (often used interchangeably with **neoliberalism**) is a narrow view of economics that refers to the idea that 'free' markets will provide the best outcomes in all spheres of society. It consistently places economic issues over social concerns (Jamrozik 2009).

Economic reforms comprise various measures 'designed to stabilise the economy, steps oriented to change its structure, and, at times, sales of public assets. The central purpose of stabilisation is to slow down inflation and improve the financial position of the state' (Bresser-Pereira, Maravall & Przeworski 1994, p. 184).

Egalitarian means economically equal (Beilharz & Hogan 2012).

Emancipation literally means 'freedom' or 'freedom promoting' and refers to an activist or social change orientation in which practice is focused on transforming processes and structures that perpetuate domination and exploitation (Healy 2005, p. 3).

Empathic solidarity takes account of the social structures that create individual hardship and social disadvantage (Banks 2012, pp. 93–4).

Empiricism refers to the principle that knowledge must be 'tested by some kind of evidence drawn from experience', preferably under controlled conditions (Abercrombie, Hill & Turner 2006, p. 130).

Engagement is regarded as the first stage of a practice process. In simple terms, engagement may involve establishing rapport and a relationship with the person, group or community with whom we work (Chenoweth & McAuliffe 2012).

Enlightenment was a movement in the 17th and 18th centuries, in which the scientific methods that proved successful in gaining control over physical nature were applied to humanity. This promoted an optimistic belief in humanism and rationalism (Beilharz & Hogan 2012).

Epistemological racism is the view that only the wisdom and knowledge of a dominant group (often white and Western) is valid. It serves to delegitimise or invisibilise other forms of knowledge, and is a view so deeply embedded as to become almost invisible and overwhelmingly accepted as the 'norm' (Scheurich & Young 1997).

Epistemology is our theory of knowledge. It addresses the question, how do we know what we know? Epistemology has to do with what we believe is the basis of knowledge (D'Cruz & Jones 2004).

Equality means to distribute resources equally (not necessarily in ways that result in equitable outcomes).

Equity means to distribute resources fairly, according to need (not necessarily equally).

Establishment social work is a **conservative** understanding of social work dominant in most welfare systems today, which uncritically accepts existing social inequalities and helps people cope with the impact of injustices instead of challenging them. It is also strongly associated with objective scientific methods for managing the marginalised in the most cost-effective and least disruptive manner possible.

Ethical decision-making models assist practitioners by providing systematic ways of thinking through ethical dilemmas, often based on a series of steps or questions (Bowles et al. 2006).

Ethical dilemmas are situations that are challenging for practitioners because it is unclear as to what interpretation, decision or action is ethically 'right' or 'wrong' (see, for example, Bowles et al. 2006).

Ethics is a domain of philosophy concerned with questions of what is right or wrong in human conduct (see, for example, McAuliffe & Chenoweth 2008).

Ethnicity is defined as a common set of values and norms, including shared patterns of seeing, thinking and acting, that constructs a group identity (Mullaly 2010, p. 96).

Evidence-based practice is based on scientific presumptions that a service user has a condition or problem that can be treated, monitored and evaluated. This results in a simplistic view of practice that doesn't address the complexities of people's lives; nor does it allow an analysis of how oppression and inequalities have contributed to service users' experiences (McDonald et al. 2011).

Existential questions concern 'the meaningfulness of one's life and sociopolitical questions about happiness ... [are transformed] into technical questions about the most effective ways of coping or managing one's emotional life and malfunction' (Rose 1996, cited in Fullagar & Gattuso 2002, p. 10).

Extreme (or absolute) poverty is defined by the World Bank as people living on US$1.25 or less per day (Ravallion, Chen & Sangraula 2008).

Family group meeting is organised by the social worker to develop a shared understanding within the family, and between the family and worker(s) about the family's concerns, and a plan of action to address these concerns (Healy 2012, p. 116).

Family therapy refers to a set of practice approaches that view problems facing a family member as produced by family dynamics that are troubling for that individual, and therefore seek to transform unhelpful family dynamics (Healy 2012. p. 116).

Femininity refers to the socially constructed characteristics of being female, including passivity, emotionality, natural caregiving, irrationality and weakness (Mullaly 2010).

Feminism is a body of theories that exposes women's oppression (patriarchal domination); it is associated with the women's movement and its struggles for women's emancipation (see, for example, Seidman 2013).

Feminists are women who advocate the rights of women to overcome patriarchal (male-dominated) inequality and oppression (Dominelli 2012).

Feminist social work 'arose out of feminist social action being carried out by women working with women in their communities. Their aim has been to improve women's wellbeing by linking their personal predicaments and often private sorrows with their social position and status in society' (Dominelli 2012, p. 6).

Feudalism refers to a hierarchal social and political system based on land ownership with a king and his lords at the top and peasant farmers and the landless at the bottom. The latter would work their lord's land in exchange for certain rights and protection (Hunt 2003).

Fieldwork placement is an educative process whereby students develop a range of professional skills under supervision in a variety of workplace settings. The aim is for students to engage with practitioners in the field, put theory into different contexts and become socialised into their profession (AASW 2012).

Frankfurt School was an influential group of unorthodox Marxist theorists whose project of 'critical theory' sought to recover the core of Marx's critique and use it to expose forces of domination in both capitalist and state-socialist societies with a view to promoting human freedom and social justice. The original Frankfurt School operated between the 1930s and 1960s. A second and third generation of Frankfurt theorists has continued under the respective leaderships of Jürgen Habermas and Axel Honneth until the present time (see, for example, Bronner 2011; Kelner 1989).

'Friendly visitors' were usually women who volunteered to visit the poor in their homes to assess their eligibility (deserving or undeserving) and needs for assistance (Horner 2012, p. 24).

Functionalist theory is associated with Emile Durkheim (1858–1917), who sought to understand modern societies and the functions of institutions and people's 'roles' within them, in terms of the metaphor of a living organism (see, for example, Yuill & Gibson 2011, p. 16). It has been a key influence on the development of systems theory in social work.

Functionally illiterate means having reading and writing skills that are inadequate to function on a daily basis and maintain employment that requires more than basic levels (Schlecty 2004).

Functionally innumerate is the inability to apply reason and comprehend basic numeracy skills. This can have a negative effect on career, health and economic choices (Reyna et al. 2009).

Gender is the social construct related to the roles, behaviours and attitudes we expect from people based on their assignment as either male or female (Mullaly 2010, p. 212).

Gendered perspective refers to the fact that most major systems in Western societies are hierarchically organised and male-dominated (Mullaly 2010). When a hierarchy becomes established, a dynamic of superiority (male)/inferiority (female) results in the superior group judging the inferior group as having less intrinsic worth and therefore assigns them roles and functions that are poorly valued, such as unpaid services (Dominelli 1998). These socially constructed roles are considered natural or inevitable (therefore, the best place for the woman is in the home – of a man) rather than male constructions that perpetuate and sustain power relations between genders.

Generalist skills underpin all social work practice (such as interpersonal communication skills and writing skills) (Compton & Galaway 1999; Trevithick 2005).

Genocide is the mass extermination of entire human populations (Bauman 1989).

Global capitalism is the extension of the dominant (capitalist) economic system to the entire world (Giddens & Sutton 2013).

Globalisation refers to large-scale changes that bring together previously separate societies into a global network, predominantly through the development of global technologies and global economies. From an economic point of view, globalisation simply means integration into the world economy, which is seen as the only means for poorer nations to develop. (For further information see Van Krieken et al. 2012.)

Government refers to a formal organisation that administers the political life of a society (Macionis 2011).

Grand narratives are abstract ideas that explain historical knowledge and experiences intended to legitimise the truth (Nola & Irzik 2005).

Great Depression (1929–38) was the extreme worldwide economic crisis that began with the collapse of the New York Stock Exchange in 1929. Its consequences were socially disastrous, rapidly creating record unemployment, mass poverty and civil unrest. (For further information see Reisch & Andrews 2001.)

Group work can be most simply understood as work with groups. This type of work can vary from being educationally orientated, therapeutic, activist in nature, or simply take the form of meeting around a particular cause. (For further information see Healy 2012.)

Hegemonic masculinity refers to the dominant social form and expectations of masculinity within a patriarchal culture. In the modern Western societies, hegemonic masculinity typically prescribes an ideal that is white, heterosexual, middle-class, able-bodied, rational and stoic in the face of adversity (see Connell 1987).

Hegemony 'is the operation of one powerful group over others, such that the consensus of the subordinated groups is achieved by convincing people it is in their interests to agree with and follow the dominant group's ideas' (Germov & Poole 2011, p. 114).

Hereditary aristocracies refers to the dominant social class emerging within feudal or agrarian societies, in which the dominance is based on the ownership of land that is inherited. Aristocratic rank is often bestowed by a monarch and enshrined in law (Hunt 2003).

Heterosexism is the form of oppression whereby heterosexuality is considered to be natural by society and all other alternatives are considered to be unnatural (Mullaly 2010, p. 212).

Homelessness can be defined as:
- 'Persons who are in improvised dwellings, tents or sleeping out
- Persons in supported accommodation for the homeless
- Persons who are staying temporarily with other households
- Persons who are staying in boarding houses
- Persons in other temporary dwellings' (Australian Bureau of Statistics 2011).

Homophobia is an irrational fear of or discomfort with homosexual people that often manifests as individual violence or structural discrimination (Mullaly 2010, p. 212).

Human rights concern the basic entitlements of every human being. Human rights are a constructed notion of universal values (i.e. they apply to everyone, everywhere) regardless of 'national origin, race, culture, age, sex or any other characteristic' (Ife 2012, p. 19).

Human services organisations 'nominate as their primary purpose the promotion of the care and well-being of people experiencing difficulties in their lives because of poverty, disability, illness, or some other life hazard' (McDonald et al. 2011, p. 4).

Human trafficking is the recruitment and transfer of people by means of threat, force, abduction, deception, abuse of power or vulnerability, or payments of benefits for the purpose of sexual exploitation, forced labour, slavery or the removal of organs (United Nations Office on Drugs and Crime 2013).

Humanitarian approach is a style of organisational management and is more aligned with social work values and approaches (in contrast to managerialism). The essence of the humanitarian approach spans three interrelated elements: relationships, culture and language (Rees 1999).

Identity refers to who we are as people. From a poststructural perspective identity is fluid and contextual, whereas previously our sense of 'self' was thought of as static or the result of fixed attributes. This interactive idea of identity formation means that we are in a constant state of change (fluidity) dependent upon time and place (context). (For further information see Sands 1996.)

Ideology is the term Marx used when referring to a system of ideas that interprets reality in the interests of a particular social class. The ideology of the ruling class will thus be the **dominant ideology** of a given society, misrepresenting the interests of that class as if these were in the interests of society as a whole (Van Krieken et al. 2012).

Imperialism refers to the domination of a powerful country over other territories and peoples beyond its borders. (For further information see Beilharz & Hogan 2012.)

Implicit assumptions are assumptions that we hold, but of which we are not necessarily aware (Fook 2012).

Individualised/Individualist/Individualistic theories view the object of (or the target for) change as the individual, with the worker's role, at a basic level, that of 'fixer' (Payne 2005, p. 45). These understandings and analyses ignore the structural factors that influence people's personal circumstances (Fook 1993).

Individualism refers to an increasingly individualist emphasis within society; this has been created by economic and social changes that have removed a mechanism of socialisation within which collectivist ideas and attitudes were once generated. Changes in the nature of the workplace, the employment relationship and management styles have all contributed to increasing individualism (Giddens & Sutton 2013).

Individualistic approaches are part of mainstream or establishment social work that understands the issue as a deficit within the individual. This analysis and explanation of social problems does not explain the persistence of problems; nor does this analysis explain why interventions and practices are ineffectual (Mullaly 2010, p. 275).

In-door relief relates to compensation for labouring in factories as opposed to 'out-door relief", which was public aid to the poor outside of institutions, such as soup kitchens and the supply of alms (Bremner 1988).

Industrial Capitalist Revolution refers to the emergence, initially in Britain in the late 18th century, of mechanised, factory-based production that replaced agriculture as the main means of production and run on a capitalist basis (Gidden & Sutton 2013).

Infantilisation involves treating an individual or group of people like babies or children (Thompson 1998).

Informed consent is the receipt of permission from a person to engage in a particular act while being fully appraised of the implications of doing so.

Institutional racism is the discriminatory behaviours embedded within organisations towards people because of their colour, culture or ethnic origin (Hollinsworth 2006).

Internalised oppression refers to the 'incorporation and acceptance by individuals within an oppressed group of the prejudices against them within the dominant society' (Pheterson 1986, p. 148).

Internationalisation refers to the development of international institutions transcending national borders (Scholte 2000, cited in Dower 2003, pp. 42–3).

Intervention refers to a method of practice applied after a professional judgement has been made, and is used to achieve 'measurable results using available resources in the most effective way' (Ife 1996, p. 52).

Invisibilisation refers to the process of making a group invisible through under-representation in public discourse (Thompson 1998).

Laissez faire, one of the guiding principles of capitalism, claims that economic systems work best when there is little government intervention. This has resulted in a great disparity of wealth in Western societies, while opposition to laissez-faire approaches led to the emergence of Keynesian economics and the growth of the welfare state early in the 20th century. However, since the emergence of the global economy in the 1970s, laissez-faire principles have informed public policy as nation states moved to deregulate financial and trade systems, reduce wages and business costs, lower taxation and reduce government spending in order to become more competitive in the global market (Dalton et al. 1996).

Law encompasses a systematic collection of principles and rules that define rights and duties, and the set of institutions that enforce them (Swain 2002).

Liaison officer is a university representative who maintains regular contact with students on fieldwork placement to clarify educational issues, monitor progress of the placement, mediate any difficulties and assess student progress (AASW 2012).

Liberal utilitarian philosophy advocates the principle of 'the greatest good for the greatest number' (Bentham [1776] 1977, p. 393). (See also **consequentialist ethics**.)

Liberalisation refers to the spread of the 'free market' in the world economy (Scholte 2000, cited in Dower 2003, pp. 42–3).

Liberals are those who favour an individualist approach to social problems, arguing that poverty is mainly the result of poor choices and that the only way out of it is for individuals to work hard and be as free as possible from state restrictions on their market exchanges (trade) (see, for example, Horner 2012).

Limits of confidentiality refers to the situations in which complete privacy (confidentiality) between the social worker and the client cannot be assured. Examples include when there is risk of serious harm to the client or another, when there is a legal requirement (court order) to disclose information, and when information is shared within an agency or team for the purposes of continuity of care (Banks 2012).

Linear models, processes or frameworks contain a number of chronological steps leading to a definitive conclusion. (For further information see Ife 2012.)

Macro interventions are focused on creating large-scale change within social and political systems.

Macro methods are collective methods of practice, such as advocacy, community development, policy development and analysis, research and social action (Allan 2009).

Macro systems examine broad social factors including the impact of global capitalism, globalisation, class inequalities and state institutions (Healy 2005).

Managerialism refers to a set of beliefs and practices that define all problems in the world (including social problems) in economic terms. It assumes that managers should be in control of all private and public organisations (including human services) and that these should be run in line with business principles and concerns (i.e. efficiency, profitability and accountancy logic) (see, for example, Evans 2009; Holscher & Sewpaul 2006).

Marginalisation is a process of decentring and/or pushing someone or something else to the margins of society (excluding them from meaningful participation) (Thompson 1998).

Marxism is a body of diverse theory associated with the work of Karl Marx that seeks to criticise, and liberate people from, economic oppression (see, for example, Seidman 2013; Van Krieken et al. 2012).

Masculinity refers to the socially constructed characteristics of being male, including strength, aggression and competitiveness (Mullaly 2010).

Mediation is an informal (not legally binding) process whereby participants engage in open discussions to resolve a dispute. The process is facilitated by a neutral third-party mediator who does not intervene, coerce or impose a particular outcome but does control the process, which calls into question the idea of 'neutrality' (Roach Anleu 2010).

Medical dominance refers to social arrangements and discourses that legitimate and sanction medical control over the definitions, management and treatment of health and illness (see, for example, Willis 1990).

Medicalisation (page 54) refers to the process of redefining normal human bodily experiences as medical problems. In other words, physical experiences that were historically seen as unproblematic suddenly become, through the intervention of the medical profession and a renaming of the experience, a problem (Holmes, Hughes & Julian 2012, p. 203).

Medicalisation (page 235) places people in the domain of the medical profession (so they are ascribed a sick or invalid status) (Thompson 1998).

Micro methods refer to direct service components of social work practice. These include methods for working with individuals, such as casework, counselling, case management and advocacy (Healy 2012).

Micro social systems is a concept derived from systems theory that looks at the individual's immediate environment (e.g. individuals, families, friends) (Healy 2005).

Migration refers to the movement of people between nation states that accompanies the movement of commodities and capital, made easier in recent times by better transportation and communication technologies. It has increased worldwide, with people migrating for a multitude of reasons, such as labour, political asylum or permanent settlement. Migration has become much more politicised, affecting domestic politics, bilateral and regional relationships and the national security policies of nation states (Castles & Miller 2003).

Modernisation refers to the modern state, bureaucracy, and so on (Scholte 2000, cited in Dower 2003, pp. 42–3).

Modernity refers to both a period in time and a set of social forms that are radically different from traditional or pre-modern societies. It can be characterised as the product of three interrelated 'revolutions' that began in Europe in the 17th century and that are now global in impact. These were (1) the Scientific Revolution and 'Enlightenment', (2) the Political Revolution and (3) the Industrial-Capitalist Revolution. (For further information see Van Krieken et al. 2012.)

Multiculturalism refers to both the discourse and federal government policy from the 1980s to the early 2000s, recognising and celebrating Australian cultural diversity and affirming that all cultural groups have equal rights to services and development. (For further information see Ife 2013.)

Multidisciplinary teams 'involve different professions working together by performing different roles in line with their own discipline' (Hughes & Wearing 2013, p. 93).

Municipal socialism refers to public enterprises at the local government level (Sawer 2003).

Nation states are a type of state that emerged around 200 years ago in which the government claims exclusive right to sovereign power (Giddens & Sutton 2013).

Neoliberalism (often used interchangeably with **economic rationalism**) is the discourse (languages, ideas and practices) used to justify global capitalism as the dominant economic system. The central tenet that all definitions of neoliberalism have in common 'is a central emphasis on the market as the organising principle of social life' (Penna & O'Brien 2013, p. 137).

Neo-Marxism is a modified version of Marxism that incorporates diverse notions of power and culture (Germov & Poole 2011).

Normalcy as used here relates to the way in which the dominant constructions of the 'family' (white, middle class, heterosexual) are seen as 'normal' while all other family structures are seen as other or deviant (Mullaly 2010).

Normalisation refers to assessing feelings and emotional responses as common and legitimate by validating and reassuring the service user that their feelings, thoughts and behaviours are entirely justified given the outside pressures of their experiences (Scott, Walker & Gilmore 1995).

Normalised refers to the process whereby many oppressed people will internalise guilt, shame and blame for their oppressive experiences because they have accepted the dominant messages that they are responsible for causing the social problems they are experiencing (Mullaly 2010, p. 238).

Normative refers to dominant cultural understandings of what is regarded as normal (e.g. 'able-bodied). Differences are seen as problematic (e.g. 'disabled), resulting in marginalisation (Barnes & Mercer 2004).

Normative consensus refers to agreement about social norms.

Nourishing terrains refers to an Indigenous Australian understanding of 'wilderness' that reflects a long history of human use and nourishment from the land (country) and that the concepts of 'country' and 'kinship' are inseparable to culture. This has resulted in Aboriginal and Torres Strait Islander people teaching their children history, supporting their kin and taking care of country (Bird 1996).

Objectivism is a paradigm that assumes there is an objective reality (that is knowable or known) and that it exists independently from the knower, and therefore it is possible and desirable to remove the subjective and intuitive dimensions of knowledge from our understandings (Meinert, Pardeck & Kreuger 2000a; Sarantakos 2005). An objectivist paradigm assumes that things have a meaning 'in themselves', independent from the person interpreting them, and from the contexts in which the person or object is situated (Crotty 1998).

Objectivity is the idea that one can stand outside of reality and observe it without any subjective interpretations or prejudices. (For further information see D'Cruz & Jones 2004.)

Oppression can be defined as the domination by powerful groups of less powerful groups in ways that restrict their rights, opportunities and access to resources (Mullaly 2010)

Organisational culture refers to the 'attitudes, beliefs, personal and cultural values shared by people and groups in an organisation that significantly impact on the way people interact with each other and with others outside of the organisation' (McDonald et al. 2011, p. 63).

Organisational practice refers to our professional purpose, which is shaped by service users' needs and expectations, our institutional context (e.g. statutory or community-based) and our professional practice base, which is the combination of theories, knowledge and values. Our choice of methods and skills and how they are applied is informed by our sense of professional purpose, which is constantly constructed by us and external sources (Healy 2012).

Othering refers to the way in which a dominant group classifies behaviour that is different from its own as 'other', enabling the othered group to be devalued and objectified (Mullaly 2010).

Out-door relief was public aid to the poor outside of institutions, such as soup kitchens and the supply of alms (Bremner 1988).

Paradigm is a set of assumptions, concepts, values and practices that provide a way of understanding the world and how it operates; for example, capitalism is considered a dominant paradigm (Mullaly 2010).

Paternalism relates to a way of working with people that provides for their needs without considering their rights or responsibilities. This form of activity is seen by some social workers as 'necessary' for those unable to take responsibility for themselves, and recipients are expected to show gratitude (Mullaly 2007, p. 82).

Pathologise means treating a perceived condition as a disease or psychologically abnormal.

Patriarchy is the term for societies that are organised on the basis of male domination, where men benefit from institutional power in ways that disadvantage women (Orme 2013). Patriarchy literally means 'rule of the father' (Ferguson 1999, p. 1048).

Philanthropic means charitable.

Pluralist approaches seek to find ways of incorporating different visions of what is morally 'good' without arriving at a single unitary position (Hugman 2013, p. 137).

Policy is a principle or rule to guide actions towards those that are most likely to achieve a desired outcome (see, for example, Jamrozik 2009).

Policy analysis involves a critical evaluation of social policies to scrutinise their impacts on society in terms of creating greater or lesser social inequality. (For further information see Jamrozik 2009.)

Policy development involves participating in the creation of new policies to meet the needs of services and people. (For further information see Jamrozik 2009.)

Political Revolution followed the Enlightenment and was strongly influenced by its ideals. If people could reason for themselves, it followed that they could govern themselves (democracy) (see, for example, Ritzer & Stepmisky 2014).

Poor Laws were enacted between 1536 and 1601 in Britain under the Tudor monarchy, which distinguished between 'deserving' (disabled, sick, orphaned, elderly) and supposedly 'undeserving' (able-bodied but unemployed or criminal) poor. (For further information see Horner 2012.)

Positivism is a theory of knowledge that claims that the only reliable form of knowledge is that which can be stated in law-like propositions and is open to empirical verification (knowledge directly observed or experienced). (For further information see D'Cruz & Jones 2004.)

Postmodernism is a theory that rejects the idea of there being a single, fixed and objective truth, and instead emphasises multiple perspectives and truths. In this view the world is not objective or mechanical, but complex, fluid, contradictory and multilayered, making it capable of different readings. Postmodernism therefore disrupts the dominant modernist view and invites us to consider alternative voices and perspectives in understanding the world and its problems (see, for example, Seidman 2013).

Poststructuralism literally means 'after structuralism' and refers to theories that reject the idea that all human activities can be totally explained as the outcome of a definite set of underlying 'social structures'. Instead of offering a singular, absolute or complete 'truth' (black and white view) about the world and its problems, poststructuralism encourages an appreciation of different understandings (multiple truths) based on differing cultural, institutional and individual standpoints and contexts. Poststructuralism originated in France in the 1970s and is generally regarded as the intellectual movement of postmodernism (see, for example, Seidman 2013).

Pragmatic activism, according to Healy (2000, p. 145) frees workers to focus on 'local, contextual and modest proposals for change', in place of grand plans, or all-or-nothing ideals.

Praxis is the term Marx used for humankind's capacity to combine theory and practice for self-reflective agency in history. Revolutionary praxis is the collective capacity to fundamentally transform oppressive social structures to further human emancipation (see Critchley 1997; Van Krieken et al. 2012).

Prejudices refer to deeply held individual beliefs or negative evaluations about others based on their membership of non-dominant groups constructed around gender, class, age, ability, sexuality, ethnicity or religion (Mullaly 2010).

Presenting problem is the most obvious and immediate concern that service users present, but not necessarily the only or most important issue.

Privatisation refers to a declining sense of community, whether for the rich or poor, in that notions of society are dominated by private individuals, private spaces and private institutions (Fisher & Karger 1997).

Professional autonomy/discretion describes the ability of social workers to work discreetly within managerialist organisational policies and practices while appearing to share professional values and at the same time advocate for their clients (Evans 2010).

Professional imperialism refers to the way that Western professional models were and are imposed and imported globally, with little recognition of local or indigenous knowledge or expertise (Faith 2008).

Professional integrity is our capacity to work in a manner consistent with our values as critically reflective practitioners. (For further information see Wagner 1990.)

Professional narrative is a term used to describe a critical approach to assessments in which the worker recognises that they are creating meanings of the service user's world and need to allow for multiple interpretations, contradictions and change, rather than assuming that issues have a cause and effect. The complexities of a situation are examined and meanings are co-constructed by workers and service users (Fook 2012, p. 135).

Professionalisation refers to a profession becoming socially recognised.

Progressive is a political stance that aims to challenge the existing social order (including its inequities and injustices) and move it towards the goal of greater freedom and equity. (For further information see Mullaly 2007.)

Projection is the imposition of unwanted feelings about oneself onto another (for example, blaming others for not keeping in contact when you don't keep in contact yourself) (Longres 1995. p. 422).

Psychodynamic theories/perspectives are individualistic theories based on the work of Sigmund Freud. They stem from the assumption that individual behaviour comes from 'movements and interactions in the mind' (Payne 2005, p. 73).

Psychosocial assessments determine the nature and extent of the person's situation and issues in their social environment (Healy 2005).

Race is a problematic term for a number of reasons. First, there is no universal agreement as to what the distinguishing criteria are for human 'races'. Second, the categories that have been employed in the past are ultimately dependent on political context and agendas, where one visibly identifiable group is contrasted with, and ranked in relation to, other groups. These differences are usually based on skin colour or some other outwardly apparent but biologically superficial characteristic. Finally, and unfortunately, since the advent of colonialism, these differences have been used by powerful groups to oppress or enslave other groups or peoples (see, for example, Holmes, Hughes & Julian 2006).

Racial bias is 'typically understood . . . in terms of individual acts of overt prejudice that are racially based' as well as other acts that are more covert; that is, hidden, subtle or not explicitly public (Scheurich & Young 1997, pp. 4–5).

Racialisation 'is the process by which race is interpreted as the primary marker of a social phemonenon' (Holmes, Hughes & Julian 2006, p. 44).

Racism is defined as beliefs, statements and acts that render certain groups inferior on the basis that they do not belong to the culture of origin of the dominant ethnic group within the state apparatus (Hollinsworth 1997).

Radical casework is a practice that 'first and foremost assumes an analysis which constantly links the causes of personal and social problems to problems in the socioeconomic structure, rather than to inadequacies inherent in individual people or in socially disadvantaged minority groups' (Fook 1993, p. 7).

Radicalism is the act of advocating for institutional change using the practice of high-risk activity to exert positive or negative influence on mainstream organisations (Cross 2012; Haines 1988).

Randomised control trials are studies in which people are allocated at random to receive one of several clinical interventions (Jadad 1998).

Rationalism holds that individuals are rational creatures and that reason, supported by observation and experiment, is the surest guide to human emancipation (Wadham, Pudsey & Boyd 2007).

Recapitulation is to believe that critical social workers' personal and professional lives would be easier if they just accepted the way things are as 'natural' or 'inevitable' and became mainstream or establishment social workers, letting go of their social change objectives (Mullaly 2010).

'Reclaim the Night' (or in some countries 'Take Back the Night') rallies encourage the 'grass roots participation in the organisation of events by as many women as possible'. These events 'draw together women from diverse backgrounds and experiences to work together in addressing issues of men's sexual violence against women and children'. The rallies are now held annually on the last Friday night in October to enable women 'to speak out against violence and to celebrate strength' (Reclaim the Night Australia 2013)

Reconciliation is a highly contested concept; however, at its simplest, it refers to estranged parties becoming friendly, harmonious and compatible. In the current Australian context, it is also a political process that, at one end of the spectrum refers to an expectation that Aboriginal and Torres Strait Islander people accept mainstream values, and at the other, an expectation and opportunity for a reinterpretation of colonial history and recognition of the self-determination and rights of Indigenous Australians. (For further discussion, see Beresford & Beresford 2006; Burridge 2009; Kaplan-Myrth 2005; Muldoon & Schaap 2012.)

Reconstruction is the process of revising unhelpful assumptions when they run counter to our intentions (Fook 2012).

Recovery concepts and discourses are often used in the context of mental health and imply not so much a cure or denial of past or current events, but a 'process [encompassing] the development of new meaning and purpose as one grown beyond the catastrophic effects of mental illness' (Anthony 1993, p. 17).

Redistributive justice principles view the state as having a role in legislating a more equal sharing of the material benefits and resources of society; the state must, therefore, act independently – and often in opposition to – market forces and promote an ethic of collective benefit rather than individual interest (Mullaly 2007, p. 126).

Reflective ethical decision-making models emphasise the importance of dialogue and the inclusion of clients in decision-making processes (McAuliffe & Chenoweth 2008).

Reflective practitioners are able to reflect on 'assumptions (hidden theory) embedded in practice, and to expose these for examination, in order to improve practice' (Fook 2012, p. 196).

Reflexivity involves locating ourselves in the picture and can be defined in three ways: (1) 'the ability of individuals to process information and create knowledge to guide life choices; (2) an individual's self-critical approach that questions how knowledge is generated and how relations of power operate in this process; and (3) a concern with the part that emotions play in social work practice' (D'Cruz, Gillingham & Melendez 2007, p. 75).

Reframing refers to a process of re-examining negative and disempowering self-concepts, through drawing on the service user's strengths and offering another way a situation can be viewed (Lundy 2004).

Registration refers to statutory regulation.

Regression involves unconsciously returning to a type of thought, feeling or behaviour associated with an earlier stage of development in order to allay fear or anxiety (for example, an older child reverting to thumb sucking when a new sibling is born) (Longres 1995, p. 422).

Relational autonomy is an ethical view of human agency that seeks an optimal balance between individual freedom and the fact that people are always underpinned and shaped by their social relations and context (Mackenzie & Stoljar 2000).

Relative confidentiality refers to the possible disclosure of records and personal information to supervisors, or by court order, or to protect a third party from a harmful situation (Geldard & Geldard 2012).

Relativism is the idea that truth depends entirely on context, that what is true for one group may not be true for another, because there are no universal criteria for settling truth claims (see Cuff, Sharrock & Francis 2006).

Repression means bottling up feelings of anxiety or distress (for example, saying things are okay when they're not) (Longres 1995, p. 422).

Research is understood in a variety of ways as it is informed by different paradigms and assumptions. From a critical perspective, research can be defined as a practice that involves generating new knowledge to understand social and environmental conditions in ways that contribute to the building of a more just, participatory and sustainable world (see, for example, Morley 2013).

Risk assessment is an organisational procedure designed to manage risk for both workers and service users in the name of accountability. The dangers in this approach are that workers can become so fixated on assessing, managing and ensuring against risk that they potentially lose sight of what is important and effective in their work with service users. Workers are often confronted with situations where risk prevails and rather than think creatively about effective solutions, they are expected to act prescriptively, which can be damaging to both themselves and the service users (Gardner 2006).

Rurality relates to non-urban communities whose economies are largely dependent on primary production, such as agriculture, which has faced increasing competition in a global economy and remains vulnerable to changing environmental patterns, such as drought. These factors have caused financial hardship, migration of young people to urban areas seeking employment, and the loss of capacity of residents and communities to determine their own futures (Alston 2012, p. 516).

Scientific philanthropy was the belief that public aid to the poor outside of institutions was undesirable and unnecessary and that charity should be organised and administered in order to compel would-be paupers to become self-supporting. This belief was based on the understanding that more consideration should be given to *who* received assistance (scientific assessment) and more attention paid to *what* types of assistance were given (application of scientific method to social problems) (Bremner 1988).

Scientific Revolution refers to the intellectual transformation that began in Europe in the 16th century through the work of Galileo, Copernicus and Isaac Newton, whose use of 'rational observation', testing, measurement and precise calculation (without reference to the supernatural) changed the way people understood the universe. Science and reason became the basis for reliable knowledge rather than 'religion and the Bible' (Wadham, Pudsey & Boyd 2007, p. 39).

Secular refers to the non-religious.

Secular humanism is the belief that human beings can direct their own *progress* towards greater freedom and equality, without religion. (For further information see Ife 2012.)

Self-determination may be defined as 'The belief that the individual or the group has the right to make decisions that affect her/himself or the group' (Berg-Weger 2013, Glossary 1–10).

Self-disclosure is a contentious practice that can be defined as 'The sharing of personal information with a client system' (Berg-Weger 2013, Glossary 1–10).

Sentient beings are living creatures who have the capacity for basic consciousness – the ability to feel or perceive pain and emotion, and experience a state of wellbeing, without necessarily being self-aware. The current scientific consensus is that all vertebrate animals are sentient beings capable of feeling pain and experiencing distress, and for this reason there are laws governing animal cruelty (Duncan 2006).

Settlement movement refers to the group that broke away from the COS. The movement developed an alternative social model for combating poverty while sowing the seeds for the group work, community development, social policy and political advocacy aspects of social work (see, for example, Ferguson 2008).

Settler capitalism is a form of capitalist development imported by a colonial elite based on livestock farming that profits from exporting agricultural produce back to the home country (Beilharz & Hogan 2012, p. xx).

Sexism refers to a set of social, economic, political and cultural beliefs, attitudes and practices that in patriarchal societies are predominantly employed to oppress women by associating a biological difference (female) with socially constructed characteristics (Mullaly 2010, p. 210).

Situated ethics involves working to exploit the gaps and contradictions within dominant discourses and 'being alert to the dominance of managerialist and neoliberal agendas ... working in the spaces between the contradictions of care and control, prevention and enforcement, empathy and equity' (Banks 2012, pp. 93–4)

Social activism (also referred to as social action) involves activities such as organising, educating and mobilising people (Baines 2007). It involves the intention to work with collective consciousness to promote, block or influence social, political, economic and/or environmental change or maintenance of the status quo.

Social or public advocacy is thinking of solutions and actions, big and small, needed for collective social change – to change the conditions that generate social problems (Baines 2007).

Social change refers to transformations of societal structures and cultural patterns, not simply of individuals' lives (Van Krieken et al. 2014, p. 4).

Social constructions refers to 'the socially created characteristics of human life based on the idea that people actively construct reality, meaning it is neither "natural" or inevitable. Therefore notions of normality/abnormality, right/wrong, and health/illness are subjective human creations that should not be taken for granted' (Germov & Poole 2011, p. 21).

Social control refers to a range of measures (both formal and informal) whereby a dominant group or institution brings other groups and individuals into conformity with its norms (Jamrozik 2009).

Social Darwinism took Charles Darwin's (1859) theory of 'natural selection' for explaining biological evolution, and misapplied it to competition between social groups and individuals (rich and poor, black and white) in which 'the strong' survive and thrive but 'the weak' die out (Woodside & McClam 2011, p. 35).

Social democracy is a form of democratic socialism that aims to extend social rights and a more equitable distribution of wealth through parliamentary reform, wage regulation, national planning and (historically) the nationalisation of strategic industries. Critics of social democracy point out that it is highly state-centred and 'top-down' in its pursuit of equity and often compromises basic socialist principles because it operates within a capitalist system. (For further information see Keman 2014.)

Social diagnosis was a form of screening developed by Mary Richmond to typify and treat the poor on a case-by-case basis (Bremner 1988).

Social or socioeconomic disadvantage refers to those who are low-income earners, temporarily unemployed or permanently excluded from the labour market resulting in lower levels of education, less access to society goods, fewer opportunities, less respect or status and less political power (Mullaly 2010, p. 207).

Social justice is an ethical norm that society is responsible for, and obliged to prevent, poverty and other extreme forms of inequality. Most definitions of social justice agree that it involves access, equity, rights and participation (see, for example, Netting, Kettner & McMurtry 2008).

Social location is how we would describe ourselves in such terms as gender, race, ethnicity, class, nationality, sexual orientation, age, disability and language as well as affiliations we may be involved in, such as religion and politics (Kirk & Okazawa-Rey 2004).

Social milieu was defined by Durkheim as the 'substratum of society' – the social environment that is composed of layers of interrelated and connected complex systems and communication mechanisms. New ideas and understandings emerge as a result of 'social life' or the interaction of individuals who have entered into diverse relationships with each other (Sawyer 2002, p. 234).

Social model focuses on the social construction of disability – access, stereotypes, conceptions of normality, ideas of difference and capacity are all defined by and embedded in the social order (Barnes & Mercer 2004).

Social movements are large collectivities of people who aim to either maintain or challenge the existing social order (Giddens & Sutton 2013).

Social policy 'is a process of authoritative allocation of material and human resources . . . for the purpose of achieving certain social, economic, cultural and political outcomes in society' (Jamrozik 2009, p. 49)

Social research, from a critical perspective, is a practice that involves generating new knowledge to understand social and environmental conditions in ways that contribute to the building of a more just, participatory and sustainable world (see, for example, Morley 2013).

Social structures (or structures) are the enduring social patterns, power divisions, institutions and inequalities that persist over time and make up a society. These can be political, economic, gendered, historical, and so on, and they exist independently of the action of any one individual (see also Germov & Poole 2011; Yuill & Gibson 2011).

Social theory examines the social sources and contexts (including social barriers and inequalities) of people's behaviours and social changes impacting on these more broadly (Joas & Knobl 2009).

Social transformationist describes the view that the major problems confronting individuals are rooted in unjust power relations and that both collective and personal action are required to change these (Healy 2000, p. 24). Strategies of transformation may be reformist or revolutionary.

Socialisation is 'the process by which an individual learns the culture of a society and internalises its norms, values and perspectives in order to know how to behave and communicate' (Germov & Poole 2011, p. 522).

Socialists favour collective approaches to problems such as poverty, which they see arising from unjust social structures. While all socialists seek the transformation of capitalism, some are reformist, attempting to gradually change the system by promoting equality from within. Others are revolutionary, seeking the complete overthrow of capitalism and its replacement by a socialist society.

Sovereign power has traditionally been understood as the unlimited rule by a state over a territory and the people in it for political, social and economic ends. Globalisation, with its emphasis on a form of multilateral global governance, has undermined the sovereign power and authority of the traditional territory state structure, and has rendered it less capable of being the vehicle of democracy and human liberation (Gills & Gray 2012). Multinational corporations are now able to shift their investments from one country to another as they search for higher profits through lower wages, lower taxes, cheap land and positional power (Dalton et al. 1996).

Specialist skills are related to expertise in particular fields of practice (Compton & Galaway 1999; Trevithick 2005).

Speciesism places a lesser value on non-human species in the web of life (Hanrahan 2011).

Standardisation refers to adopting a 'one-size-fits-all' approach instead of aiming to cater for the individual needs of diverse populations; this fits well with neoliberal management models aimed at cost cutting and reducing the range and complexity of social work skills (Baines 2007).

Status quo literally refers to maintenance of the existing order.

Stereotyping refers to an oversimplified, biased and inflexible conception of a social group (Thompson 1998).

Stigma refers to the socially constructed characteristics and attributes associated with marginalised groups. Members of these groups will often internalise their guilt and shame, accepting the dominant construction and believing that they are to blame for the social problems they are experiencing (Mullaly 2010).

Structural analysis recognises that there are structural explanations (rather than individual explanations) for social issues and that some groups are excluded from, marginalised within or exploited by social, economic and political power. Poor people did not invent poverty; people of colour did not create racism – these are structural problems that can only be resolved by structural change. (Mullaly 2010, p. 276).

Structural context is the way in which social institutions, laws, policies and practices allocate goods and services with positive social value (good health care, decent housing, high social status) to dominant group members within the constructions of race, class, gender, sexuality, ethnicity, age, religion and ability, while allocating goods and services with negative social value (inadequate housing, low social status, incarceration) to members of the marginalised groups (Mullaly 2010, p.150).

Structural inequalities refer to inequalities in power and resources resulting from people's positioning in social structures (class, gender, ethnicity, age, and so on) and not their personal or physical abilities. Those with less power and fewer resources generally suffer greater social disadvantage and face more barriers in meeting needs and pursuing goals (Fook & Morley 2005; Davis 2007).

Structures See **social structures**.

Subject position refers to the social role constructed for an individual through a discourse; for example, the way in which people are turned into 'patients' by medical discourse (Gray 2007).

Subjectivity is the personal experience, judgements, feelings and perceptions of the world shaped by culture and language but specific to an individual person (subject). In Western thought, subjectivity is contrasted with 'objectivity', which is said to be knowledge of things (objects) independent from any individual's perception and therefore more reliable (see, for example, Fook 2012).

Subjugated views are those that differ from, or are alternative positions to, those of the dominant group. When particular views are adopted by the dominant group, they are given legitimacy, whereas alternative views are discounted. This is often seen in the media, which promotes the views of the dominant group (Mullaly 2010).

Sublimation involves converting a socially objectionable thought, feeling or behaviour into a socially acceptable one (for example, yelling at the television during a football game rather than hitting someone) (Longres 1995, p. 422).

Suffragettes were activists who campaigned for women's right to vote.

Supervision in social work involves 'the forming of a partnership to explore shared and different meanings of practice, with a view to jointly creating meanings which might grapple with some of the dilemmas of practice' (Fook 2012, p. 173).

Sustainability means that systems must be able to be maintained in the long term (therefore, resources should only be used at the rate at which they can be replenished) and that outputs to the environment should be limited to the level at which they can adequately be absorbed. Ideally, consumption would be minimised rather than maximised (Ife 2013, p. 51).

Systems theory refers to a diverse range of theoretical approaches that are centred on the idea of a 'system', which refers to a specific set of interrelated parts that make up a larger whole (Payne 2005).

Technicism is the over-reliance on techniques, skills and competencies. Technicist approaches focus on how to do practice as if it is a purely technical exercise and assume that practice can be adequate without theory thus perpetuating an artificial division between practice and context. (For further information see Dominelli 2009; Fook 2012.)

Technocratic means over-reliance on technology, which poses a threat to 'professional expertise and autonomy' (Fook 2012, p. 24).

Termination is a term used by mainstream social work to mark the end of a working relationship or formal disengagement of the service user from the service (Chenoweth & McAuliffe 2012).

Theory is a 'way of looking' that helps us understand or make sense of some aspect of the world. It interprets the things we (and others) experience that would otherwise not make sense as isolated events or observations (see, for example, Joas & Knobl 2009).

Therapeutic interventions involve working with individuals, families or small groups in order to bring about change at a personal or relational level (Chenoweth & McAuliffe 2012, p. 195).

Trade unions are organisations formed by employees in a particular trade or industry to collectively negotiate and advance the working conditions and income security of their members. (For further information see Giddens 2006, pp. 748–51.)

Transformative learning is deep learning that potentially challenges and changes how one sees the world (Ramsdem 1998).

Trivialisation entails not taking a group of people's views, issues and self-definitions seriously (Thompson 1998).

Underclass is a derogatory term used to represent a group of people with no past or future attachment to the labour market – for example, the long-term unemployed, homeless people, those with a lived experience of mental illness or a disability (Mullaly 2010, p. 207).

Undeserving is a term derived from dominant discourses that is used to invalidate the needs of service users by declaring them unworthy recipients of services and/or resources.

Universal means concepts, assumptions, and so on can be applied to entire populations regardless of culture, gender and socioeconomic status, for example (see, for example, Ife 2012).

Universal provision refers to social services given to everyone in society (not means-tested or targeted to a particular group) on the basis of comprehensive risk coverage, generous benefit levels, egalitarianism and full employment (Fawcett et al. 2009).

Universal truths refers to knowledge that seeks to provide explanation and understanding about human behaviour and society that will apply to everyone, no matter what culture or society they live in (Payne & Askeland 2008).

Universalisation refers to the imposition of the same images and ideas across the world (Scholte 2000, cited in Dower 2003, pp. 42–3).

Universalising refers to the feminist/anti-oppressive counselling skill that encourages the service user to see their experience in light of structural inequalities that are shared by others (Scott, Walker & Gilmore 1995).

Utopia is an imagined future of complete wellbeing. It literally means 'no-place-land' or 'good-place-land' (More [1516] 2001) but is commonly used to refer to an ideal society.

Validation refers to the skill of affirming the 'truth' of a person's subjective experience, affirming their telling of their story and what has occurred (Harms 2007; Scott, Walker & Gilmore 1995).

Virtue ethics are premised on the notion of the virtuous practitioner: that by cultivating and enacting particular character traits or personal qualities one will inherently be guided to practise ethically (Bowles et al. 2006).

'Welfare dependence' is a derogatory term perpetuated by proponents of neoliberalism to blame and stigmatise people who are receiving government entitlements.

Welfare state is the means by which governments, through social and economic policies (e.g. education and labour market policies), facilitate or restrict access to resources and opportunities that assist people to live independent and meaningful lives. In this way the state maintains social order and control of its citizens in a way that ensures their survival and enhances their social functioning (see, for example, Janrozik 2009; O'Connor et al. 2008).

White privilege refers to superiority presumed by those with white skin as dominant members of society, thus affording benefits over those with non-white skin. This attitude contributes to racism (Hollinsworth 2006).

Worldview is the overall beliefs and assumptions that inform our interpretation of life and the world. Sire (2004, p. 19) defines a worldview as 'a set of presuppositions (assumptions which may be true, partially true or entirely false) which we hold (consciously or subconsciously, consistently or inconsistently) about the basic makeup of our world'.

References

Abercrombie, N., Hill, S. and Turner, B., 2006, *Dictionary of Sociology*, 5th edn, Penguin Books, London.

Addams, J., 1912, *Twenty Years at Hull House: With Autobiographical Notes*, Macmillan, New York, http://digital.library.upenn.edu/women/addams/hullhouse/hullhouse.html.

Agger, B., 2013, *Critical Social Theories: An Introduction*, 3rd edn, Oxford University Press, Oxford.

Alia, V and Bull, S., 2005, *Media and Ethnic Minorities*, Edinburgh University Press, Edinburgh.

Alinsky, S., 1971, *Rules for Radicals. A Pragmatic Primer for Realistic Radicals*, Random House, New York.

Allan, J., 2009, 'Doing critical social work' in J. Allan, L. Briskman and B. Pease, eds, *Critical Social Work: Theories and Practices for a Socially Just World*, 2nd edn, Allen & Unwin, Crows Nest, NSW.

Allan, J., Briskman, L. and Pease, B., eds, 2009, *Critical Social Work: Theories and Practices for a Socially Just World*, 2nd edn, Allen & Unwin, Crows Nest, NSW.

Alston, M., 2012, 'Rural male suicide in Australia', *Social Science and Medicine*, 74 (4): 515–22.

Alston, M. and Kent, J., 2008, 'The big dry: The link between rural masculinities and poor health outcomes for farming men', *Journal of Sociology*, 44 (2): 133–47.

Alvaro, C., Jackson, L., Kirk, S., McHugh, T., Hughes, J., Circop, A. and Lyons, R., 2010, 'Moving Canadian governmental policies beyond a focus on individual lifestyle: Some insights from complexity and critical theories', *Health Promotion International*, 26 (1): 91–9.

American Psychiatric Association, 2013, *Diagnostic and Statistical Manual of Mental Disorders, Volume V*, American Psychiatric Association, Arlington, VA.

Amsler, S., 2011, 'From "therapeutic" to political education: The centrality of affective sensibility in critical pedagogy', *Critical Studies in Education*, 52 (1): 47–63.

Anthony, W., 1993, 'Recovery from mental illness: The guiding vision of the mental health service system in the 1990s', *Psychosocial Rehabilitation Journal*, 16 (4): 11–23.

Astbury, J., 1996, *Crazy for You: The Making of Women's Madness*, Oxford University Press, Melbourne.

Attlee, C., 1920, *The Social Worker*, G. Bell, London.

Australian Association of Social Workers (AASW), 2002, *Code of Ethics 1999*, 2nd edn, Barton, ACT, http://www.aasw.asn.au/document/item/92.

— 2010, *Code of Ethics 2010*, Barton, ACT, http://www.aasw.asn.au/practitioner-resources/code-of-ethics.

— 2011, *Consultation Paper: Options for Regulation of Unregistered Health Practitioners*, Australian Health Ministers'Advisory Council, Melbourne.

— 2012, *Australian Social Work Education and Accreditation Standards*, Barton, ACT.

Australian Bureau of Statistics, 2011, *ABS Review of Counting the Homeless Methodology*, August 2011, cat. no. 2050.0.55.002, Canberra, ACT.

— 2012a, *Average Weekly Earnings*, November, cat no. 6302.0, Canberra, ACT.

— 2012b, *Education and Work, Australia*, May, cat. no. 6227.0, Canberra, ACT.

Australian Community Workers Association, 2010, *Code of Ethics*, http://www.acwa.org.au/about/code-of-ethics.

Australian Human Rights Commission, 2012, *Face the Facts 2012: Some Questions and Answers about Indigenous Peoples, Migrants and Refugees and Asylum Seekers*, ch. 3, https://www.humanrights.gov.au/publications/face-facts-2012/2012-face-facts-chapter-3.

Australian Institute of Health and Welfare (AIHW), 2008, *Australia's Health 2008*, Australian Institute of Health and Welfare, Canberra.

Australian Law Reform Commission (ALRC), 2010, *Family Violence – A National Legal Response: Final Report*, Australian Law Reform Commission, Sydney.

Australian Securities and Investments Commission (ASIC), 2013, 'Credit card debt clock', https://www.moneysmart.gov.au/borrowing-and-credit/credit-cards/credit-card-debt-clock#about.

Bacchi, C., 2009, *Analysing Policy: What's the Problem Represented to Be?*, Pearson, Frenchs Forest, NSW.

Badham, V., 2013, 'Illiteracy rates: Australia's national shame', *The Guardian*, 27 September.

Bailey, A., 2004, 'Privilege: Expanding on Marilyn Fry's oppression' in L. Heldke and P. O'Connor, eds, *Oppression, Privilege and Resistance: Theoretical Perspectives on Racism, Sexism and Heterosexism*, McGraw-Hill, Boston.

Bailey, R. and Brake, M., eds, 1975, *Radical Social Work*, Pantheon Books, New York.

Bainbridge, L., 1999, 'Competing paradigms in mental health practice and education' in B. Pease and J. Fook, eds, *Transforming Social Work Practice: Postmodern Critical Perspectives* Allen & Unwin, Crows Nest, NSW.

Baines, D., 2006, '"If you could change one thing": Social service workers and restructuring', *Australian Social Work*, 59 (1): 20–34.

— 2007, 'Bridging the practice-activism divide in mainstream social work: Organizing and social movements' in D. Baines, ed, *Doing Anti-Oppressive Practice: Building Transformative Politicized Social Work*, Fernwood Publishing, Halifax, BC.

— 2010, '"If we don't get back to where we were before": Working in the restructured non-profit social services', *British Journal of Social Work*, 40: 928–45.

— ed., 2011, *Doing Anti-Ooppressive Practice: Social Justice and Social Work*, 2nd edn, Fernwood Publishing, Halifax, BC.

Banks, S., 2012, *Practical Social Work – Ethics and Values in Social Work*, 4th edn, Palgrave Macmillan, Hampshire.

Barker, R., 1995, *The Social Work Dictionary*, 3rd edn, National Association of Social Workers, Washington, DC.

Barnes, C. and Mercer, G., 2004, 'Theorising and research disability from a social model perspective' in C. Barnes and G. Mercer, eds, *Implementing the Social Model of Disability: Theory and Research*, Disability Press, Leeds.

Barnes, M. and Bowl, R., 2001, *Taking Over the Asylum: Empowerment and Mental Health*, Palgrave Macmillan, Basingstoke.

Barrett, C., 2008, *My People: A Project Exploring the Experiences of Gay, Lesbian, Bisexual, Transgender and Intersex Seniors in Aged-Care Services*, Matrix Guild, Melbourne.

Barton, J., 2003, *Understanding Old Testament Ethics: Approaches and Explorations*, John Knox Press, Louisville.

Baskin, C., 2006, 'Aboriginal world views as challenges and possibilities in social work education', *Critical Social Work*, 7 (2).

Bauman, Z., 1989, *Modernity and the Holocaust*, Cornell University Press, New York.

Bay, U. and Macfarlane, S., 2011, 'Teaching critical reflection: A tool for transformative learning in social work?', *Social Work Education*, 30 (7): 745–58.

Baylis, J. and Smith, S., 1997, *The Globalization of World Politics*, Oxford University Press, Oxford.

Beckett, C. and Maynard, A., 2005, *Values and Ethics in Social Work*, Sage, London.

Beddoe, L., 2009, 'Creating continuous conversation: Social work and learning organizations', *Social Work Education: The International Journal*, 28 (7): 722–36.

Beilharz, P. and Hogan, T., 2012, *Sociology: Antipodean Perspectives*, 2nd edn, Oxford University Press, New York.

Bell, D. and Klein, R., 1996, *Radically Speaking: Feminism Reclaimed*, Spinifex Press, Melbourne.

Bell, K., 2013, 'Protecting public housing tenants in Australia from forced eviction: The fundamental importance of the human right to adequate housing and home', *Monash University Law Review*, 39 (1): 1–37.

Bennett, B., 2013, 'Stop deploying your white privilege on me! Aboriginal and Torres Strait Islander engagement with the Australian Association of Social Workers', *Australian Social Work*, http://www.tandfonline.com/doi/abs/10.1080/0312407X.2013.840325#.U0TOFqLm7Sd.

Bennett, B., Green, S., Gilbert, S. and Bessarab, D., 2013, *Our Voices: Aboriginal and Torres Strait Islander Social Work*, Palgrave Macmillan, South Yarra.

Bentham, J., [1776] 1977, 'A comment on the Commentaries and A Fragment on Government' in J. H. Burns and H. L. A. Hart, eds, *The Collected Works of Jeremy Bentham*, London.

Beresford, P., 2005, 'Developing self-defined social approaches to madness and distress' in S. Ramon and J. Williams, eds, *Mental Health at the Crossroads: The Promise of the Psychosocial Approach*, Ashgate, Aldershot.

Beresford, Q. and Beresford, M., 2006, 'Race and reconciliation: The Australian experience in international context', *Contemporary Politics*, 12 (1): 65–78.

Berg-Weger, M., 2013, *Social Work and Social Welfare: An Invitation*, Routledge, New York.

Berlinski, M., 2008, *There Is No Alternative: Why Margaret Thatcher Matters*, Basic Books, New York.

Berthoin, A. and Friedman, V., 2003, *Negotiating Reality as an Approach to Intercultural Competence*, Discussion Paper No. SPIII 2003–101, Wissenschaftszentrum Berlin fur Sozialforschung.

Bessarab, D. and Crawford, F., 2010, 'Aboriginal practitioners speak out: Contextualising child protection interventions', *Australian Social Work*, 6 (2): 179–93.

Bird, R., 1996, *Nourishing Terrains: Australian Aboriginal View of Landscape and Wilderness*, Australian Heritage Commission, Canberra.

Black, B., 2009, 'Empowering and rights-based approaches to working with older people' in J. Allan, L. Briskman and B. Pease, eds, *Critical Social Work: Theories and Practices for a Socially Just World*, 2nd edn, Allen & Unwin, Crows Nest, NSW.

Bonner, C., 2011, 'My school, PISA and Australia's equity gap', *Inside Story: Current Affairs and Culture from Australia and Beyond*, http://inside.org.au/equity/.

Bottomly, A. and Judge, C., 2012, 'Still fighting for equal pay', *Marxist Left Review*, 4, Winter.

Bottrell, D. and Armstrong D., 2007, 'Changes and exchanges in marginal youth transitions', *Journal of Youth Studies*, 10 (3): 353–71.

Bowen, M., 1978, *Family Therapy in Clinical Practice*, Aronson, New York.

Bowles, W., Collingridge, M., Curry, S. and Valentine, B., 2006, *Ethical Practice in Social Work: An Applied Approach*, Allen & Unwin, Crows Nest, NSW.

Boyle, M., 2007, 'The problem with diagnosis', *The Psychologist*, 20 (5): 290–2.

Braybrooke, M., 2009, *Beacons of the Light: 100 Holy People Who Have Shaped the History of Humanity*, O Books, London.

Bremner, R., 1988, *American Philanthropy*, 2nd edn, University of Chicago Press, Chicago.

Bresser-Pereira, L., Maravall, J. and Przeworski, A., 1994, 'Economic reforms in new democracies: A social-democratic approach' in W. Smith, C. Acuna and E. Gamarra, eds, *Theoretical and Comparative Perspectives for the 1990s*, Transaction Books, New Brunswick, USA.

Briskman, L., 2003, 'Indigenous Australians: Towards Postcolonial Social Work?' in J. Allan, L. Briskman and B. Pease, eds, *Critical Social Work: Theories and Practices for a Socially Just World*, Allen & Unwin, Crows Nest, NSW.

— 2014, *Social Work with Indigenous Communities: A Human Rights Approach*, 2nd edn, The Federation Press, Annandale.

Briskman, L., Latham, S. and Goddard, C., 2008, *Human Rights Overboard: Seeking Asylum in Australia*, Scribe, Melbourne.

Briskman L., Pease B. and Allan, J., 2009, 'Introducing critical theories for social work in a neo-liberal context' in J. Allan, L. Briskman and B. Pease, eds, *Critical Social Work: Theories and Practices for a Socially Just World*, 2nd edn, Allen & Unwin, Crows Nest, NSW.

Bronfenbrenner, U., 1979, *The Ecology of Human Development: Experiments by Nature and Design*, Harvard University Press, Cambridge, Mass.

Bronner, E., 2011, *Critical Theory: A Very Short Introduction*, Oxford University Press, Oxford.

Brookfield, S., 1995, *Becoming a Critically Reflective Teacher*, Jossey-Bass, San Francisco.

Brown, J., 2007, 'Sex crimes in suburbia: The recent legal and scientific advances in the assistance given to victims of sexual assault', *On Crime and Law*, 66 (3): 111–17.

Brown, T., 2003, 'Critical race theory speaks to the sociology of mental health: Mental health problems produced by racial stratification', *Journal of Health and Social Behaviour*, 44 (3): 292–301.

— 2008, 'Race, racism and mental health: Elaboration of critical race theory's contributions to the sociology of mental health, *Contemporary Justice Review*, 11(1): 53–62.

Brynjolfsson, E. and McAfee, A., 2011, *Race Against the Machine: How the Digital Revolution is Accelerating Innovation, Driving Productivity and Irreversibly Transforming Employment and the Economy*, Digital Frontiers Press, Lexington, MA.

Burkett, P., 2005, 'Marx's vision of sustainable human development', *Monthly Review*, 57(5): 34–62.

Burridge, N., 2009, 'Perspectives on reconciliation and Indigenous rights', *Cosmopolitan Civil Societies Journal*, 1 (2): 111–28.

Butler, J., 1990, *Gender Trouble: Feminism and the Subversion of Identity*, Routledge, London.

Campbell, C., 2002, 'The search for congruency: Developing strategies for anti-oppressive social work pedagogy', *Canadian Social Work Review*, 19(1): 25–42.

Canaan, J., 2005, 'Developing a pedagogy of critical hope', *Learning and Teaching in the Social Sciences*, 2 (3): 159–74.

Carniol, B., 1991, *Case Critical: Challenging Social Work in Canada*, Between the Lines, Toronto.

— 1992, 'Structural social work: Maurice Moreau's challenge to social work practice', *Journal of Progressive Human Services*, 3 (1): 1–20.

Caro, D., 2009, 'Socio-economic status and academic achievement trajectories from childhood to adolescence', *Canadian Journal of Education*, 32 (3): 558–90.

Carter, B. and McGoldrick, M., 2005, 'Overview: the expanded family life cycle – individual, family and social perspectives' in B. Carter and M. McGoldrick, *The Expanded Family Life Cycle: Individual, Family and Social Perspectives*, Person Allyn & Bacon, NY.

Cassells, R., Miranti, R., Nepal, B. and Tanton, R., 2009, *She Works Hard for Her Money: Australian Women and the Gender Divide*, National Centre Social and Economic Modelling NATSEM, University of Canberra, Canberra, ACT.

Castles, F., 1985, *The Working Class and Welfare: Reflections on the Political Development of the Welfare State in Australia and New Zealand, 1890–1980*, Allen & Unwin, Sydney.

Castles, S. and Miller, M., 2003, *The Age of Migration: International Population Movements in the Modern World*, The Guilford Press, New York.

Chambers, P., 2004, 'The case for critical social gerontology in social work education and older women', *Social Work Education*, 23 (6): 745–58.

Chambon, A., 1999, 'Foucault's approach: Making the familiar visible' in A. Chambon, A. Irving and L. Epstein, eds, *Reading Foucault for Social Work*, Columbia University Press, New York.

Chambon, A., Irving, A., and Epstein, L., eds, 1999 *Reading Foucault for Social Work*, Columbia University Press, New York.

Cheal, D., 2005, *Dimensions of Sociological Theory*, Palgrave Macmillan, Basingstoke.

Chenoweth, L. and McAuliffe, D., 2012, *The Road to Social Work and Human Service Practice*, 2nd edn, Cengage Learning, Melbourne.

Collings, S. and Davies, L., 2008, '"For the sake of the children": Making sense of children and childhood in the context of child protection', *Journal of Social Work Practice*, 22 (2): 181–93.

Commonwealth of Australia, 2008, *The Long Road Home: A National Approach to Reducing Homelessness*, Homelessness Task Force, Department of Families, Housing, Community Services and Indigenous Affairs, Canberra, ACT.

Compton, B. and Galaway, B., 1999, *Social Work Processes*, 6th edn, Brooks/Cole Publishing Company, Pacific Grove, CA.

Connell, R. W., 1987, *Gender and Power: Society, the Person and Sexual Politics*, Allen & Unwin, Sydney.

Cook, B. 2008, *National, Regional and Local Employment Policies in Sweden and the United Kingdom*, Centre for Full Employment and Equity, University of Newcastle, Callahan.

Cooper, L., 2009, 'Edna Chamberlain (1921–2005): A leader through times of transition and change', *Social Work and Society, International Online Journal*, 17 (1).

Coorey, P., 2011, 'Gillard's $2bn equal pay push to see lowest-paid workers' salaries soar', *Sydney Morning Herald*, 10 November.

Coppock, V. and Dunn, B., 2010, *Understanding Social Work Practice in Mental Health*, Sage, London.

Corrigan, P. and Leonard, P., 1978, *Social Work Practice under Capitalism: A Marxist Approach*, Macmillan, London.

Cort, J., 1988, *Christian Socialism: An Informed History*, Orbis Books, New York.

Cosgrove, L., 2005, 'When labels mask oppression: implications for teaching psychiatric taxonomy to health counsellors', *Journal of Mental Health Counselling*, 27 (4): 283–97.

Cox, E., 1996, *Leading Women: Tactics for Making a Difference*, Random House, Sydney.

Craig, G., 2002, 'Poverty, social work and social justice', *British Journal of Social Work*, 32 (6): 669–82.

— 2010, 'Private schools rake in profit', *The Age*, 12 September.

Crain, W., 2014, *Theories of Development: Concepts and Applications*, 6th edn, Pearson Education, Harlow.

Critchley, P., 1997, 'The philosophy of praxis' in P. Critchley, *Beyond Modernity and Postmodernity: Volume 2, Active Materialism* (ebook), http://mmu.academia.edu/PeterCritchley/Books.

Cross, R., 2012, 'Radicalism' in D. Snow, D. della Porta, B. Klandermans and D. McAdam, eds, *The Blackwell Encyclopedia of Social and Political Movements*, Wiley/Blackwell, Oxford.

Crotty, M., 1998, *The Foundations of Social Research: Meaning and Perspective in the Research Process*, Allen & Unwin, St Leonards, NSW.

Cuff, E., Sharrock, W. and Francis, D., 2006, *Perspectives in Sociology*, 5th edn, Routledge, London.

Cullum, P., 1992, '"And hir name was Charite": Charitable giving by and for women in late Medieval Yorkshire' in *Woman is a Worthy Wight: Women in English Society c. 1200–1500*, Alan Sutton, Stroud.

Dalrymple, B. and Burke, B., 1995, *Anti-Oppressive Practice: Social Care and the Law*, Open University Press, Buckingham.

Dalton, T., Draper, M., Weeks, W. and Wiseman, J., 1996, *Making Social Policy in Australia: An Introduction*, Allen & Unwin, Sydney.

Darling, D., 2013, *A History of Social Justice and Political Power in the Middle East: The Circle of Justice from Mesopotamia to Globalization*, Routledge, Abingdon.

Davies, L. and Leonard, P., eds, 2004, *Social Work in a Corporate Era: Practices of Power and Resistance*, Ashgate, Aldershot.

Davis, A., 2007, 'Structural Approaches to Social Work' in J. Lishman, *Handbook for Practice Learning in Social Work and Social Care*, 2nd edn, Jessica Kingsley Publications, London.

D'Cruz, H., Gillingham, P. and Melendez, S., 2007, 'Reflexivity, its meanings and relevance for social work: A critical review of the literature', *British Journal of Social Work*, 37 (1): 73–90.

D'Cruz, H. and Jones, M., 2004, *Social Work Research: Ethical and Political Contexts*, Sage, London.

de Beauvoir, S., [1949] 1993, *The Second Sex*, Everyman, London.

Dean, R., 1993, 'Teaching a constructivist approach to clinical practice' in J. Laird, ed, *Revisioning Social Work Education: A Social Constructionist Approach*, Haworth Press, New York.

— 2011, 'Becoming a social constructionist: From Freudian beginnings to narrative endings' in S. L. Witkin, ed, *Social Construction and Social Work Practice: Interpretations and Innovations*, Columbia University Press, New York.

Deegan, P., 1988, 'Recovery: The lived experience of rehabilitation', *Psychosocial Rehabilitation Journal*, 11 (4): 11–19.

— 1996, 'Recovery as a journey of the heart', *Psychiatric Rehabilitation Journal*, 11 (4): 91–7.

Deepak, A., 2012, 'Globalization, power and resistance: Postcolonial and transnational feminist perspectives for social work practice', *International Social Work*, 55 (6): 779–93.

Derrida, J., 1978, *Writing and Difference*, University of Chicago Press, Chicago.

DiAngelo, R., 1997, 'Heterosexism: Addressing internalized dominance', *Journal of Progressive Human Services*, 8 (1): 5–21.

Di Marco, K., Pirie, P. and Au-Yeung, W., 2011, *A History of Public Debt in Australia*, Treasury, Commonwealth of Australia, Canberra, ACT.

Dominelli, L., 1998, 'Anti-oppressive practice in context' in R. Adams, L. Dominelli and M. Payne, eds, *Social Work: Themes, Issues and Critical Debates*, Palgrave Macmillan, Basingstoke.

— 2002a, *Anti-Oppressive Social Work Theory and Practice*, Palgrave Macmillan, Basingstoke.

— 2002b, *Feminist Social Work Theory and Practice*, Palgrave Macmillan, Basingstoke.

— 2009, *Introducing Social Work*, Polity Press, Cambridge.

— 2012, *Green Social Work: From Environmental Crises to Environmental Justice*, Polity Press, Cambridge.

Dominelli, L. and McLeod, E., 1989, *Feminist Social Work*, Macmillan Press, London.

Dower, N., 2003, *An Introduction to Global Citizenship*, Edinburgh University Press, Edinburgh.

Drakeford, M., 2002, 'Social Work and Politics' in M. Davies, ed, *The Blackwell Companion to Social Work*, Blackwell, Oxford.

Duncan, B., 1998, 'Stepping off the throne' reprinted in the *Richmond Fellowship of Victoria Newsletter*, 10 August, Melbourne.

Duncan, I., 2006, 'The changing concept of animal sentience', *Applied Animal Behaviour Science*, 100 (1): 11–19.

Dustin, D., 2007, *The McDonaldization of Social Work*, Ashgate, Aldershot.

Dutton, D. and Kropp, R., 2000, 'A review of domestic violence risk assessments', *Trauma, Violence and Abuse*, 1 (2): 171–81.

Edwards, S., 2010, 'Matauranga Maori literacies: Indigenous literacy as epistemological freedom v Eurocentric imperialism' in World Indigenous Nations Higher Education Consortium, eds, *Indigenous Voices, Indigenous Research*, Deakin University Printery, Waurn Ponds, Victoria.

EIROnline: European Industrial Relations Observatory On-line, 2013, http://www.eurofound.europa.eu/eiro/2003/11/tfeature/se0311104t.htm.

Engels, F., [1887] 2009, *The Condition of the Working Class in England*, D. McLellan, ed, Oxford University Press, Oxford.

Erikson, E., 1959, *Identity and the Life Cycle*, International University Press, New York.

Estes, C., 2005, 'Women, ageing and inequality: a feminist perspective' in M. L. Johnson, ed, *The Cambridge Handbook of Age and Ageing*, Cambridge University Press, Cambridge.

Evans, T., 2009, 'Managing to be professional? Team managers and practitioners in modernised social work' in J. Harris and V. White, eds, *Modernising Social Work: Critical Considerations*, The Policy Press, Bristol.

— 2010, *Professional Discretion in Welfare Services: Beyond Street-Level Bureaucracy*, Ashgate Publishing, Surrey.

Fabrega, H., 2008, 'On the postmodernist critique and reformation of psychiatry', *Psychiatry*, 71 (2): 183–96.

Fahmi, K., 2004, 'Social work practice and research as an emancipatory process' in L. Davies and P. Leonard, eds, *Social Work in a Corporate Era: Practices of Power and Resistance*, Ashgate, Aldershot.

Faith, E., 2008, 'Indigenous social work education: A project for all of us?' in M. Gray, J. Coates and M. Yellow Bird, eds, *Indigenous Social Work Around the World*, Ashgate, Aldershot.

Fausto-Sterling, A., 1999, 'Menopause: the storm before the calm' in J. Price and M. Shildrick, eds, *Feminist Theory and the Body: A Reader*, Edinburgh University Press, Edinburgh.

Fawcett, B., Goodwin, S., Meagher, G. and Phillips, R., 2009, *Social Policy for Social Change*, Palgrave Macmillan, South Yarra.

Featherstone, B. and Green, L., 2013, 'Judith Butler' in M. Gray and S. Webb, eds, *Social Work: Theories and Methods*, 2nd edn, Sage, London.

Feenberg, A., Pippin, R. and Webel, C., 1987, *Marcuse: Critical Theory and the Promise of Utopia*, Macmillan, London.

Ferguson, I., 2008, *Reclaiming Social Work: Challenging Neoliberalism and Promoting Social Justice*, Sage, London.

— 2009, 'Another social work is possible!' in V. Leskošek, ed, *Theories and Methods of Social Work: Exploring Different Perspectives*, University of Ljubljana, Ljubljana.

— 2011, 'Why class (still) matters' in M. Lavalette, ed., *Radical Social Work Today: Social Work at the Crossroads*, Policy Press, Bristol.

Ferguson, I. and Woodward, R., 2009, *Radical Social Work in Practice: Making a Difference*, Policy Press, Bristol.

Ferguson, K., 1999, 'Patriarchy' in H. Tierney, ed, *Women's Studies Encyclopedia*, Vol 2, Greenwood Publishing, New York.

Ferrari, J., 2013, 'Double the poor at public schools', *The Australian*, 11 April.

Festinger, L., 1957, *A Theory of Cognitive Dissonance*, Stanford University Press, Stanford, CA.

Figley, C., 2002, 'Compassion fatigue: Psychotherapists' chronic lack of self care', *Journal of Clinical Psychology*, 58 (11): 1433–41.

Fisher, R. and Karger, H., 1997, *Social Work and Community in a Private World*, Longman, New York.

Flannery, K. and Marcus, J., 2012, *The Creation of Inequality: How Our Prehistoric Ancestors Set the Stage for Monarchy, Slavery and Empire*, Harvard University Press, USA.

Fook, J., 1993, *Radical Casework: A Theory of Practice*, Allen & Unwin, Sydney.

— ed, 1996, *The Reflective Researcher: Social Workers' Theories of Practice Research*, Allen & Unwin, Sydney.

— 1999, *Reflexivity as Method*, La Trobe University, Bundoora.

— 2000, 'The lone crusader: Constructing enemies and allies in the workplace' in L. Napier and J. Fook, eds, *Breakthroughs in Practice: Theorising Critical Moments in Social Work*, Whiting and Birch, London.

— 2004, 'Critical reflection and transformative possibilities' in L. Davies and P. Leonard, eds, *Social Work in a Corporate Era: Practices of Power and Resistance*, Ashgate, Aldershot.

— 2012, *Social Work: A Critical Approach to Practice*, 2nd edn, Sage, London.

Fook, J. and Gardner, F., 2007, *Practising Critical Reflection: A Resource Handbook*, Open University Press, Maidenhead.

Fook, J. and Morley, C., 2005, 'Empowerment: A contextual perspective' in S. Hick, J. Fook and R. Pozzuto, eds, *Social Work: A Critical Turn*, Thompson, Toronto.

Fook, J., Ryan, M. and Hawkins, L., 2000, *Professional Expertise: Practice, Theory and Education for Working in Uncertainty*, Whiting and Birch, London.

Foucault, M., 1977, *Discipline and Punish: The Birth of the Prison*, Allen Lane, London.

— 1980, *Power/Knowledge: Selected Interviews and Other Writings 1972–1977*, Harvester Press, Brighton.

Freeman, S., 2005, 'Attachment theory' in *Grief and Loss: Understanding the Journey*, Brooks/Cole, Victoria.

Freud, S., 1953, *Three Essays on the Theory of Sexuality*, Hogarth, London.

Fullagar, S. and Gattuso, S., 2002, 'Rethinking gender, risk and depression in Australian mental health policy', *Australian e-Journal for the Advancement of Mental Health*, 1 (3).

Galper, J., 1975, *The Politics of Social Services*, Englewood Cliffs, Prentice-Hall, NJ.

Gandhi, L., 1998, *Postcolonial Theory: A Critical Introduction*, Columbia University Press, New York.

Gardiner-Garden, J., 1999, *From Dispossession to Reconciliation*, Research Paper No. 27 1998–99, Parliamentary Library, Canberra.

Gardner, F., 2006, *Working with Human Service Organisations*, Oxford University Press, South Melbourne.

Garrett, P., 2013, *Social Work and Social Theory: Making Connections*, Policy Press, Bristol.

Garvey, D., 2008, 'Review of the social and emotional wellbeing of Indigenous Australian peoples', Australian Indigenous Health *Infonet*, http://www.healthinfonet.ecu.edu.au/sewb_review.

Garvin, C., Gutierrez, L. and Galinsky, M., 2004, *Handbook of Social Work with Groups*, Guilford Press, New York.

Geldard, D. and Geldard, K., 2012, *Basic Personal Counselling: A Training Manual For Counsellors*, 7th edn, Prentice Hall, Frenchs Forest, NSW.

Germov, J. and Poole, M., 2011, *Public Sociology: An Introduction to Australian Society*, 2nd edn, Allen & Unwin, Crows Nest, NSW.

Gibbs, A., 2001, 'The changing nature and context of social work research', *British Journal of Social Work*, 31 (5): 687–704.

Giddens, A. and Sutton, P., 2013, *Sociology*, 6th edn, Polity Press, Cambridge.

Gills, B. K. and Gray, K., 2012, 'People power in the era of global crisis: Rebellion, resistance and liberation', *Third World Quarterly*, 33 (2): 205–24.

Giroux, H., 2001, '"Something's missing": Cultural studies, neoliberalism and the politics of educated hope', *Strategies*, 14 (2): 227–52.

— 2004, 'When hope is subversive', *Tikkun*, 19 (6): 38–9.

— 2011, *On Critical Pedagogy*, Continuum, New York.

Gleeson, D., 2006, 'The professionalisation of Australian Catholic social welfare, 1920–1985', PhD thesis, University of New South Wales, Sydney.

Goddard, C., Saunders, J., Stanley, J. and Tucci, J., 1999, 'Structured risk assessment procedures: Instruments of abuse?', *Child Abuse Review*, 8: 251–63.

Goldstein, H., 1987, 'The neglected moral link in social work practice', *Social Work*, 32: 181–7.

Golightley, M., 2008, *Social Work and Mental Health*, 3rd edn, Learning Matters Ltd, Exeter.

Gowdy, J., 1997, *Limited Wants, Unlimited Means: A Reader on Hunter-Gatherer Economics and the Environment*, Island Press, Washington.

Gramsci, A., 1971, *Selections from the Prison Notebooks of Antonio Gramsci*, Lawrence & Wishart, London.

Gratz, B., 1988, 'The reproduction of privilege in Australian education', *British Journal of Sociology*, 39 (3): 358–76.

Gray, J., 2007, '(Re)considering voice', *Qualitative Social Work*, 6: 411–30.

Gray, M., 2008, 'Postcards from the West: Mapping the vicissitudes of Western social work', *Australian Social Work*, 61 (1): 1–6.

Gray, M. and Coates, J., 2012, 'Environmental ethics for social work: social work's responsibility to the non-human world', *International Journal of Social Welfare*, 21: 239–47.

Gray, M. and Gibbons, J., 2007, 'There are no answers, only choices: Teaching ethical decision making in social work', *Australian Social Work*, 60 (2): 222–38.

Green, R., 2007, 'Gay and lesbian couples in therapy – A social justice perspective' in E. Aldarondo, ed, *Advancing Social Justice Through Clinical Practice*, Lawrence Erlbaum Associates, Mahwah, NJ.

Green, S. and Baldry E., 2008, 'Building Indigenous social work', *Australian Social Work*, 61 (4): 389– 402.

Greene, R., 2008, *Human Behavior Theory and Social Work Practice*, 3rd edn, Aldine Transaction, New Brunswick, USA.

Grenier, A., 2008, 'Recognising and responding to loss and "rupture" in older women's accounts', *Journal of Social Work Practice*, 22(2): 195–209.

Gurney, O. and Kramer, S., 1965, 'Two fragments of Sumerian laws', *Assyriological Studies*, 16: 13–9.

Habermas, J., 1990, 'Discourse ethics: Notes on a program of philosophical justification' in S. Benhabib and F. Dallmayr, eds, *The Communicative Ethics Controversy*, MIT Press, Cambridge, MA.

Haebich, A., 2000, *Broken Circles: Fragmenting Indigenous Families 1800–2000*, Fremantle Press, Fremantle.

Haines, H., 1988, *Black Radicals and the Civil Rights Mainstream, 1954–1970*, The University of Tennessee Press, Knoxville, TN.

Hamington, M., 2010, 'Community organizing: Addams and Alinsky' in M. Hamington, ed, *Feminist Interpretations of Jane Addams*, Pennsylvania State University Press, University Park, Pennsylvania.

Hanrahan, C., 2011, 'Challenging anthropocentricism in social work through ethics and spirituality: Lessons from studies in human–animal bonds', *Journal of Religion and Spirituality in Social Work: Social Thought*, 30: 3: 272–93.

Harms, L., 2007, *Working with People*, Oxford University Press, South Melbourne.

— 2010, *Understanding Human Development: A Multidimensional Approach*, 2nd edn, Oxford University Press, Melbourne.

Harris, J. and White, V., 2009, 'Intensification, individualisation, inconvenience, interpellation' in J. Harris and V. White, eds, *Modernising Social Work: Critical Considerations*, Policy Press, Bristol.

Hart, N., 2007, 'Disciplining through depression: An analysis of contemporary discourse on women and depression', *Women's Studies in Communication*, 30(3): 284–309.

Hartman, A., 1991, 'Words create worlds', *Social Work*, 36 (4): 275.

Healy, B. and Renouf, N., 2005, 'Contextualised social policy: An Australian perspective' in S. Ramon and J. Williams, eds, *Mental Health at the Crossroads: The Promise of the Psychosocial Approach*, Ashgate, Aldershot.

Healy, K., 1999, 'Power and activist social work' in B. Pease, and J. Fook, eds, *Transforming Social Work Practice: Postmodern Critical Perspectives*, Allen & Unwin, St Leonards, NSW.

— 2000, *Social Work Practices: Contemporary Perspectives on Change*, Sage, London.

— 2005, *Social Work Theories in Context: Creating Frameworks for Practice*, Palgrave Macmillan, London.

— 2012, *Social Work Methods and Skills: The Essential Foundations of Practice*, Palgrave Macmillan, London.

Healy, K. and Lonne, B., 2010, *The Social Work and Human Services Workforce: Report from a National Study of Education, Training and Workforce Needs*, Australian Learning and Teaching Council, Strawberry Hills, NSW.

Heinsch, M., 2012, 'Getting down to earth: Finding a place for nature in social work practice', *International Journal of Social Welfare*, 21: 309–18.

Henderson, C., 2008, 'Gaols or de facto mental institutions? Why individuals with a mental illness are over-represented in the criminal justice system in New South Wales, Australia', *Journal of Offender Rehabilitation*, 45(1): 69–80.

Henderson, G., Robson, C., Cox, L., Dukes, C., Tsey, K. and Haswell, M., 2004, 'Social and emotional wellbeing of Aboriginal and Torres Strait Islander people within the broader context of the social determinants of health' in I. Anderson, F. Baum and M. Bentley, eds, *Beyond Bandaids: Exploring the Underlying Social Determinants of Aboriginal Health*, papers from the Social Determinants of Aboriginal Health workshop, Adelaide.

Hennig, C., 1975, 'Introduction' in *Inside Welfare: Revolutionary Welfare Workers*, Working Paper No. 1, University of Queensland, Brisbane.

Hennum, N., 2012, 'Children's confidences, parents' confessions: Child welfare dialogues as technologies of control', *Qualitative Social Work*, 11 (5): 535–49.

Herbert, J., 2003, 'Indigenous research: A communal act', proceedings of the NZARE/AARE Joint Conference, 29 November – 3 December 2003, Auckland, NZ.

Hick, S., Fook, J. and Pozzuto, R., eds, 2005, *Social Work: A Critical Turn*, Thompson Education Publishing, Toronto.

Hickel, J., 2013, 'Global wealth inequality: What you never knew you never knew', http://blogs.lse.ac.uk/indiaatlse/2013/04/11/global-wealth-inequality-what-you-never-knew-you-never-knew/.

Hirst, J., 1984, 'Keeping colonial history colonial: The Hartz thesis revisited', *Historical Studies*, 21 (28): 85–104.

Hollinsworth, D., 1997, *The Resurgence of Racism: Howard, Hanson and the Race Debate*, Monash Publications in History, No. 24, Monash University, Melbourne.

— 2006, *Race and Racism in Australia*, 3rd edn, Social Science Press, South Melbourne.

Holmes, D., Hughes, K and Julian, R., 2012, *Australian Sociology: A Changing Society*, Pearson, Frenchs Forest, NSW.

Holscher, D. and Sewpaul, V., 2006, 'Ethics as a site of resistance: The tension between social control and critical reflection', *Research Reports*, 1: 251–72.

Horner, N., 2012, *What is Social Work?*, 4th edn, Sage, London.

Howe, D., 2009, *A Brief Introduction to Social Work Theory*, Palgrave Macmillan, London.

Hudson, L., 2011, 'A species of thought: Bare life and animal being', *Antipode*, 43: 5: 1659–78.

Hughes, M. and Wearing, M., 2013, *Organisations and Management in Social Work*, 2nd edn, Sage, London.

Hugman, R., 2013, *Culture, Values and Ethics in Social Work: Embracing Diversity*, Routledge, Oxford.

Hulse, K. and Saugeres, L., 2008, *Housing Insecurity and Precarious Living: An Australian Exploration*, AHURI (Australian Housing and Urban Research Institute), Final Report No. 24, Swinburne-Monash Research Centre, Melbourne.

Hulse, K., Miligan, V and Easthope, H., 2012, *Secure Occupancy in Rental Housing: Conceptual Foundations and Comparative Perspectives*, Australian Housing and Urban Research Institute, Melbourne.

Human Rights and Equal Opportunity Commission (HREOC), 1993, *First Report 1993*, *Aboriginal and Torres Strait Islander Social Justice Commission*, HREOC, Sydney.

Humphries, B., 2008, *Social Work Research for Social Justice*, Palgrave Macmillan, Basingstoke.

Hunt, F., 2003, *Property and Prophets: The Evolution of Economic Institutions and Ideologies*, M. E. Sharpe, New York.

Hurst, M., 1995, 'Counselling women from a feminist perspective' in W. Weeks and J. Wilson, eds, *Issues Facing Australian Families*, 2nd edn, Longman, Melbourne.

Ife, J., 1996, *Rethinking Social Work*, Longman, South Melbourne.

— 2012, *Human Rights and Social Work: Towards Rights-Based Practice*, 3rd edn, Cambridge University Press, Cambridge.

— 2013, *Community Development in an Uncertain World*, Cambridge University Press, Cambridge.

Irani, K. and Silver, M., eds, 1995, *Social Justice in the Ancient World*, Greenwood Press, Connecticut.

Jadad, A., 1998, *Randomised Controlled Trials: A User's Guide*, BMJ Books, London.

Jamrozik, A., 2009, *Social Policy in the Post-Welfare State: Australian Society in a Changing World*, 3rd edn, Pearson, Frenchs Forest, NSW.

Jarman-Rohde, L., McFall, J., Kolar, P. and Strom, G., 1997, 'The changing context of social work practice: Implications and recommendations for social work educators', *Journal of Social Work Education*, 33 (1): 29–46.

Joas, H. and Knobl, W., 2009, *Social Theory: Twenty Introductory Lectures*, Cambridge University Press, Cambridge.

Jones, C., 2005, 'The neo-liberal assault: Voices from the front line of British state social work' in I. Ferguson, M. Lavalette and E. Whitmore, eds, *Globalisation, Global Justice and Social Work*, Routledge, London.

Jordan, J., 2012, 'Silencing rape, silencing women' in J. Brown and S. Walklate, eds, *Handbook on Sexual Violence*, Routledge, London and New York.

Kaplan-Myrth, N., 2005, 'Sorry mates: Reconciliation and self-determination in Australian Aboriginal health', *Human Rights Review*, July–September: 69–83.

Karenga, M., 2004, *Maat, The Moral Ideal in Ancient Egypt*, Routledge, London.

Kellner, D., 1989, *Critical Theory, Marxism and Modernity*, Johns Hopkins University Press, Baltimore.

Keman, H., 2014, *Social Democracy: A Comparative Account of the Left Wing Party Family*, Routledge, London.

Kenny, M., 2013, 'Afghanistan's cabinet has more women', *Sydney Morning Herald*, 17 September.

Kenny, S., 2010, *Developing Communities for the Future: Community Development in Australia*, 4th edn, Cengage, Melbourne.

Kessaris, T. N., 2006, 'About being Mununga (whitefella): Making covert group racism visible', *Journal of Community and Applied Social Psychology*, 16: 347–62.

Kessl, F., 2009, 'Critical reflexivity, social work, and the emerging European post-welfare states', *European Journal of Social Work*, 12 (3): 305–17.

Kirk, G. and Okazawa-Rey, M., 2004, *Women's Lives: Multicultural Perspectives*, 3rd edn, McGraw-Hill, New York.

Kirk, S., 2005, 'Introduction: Critical perspectives' in S. Kirk, ed, *Mental Disorders in the Social Environment: Critical Perspectives*, Columbia University Press, New York.

Kunnen, N. and MacKay, S., 2009, 'Housing and homelessness' in P. Swain and S. Rice, eds, *In the Shadow of the Law: The Legal Context of Social Work Practice*, 3rd edn, The Federation Press, Annandale.

Kutchins, H. and Kirk, S., 1997, *Making Us Crazy: DSM – The Psychiatric Bible and the Creation of Mental Disorders*, Free Press, New York.

LaPan, A. and Platt, T., 2005, '"To stem the tide of degeneracy": The eugenic impulse in social work' in S. A. Kirk, ed, *Mental Disorders in the Social Environment*, Columbia University Press, New York.

Lathouras, A., 2010, 'Developmental Community Work – A Method' in A. Ingamells, A. Lathouras, R. Wiseman, P. Westoby and F. Caniglia, eds, *Community Development Practice: Stories, Method and Meaning*, Common Ground, Altona.

Lavalette, M., ed, 2011, *Radical Social Work Today: Social Work at the Crossroads*, Policy Press, University of Bristol.

Lazzarato, M., 2012, *The Making of Indebted Man: Essay on the Neoliberal Condition*, MIT Press, Cambridge, MA.

Leibrich, J., 1998, 'The healer within: A personal view of recovery' in S. Romans, ed, *Folding Back the Shadows: A Perspective on Women's Mental Health*, University of Otago Press, Dunedin.

Leigh, A., 2013, *Battlers and Billionaires: The Story of Inequality in Australia*, Redback, Melbourne.

Lengermann, P. and Niebrugge-Brantley, J., 2014, 'Contemporary feminist theory' in G. Ritzer and J. Stepnisky, *Sociological Theory*, 9th edn, McGraw Hill, New York.

Leonard, P., 1994, 'Knowledge/power and postmodernism: Implications for the practice of a critical social work education', *Canadian Social Work Review/Revue Canadienne de Service Social*, 11 (1): 11–26.

— 1997, *Postmodern Welfare: Reconstructing an Emancipatory Project*, Sage, London.

Lerner, G., 1986, *The Creation of Patriarchy*, Oxford University Press, New York.

Liddell, H. and Scott, R. 1940, *A Greek-English Lexicon*, Clarendon Press, Oxford.

Lloyd, C., King, R. and Chenoweth, L., 2002, 'Social work, stress and burnout: A review', *Journal of Mental Health*, 11 (3): 255–65.

Loftus, S., Higgs, J. and Trede, F., 2011, 'Researching living spaces: Trends in creative qualitative research' in J. Higgs, A. Titches, D. Horsfall and D. Bridges, eds, *Critical Spaces for Qualitative Researching: Living Research*, Sense Publishers, Rotterdam.

Longres, J., 1995, 'Three psychological perspectives' in *Human Behaviour in the Social Environment*, 2nd edn, Peacock Publishers, Itasca, Illinois.

Lovejoy, M., 1984, 'Recovery from schizophrenia: A personal odyssey', *Hospital and Community Psychiatry*, 35 (8): 807–12.

Lundy, C., 2004, *Social Work and Social Justice*, Broadview Press, Ontario.

MacCunn, J., 1911, *Liverpool Address on Ethics of Social Work*, The University Press, London.

Macfarlane, S., 2006, 'Support and recovery in a therapeutic community', PhD thesis, RMIT University, Melbourne.

— 2009, 'Opening spaces for alternative understandings in mental health practice' in J. Allan, L. Briskman and B. Pease, eds, *Critical Social Work: Theories and Practices for a Socially Just World*, 2nd edn, Allen & Unwin, Crows Nest, NSW.

— 2014, 'Mental health, social work and professionalism' in L. Beddoe and J. Maidment, eds, *Social Work Practice for Promoting Health and Wellbeing: Critical Issues*, Routledge, Abingdon, UK.

Macionis, J., 2011, *Sociology*, Pearson Higher Education, NJ.

Mackenzie, C. and Stoljar, N., eds, 2000, *Relational Autonomy*, Oxford University Press, New York and Oxford.

Maddison, S. and Scalmer, S., 2006, *Activist Wisdom: Practical Knowledge and Creative Tension in Social Movements*, UNSW Press, Sydney.

Madhu, P., 2011, 'Praxis intervention: Towards a new critical social work practice', *SSRN eLibrary*, http://ssrn.com/paper=1765143.

Maidment, J. and Macfarlane, S., 2011, 'Crafting communities: Promoting inclusion, empowerment and learning between older women', *Australian Social Work*, 64 (3): 283–98.

Mandela, N., 1995, *A Long Walk to Freedom: The Autobiography of Nelson Mandela*, Abacus, London.

— 2013. *Madiba: The Wisdom of Nelson Mandela*, Lemur Books, Alberton.

Mandell, D., 2008, 'Power, care and vulnerability: Considering use of self in child welfare work', *Journal of Social Work Practice*, 22 (2): 235–48.

Marchant, H., 1985, 'A feminist perspective on the development of the social work profession in New South Wales', *Australian Social Work*. 38 (1): 35–43.

Marchant, H. and Wearing, B., 1986, *Gender Reclaimed: Women and Social Work*, Hale & Iremonger, Sydney.

Marcuse, H., 1972, *One-Dimensional Man*, Abacus, London.

Marginson, S., 2006, 'Hayekian neo-liberalism and academic freedom', Keynote Address, proceedings of the 35th Conference of the Philosophy of Education Society of Australasia, University of Sydney, Australia.

Martin, J., 2003, 'Mental health: Rethinking practices with women' in J. Allan, B. Pease and L. Briskman, eds, *Critical Social Work: An Introduction to Theories and Practices*, Allen & Unwin, Crows Nest, NSW.

Martin, K. and Mirraboopa, B., 2007, 'Ways of knowing, being and doing: A theoretical framework and methods for indigenous and indigenist re-search', *Journal of Australian Studies*, Jan 2003: 203–18.

Marx, K., [1843] 1977, *Critique of Hegel's Philosophy of Right*, J. O'Malley, ed, Cambridge University Press, Cambridge.

— [1845] 1888, 'Theses against Feuerbach' in *The Marx/Engels Selected Works*, vol. 1, Progress Publishers, Moscow.

— [1875] 1970, 'The critique of the Gotha program' in *Marx/Engels Selected Works*, vol. 3, Progress Publishers, Moscow.

Marx, K. and Engels, F., [1848] 1969, 'The Communist Manifesto' in *The Marx/Engels Selected Works*, vol. 1, Progress Publishers, Moscow.

May, R., 2007, 'Working outside the diagnostic frame', *The Psychologist*, 20 (5): 300–1

McAuliffe, D. and Chenoweth, L., 2008, 'Leave no stone unturned: The inclusive model of ethical decision making', *Ethics and Social Welfare*, 2 (1): 38–49.

McDonald, C., Craik, C., Hawkins, L. and Williams, J., 2011, *Professional Practice in Human Service Organisations*, Allen & Unwin, Crows Nest, NSW.

McIntosh, P., 1998, 'White privilege: Unpacking the invisible knapsack' in M. McGoldrick, ed, *Re-visioning Family Therapy: Race, Culture and Gender in Clinical Practice*, The Guildford Press, New York.

McIntyre, S., 2012, '1880–1914' in P. Beilharz and T. Hogan, *Sociology: Antipodean Perspectives*, 2nd edn, Oxford University Press, New York.

McKendrick B., 2001, 'The promise of social work: Directions for the future', *Social Work/ Maatskaplike Werk*, 37: 105–11.

McKinnon, J., 2008, 'Exploring the nexus between social work and the environment', *Australian Social Work*, 61, 3: 256–68.

McLaughlin, H., 2009, 'What's in a name: "client", "patient", "customer", "expert by experience", "service user" – what's next?', *British Journal of Social Work*, 39: 1101–17.

McMahon, A., 2003, 'Redefining the beginnings of social work in Australia', *Advances in Social Work and Welfare Education*, 5 (1): 83–94.

Meagher, G. and Parton, N., 2004, 'Modernising social work and the ethics of care', *Social Work and Society*, 2 (1): 10–27.

Meinert, R., Pardeck, J. and Kreuger, L., 2000a, *Social Work: Seeking Relevancy in the Twenty-First Century*, Hapworth Press, Binghampton.

— 2000b, 'The Victorian AASW's first major social action challenge: The 1965 approach from the Australian Labor Party Social Services Committee', *Victorian Social Work*, 9 (2): 19–20.

— 2003, 'Social workers and social action: A case study of the Australian Association of Social Workers Victorian branch', *Australian Social Work*, 56 (1): 121–31.

— 2009, 'Tracing the origins of critical social work practice' in J. Allan, L. Briskman and B. Pease, eds, *Critical Social Work: Theories and Practices for a Socially Just World*, 2nd edn, Allen & Unwin, Crows Nest, NSW.

Mendes, P., 2003, 'Social workers and social action: A case study of the Australian Association of Social Workers' Victorian branch', *Australian Social Work*, vol. 56, no. 1, pp. 16–27.

Mental Health Council of Australia, 2005, *Not for Service: Experiences of Injustice and Despair in Mental Health Care in Australia*, Mental Health Council of Australia, Canberra, ACT.

Menzies, K. and Gilbert, S., 2013, 'Engaging communities' in B. Bennett, S. Green Gilbert and D. Bessarab, eds, *Our Voices: Aboriginal and Torres Strait Islander Social Work*, Palgrave Macmillan, South Yarra, Melbourne.

Meyer, M., 2003, *Ho'oulu: Our Time of Becoming – Hawaiian Epistemology and Early Writings*, 'Ai Pohaku Press, Native Books, Honolulu, Hawai'i.

Middleman, R. and Wood, G., 1990, *Skills for Direct Practice in Social Work*, Columbia University Press, New York.

Millenium Campaign, 2007, *MDG 1: Cut Extreme Poverty and Hunger in Half by 2015*, http://www.un-kampagne.de/fileadmin/downloads/ziele/factsheet_englisch.pdf.

Miller, S., Hayward, R. and Shaw, T., 2012, 'Environmental shifts for social work: A principles approach', *International Journal of Social Welfare*, 21: 270–7.

Mills, C. W., 1959, *The Sociological Imagination*, Oxford University Press, New York.

Mitra, A., Bhatia, M. and Chatterjee, S., 2013, 'Perspectives on women's studies from India: Strengths, struggles and implications for programs in the US', *Journal of International Women's Studies*, 14 (3): 194–209.

Moncrieff, J., 2006, 'The politics of psychiatric drug treatment' in D. Double, ed, *Critical Psychiatry: The Limits of Madness*, Palgrave Macmillan, Basingstoke.

More, T., [1516] 2001, *Utopia*, Yale University Press, New Haven.

Moreau, M., 1979, 'A structural approach to social work practice', *Canadian Journal of Social Work Education*, 5 (1): 78–94.

— [in collaboration with P. Leonard], 1989, *Empowerment: Through a Structural Approach to Social Work. A Report from Practice*, National Welfare Grants Program, Health and Welfare Canada, Ottawa.

Morgan, M., 2011, 'Greek and Hebrew: Religion, ethics, and Judaism' in *The Cambridge Introduction to Emmanuel Levinas*, Cambridge University Press, Cambridge.

Morley, C., 2003a, 'The dominance of risk assessment in child protection: Is it risky?', *Social Work Review*, XV (1&2): 33–6.

— 2003b, 'Towards critical social work practice in mental health: A review', *Journal of Progressive Human Services*, 14 (1): 61–84.

— 2005, 'Collaborative social work practice in opposing paradigms: Issues to emerge from a sexual assault and mental health project', *Women Against Violence: An Australian Feminist Journal*, 16: 4–14.

— 2013, 'Some methodological and ethical tensions in using critical reflection as a research methodology' in J. Fook and F. Gardner, eds, *Critical Reflection in Context: Applications in Health and Social Care*, Routledge, London.

— 2014, *Practising Critical Reflection to Develop Emancipatory Change*, Ashgate, Aldershot, UK.

— (unpub), 'What is the capacity of critical reflection to enhance practitioner agency to work towards emancipatory outcomes?', An evaluation of training undertaken on behalf of The Workforce Council, Inc, University of the Sunshine Coast, 2012.

Morley, C. and Ablett, P. (unpub1), 'The impact of a group presentation/performance assessment on first year social work and human service students: Identity, learning and connection', Open Learning and Teaching Grants Program, University of the Sunshine Coast, 2011.

— (unpub2), 'The impact of facilitated live examined role-plays on student learning regarding the links between critical theory and social work practice', Open Learning and Teaching Grants Program, University of the Sunshine Coast, 2012.

Morley, C. and Fook, J., 2005, 'The importance of pet loss and some implications for services', *Mortality*, 10 (2): 127–43.

Morley, C. and Macfarlane, S., 2008, 'The continued importance of a feminist analysis: Making gendered inequalities visible through a critique of Howard government policy on domestic violence', *Just Policy: A Journal of Australian Social Policy*, 47: 31–8.

— 2012, 'The nexus between feminism and postmodernism: Still a central concern for critical social work', *British Journal of Social Work*, 42 (4): 687–705.

— (unpub), 'Critical social work as ethical social work using critical reflection to research students' resistance to neoliberalism'.

Morrow, L., Verins, I. and Willis, E., 2002, 'Introduction' in L. Morrow, I. Verins and E. Willis, eds, *Mental Health and Work: Issues and Perspectives*, AUSEINET: The Australian Network for Promotion, Prevention and Early Intervention for Mental Health, Adelaide.

Morton, A., 2009, 'First climate refugees move to new home', *The Age*, 29 July.

Mostov, J., 1989, 'Karl Marx as democratic theorist', *Polity*, 22 (2): 195–212.

Muldoon, P. and Schaap, A., 2012, 'Aboriginal sovereignty and the politics of reconciliation: The constituent power of the Aboriginal Embassy in Australia', *Environment and Planning D: Society and Space*, 30, 534–50.

Mullaly, B., 1993, *Structural Social Work: Ideology, Theory, and Practice*, McClelland and Stewart, Toronto.

— 2002, *Challenging Oppression: A Critical Approach to Social Work*, Oxford University Press, Toronto.

— 2007, *The New Structural Social Work*, 3rd edn, Oxford University Press, Ontario.

— 2010, *Challenging Oppression and Confronting Privilege*, 2nd edn, Oxford University Press, Ontario.

Nagle, D., 2010, *The Ancient World: A Social and Cultural History*, 7th edn, Prentice Hall, Upper Saddle River, NJ.

Napier, L. and Fook, J., 2000, 'Reflective practice in social work' in L. Napier and J. Fook, ed, *Breakthroughs in Practice: Theorising Critical Moments in Social Work*, Whiting and Birch, London.

Netting, F., Kettner, P. and McMurtry, S., 2008, *Social Work Macro Practice*, 4th edn, Pearson, Melbourne.

Nichol, W., 1985, 'Medicine and the labour movement in New South Wales, 1788–1850', *Labour History*, 49: 19–37.

Nichols, J., 1977, 'Social work education and women's lib . . . A dead issue?' *Contemporary Social Work Education*, 1 (2): 52–44.

Nola, R. and Irzik, G., 2005, *Philosophy, Science, Education and Culture*, Springer, Netherlands.

Norton, C., 2012, 'Social work and the environment: An ecosocial approach', *International Journal of Social Welfare*, 21: 299–308.

O'Connor, I., Wilson, J., Setterlund, D. and Hughes, M., 2008, *Social Work and Human Service Practice*, 5th edn, Pearson Longman, Frenchs Forest, NSW.

Orme, J., 2013, 'Feminist social work' in M. Gray and S. Webb, eds, *Social Work: Theories and Methods*, 2nd edn, Sage, London.

O'Sullivan, M. and Kersley, R., 2012, 'Global trends: Global wealth 2012: The year in review', https://www.credit-suisse.com/ch/en/news-and-expertise/news/economy/global-trends.article.html/article/pwp/news-and-expertise/2012/10/en/global-wealth-2012-the-year-in-review.html.

Oxfam 2013, 'The cost of inequality: How wealth and income extremes hurt us all', http://www.oxfam.org/sites/www.oxfam.org/files/cost-of-inequality-oxfam-mb180113.pdf.

Pack, M., 2013, 'An evaluation of critical-reflection on service-users and their families: Narratives as a teaching resource in a post-graduated allied mental health program – an integrative approach', *Social Work in Mental Health*, 11 (2): 154–66.

Pare, A., 2004, 'Texts and power: Toward a critical theory of language' in L. Davies and P. Leonard, eds, *Social Work in a Corporate Era: Practices of Power and Resistance*, Ashgate, Aldershot.

Parker, S., Fook, J. and Pease, B., 1999, 'Empowerment: The modernist social work concept par excellence' in B. Pease and J. Fook, eds, *Transforming Social Work Practice: Postmodern Critical Perspectives*, Allen & Unwin, St Leonards, NSW.

Parton, N. and O'Byrne, P., 2000, *Constructive Social Work: Towards a New Practice*, Allen & Unwin, St Leonards, NSW.

Patkar, M., 1991, 'The Right Livelihood Award', http://www.rightlivelihood.org/narmada.html.

Payne, M., 2005, *Modern Social Work Theory*, 3rd edn, Palgrave Macmillan, Basingstoke.

— 2006, *What is Professional Social Work?*, 2nd edn, Policy Press, Bristol.

Payne, M. and Askeland, G., 2008, *Globalization and International Social Work: Postmodern Change and Challenge*, Ashgate, Aldershot.

Pease, B., 2010, *Undoing Privilege: Unearned Advantage in a Divided World*, Zed Books, London.

Pease, B. and Fook, J., 1999, eds, *Transforming Social Work Practice: Postmodern Critical Perspectives*, Routledge, London.

Peel, M., 2008, 'Charity Organisation Society' in *Melbourne: The City Past and Present*, School of Historical Studies, University of Melbourne, Parkville.

Penna, S. and O'Brien, M., 2013, 'Neoliberalism' in M. Gray and S. Webb, eds, *Social Work Theories and Methods*, 2nd edn, Sage, London.

Perlman, H., 1957, *Social Casework: A Problem-Solving Process*, University of Chicago Press, Chicago.

Pheterson, G., 1986, 'Alliances between women: Overcoming internalised oppression and internalised domination', *Signs: Journal of Women in Culture and Society*, 12 (1): 146–60.

Phillips, J., 2000, *Contested Knowledge: A Guide to Critical Theory*, Zed Books, London and New York.

Pierson, J., 2011, *Understanding Social Work: History and Context*, Open University Press, Maidenhead.

Pinkerton, J., 2002, 'Child protection' in R. Adams, L. Dominelli and M. Payne, eds, *Critical Practice in Social Work*, Palgrave Macmillan, Basingstoke.

Plath, D., 2013, 'Evidence-based practice' in M. Gray and S. Webb, eds, *Social Work Theories and Methods*, 2nd edn, Sage, London.

Plionis, E., 2004, 'Teaching students how to avoid errors in theory application', *Brief Treatment and Crisis Intervention*, 4 (1): 49–56.

Pope, G., Drew, W., Lazaruz, J. and Ellis, F., [1886] 1982, *Tirukkural: English Translation and Commentary*, The South India Saiva Siddhantha Works Publishing Society, Tinnevelly Limited, India.

Powell, J., 2013, 'Michel Foucault' in M. Gray and S. Webb, eds, *Social Work Theories and Methods*, 2nd edn, Sage, London.

Pozzuto, R., 2000, 'Notes on a possible critical social work', *Critical Social Work*, 1 (1).

Pozzuto, R., Brent Angell, G. and Dezendorf, P., 2005, 'Therapeutic critique: Traditional versus critical perspectives' in S. Hick, J. Fook and R. Pozzuto, eds, *Social Work: A Critical Turn*, Thompson Educational Publishing, Toronto.

Prasad, M., 1995, 'Social Justice in Ancient India: in Arthaśāstra' in K. D. Irani and M. Silver, eds, *Social Justice in the Ancient World*, Greenwood Press, Connecticut.

Pratt, N., 2004, 'Bringing politics back in: Examining the link between globalization and democratization', *Review of International Political Economy*, 11 (2): 311–36.

Pritchard, C. and Taylor, R., 1978, *Social Work: Reform or Revolution?*, Routledge and Kegan Paul, London.

Queensland Government, 2013, 'What is child abuse?', http://www.communities.qld. gov.au/childsafety/protecting-children/what-is-child-abuse.

Quinn, M., 2009, 'Towards anti-racist and culturally affirming practices' in J. Allan, L. Briskman and B. Pease, eds, *Critical Social Work: Theories and Practices for a Socially Just World*, 2nd edn, Allen & Unwin, Crows Nest, NSW.

Ramsden, P., 1998, *Learning to Lead in Higher Education*, Routledge, London.

Ravallion, M., Chen, S. and Sangraula, P., 2008, *Dollar a Day Revisited*, Policy Research Working Paper 4640, World Bank, Washington, DC.

Ray, R. and Phillips, J., 2002, 'Older people' in R. Adams, L. Dominelli and M. Payne, eds, *Critical Practice in Social Work*, Palgrave Macmillan, Basingstoke.

Read, J., 2004, 'Poverty, ethnicity and gender' in J. Read, L. Mosher and R. Bentall, eds, *Models of Madness: Psychological, Social and Biological Approaches to Schizophrenia*, Routledge, London and New York.

Reamer, F., 2006, *Social Work Values and Ethics*, 3rd edn, Colombia University Press, New York.

Reclaim the Night Australia, 2013, http://www.isis.aust.com/rtn/.

Rees, S., 1991, *Achieving Power*, Allen & Unwin, Sydney.

— 1999, 'Managerialism in social welfare: Proposals for a humanitarian alternative', *European Journal of Social Work*, 2 (2): 193–202.

Reisch, M., 2002, 'Defining social justice in a socially unjust world', *Families in Society: The Journal of Contemporary Human Services*, 83(4): 434–54.

Reisch, M. and Andrews, J., 2001, *The Road Not Taken: A History of Radical Social Work in the Untied States*, Brunner-Routledge, Philadelphia.

Reyna, V., Nelson, W., Han, P. and Dieckmann, N., 2009, 'How numeracy influences risk comprehension and medical decision making', *Psychological Bulletin*, 135 (6): 943–73.

Reynolds, B., 1963, *An Uncharted Journey: Fifty Years of Growth in Social Work*, The Citadel Press, New York.

Rifkin, J., 2004, *The End of Work: The Decline of the Global Labour Force and the Dawn of the Post Market Era*, 2nd edn, Tarcher/Penguin, New York.

Ritzer, G. and Stepnisky, J., 2014, *Sociological Theory*, 9th edn, McGraw Hill, New York.

Roach Anleu, S., 2010, *Law and Social Change*, Sage, London.

Rogers, A. and Pilgrim, D., 2003, *Mental Health and Inequality*, Palgrave Macmillan, Basingstoke.

Rogers, D., 2008, 'Out of sight, out of mend: mentally ill in Queensland correctional centres' *Queensland Law Student Review*, 1 (2): 88–100.

Rogowski, S., 2010, *Social Work: The Rise and Fall of a Profession?*, Policy Press, Bristol.

Rojek, C., Peakcock, G. and Collins, S., 1988, *Social Work and Received Ideas*, Routledge, London.

Rossiter, A., 1996, 'A perspective on critical social work', *Journal of Progressive Human Services*, 7 (2): 23– 41.

— 2005, 'Discourse analysis in critical social work: From apology to question', *Critical Social Work*, 6 (1).

— 2011, 'Unsettled social work: The challenge of Levinas's ethic', *British Journal of Social Work*, 41 (5): 980–95.

Rousseau, J., [1762] 2012, *The Social Contract* (ebook), http://ebooks.adelaide.edu.au/r/rousseau/jean_jacques/r864s/.

Rowe, W., Hanley, J., Moreno, E. and Mould, J., 2000, 'Voices of social work practice: International reflections on the effects of globalisation' in B. Rowe, ed, *Social Work and Globalisation*, Joint Conference of the International Federation of Social Workers and International Association of Schools of Social Work, Quebec.

Ryan, F., 2011, 'Kanyininpa (holding): A way of nurturing children in Aboriginal Australia, *Australian Social Work*', 64 (2): 183–97.

Ryan, T., 2011, *Animals and Social Work: A Moral Introduction*, Palgrave Macmillan, London.

Sahlins, M., 2004, *Stone-Age Economics*, 2nd edn, Routledge, London, University of Chicago Press, Chicago.

Salas, L., Soma, S. and Segal, E., 2010, 'Critical theory: Pathway from dichotomous to integrated social work practice', *Families in Society: The Journal of Contemporary Social Services*, 91 (1): 91–6.

Sands, R., 1996, 'The elusiveness of identity in social work practice with women', *Clinical Social Work Journal*, 24 (2): 167–86.

Saraga, E., 1993, 'The abuse of children' in R. Dallos and E. Mclaughlan, *Social Problems and the Family*, Sage, London.

Sarantakos, S., 2005, *Social Research*, 3rd edn, Palgrave Macmillan, Basingstole.

Sargent, M., Nilan, P. and Winter, G., 1997, *The New Sociology for Australians*, 4th edn, Longman, Melbourne.

Sawer, M., 2003, *The Ethical State?: Social Liberalism in Australia*, Melbourne University Press, Melbourne.

Sawyer, K., 2002, 'Durkheim's dilemma: Toward a sociology of emergence', *Sociological Theory*, 20 (2): 227–47.

Scheurich, J. and Young, M., 1997, 'Coloring epistemologies: Are our research epistemologies racially biased?', *Educational Researcher*, 26 (4): 4–16.

Scheyett, A. and Diehl, M., 2004, 'Walking our talk in social work education: partnering with consumers of mental health services', *Social Work Education*, 23 (4): 435–50.

Schlecty, P., 2004, *Shaking up the Schoolhouse: How to Support and Sustain Educational Innovation*, Jossey-Bass, New Jersey.

Schon, D. 1987, *Educating the Critically Reflective Practitioner: Toward a New Design for Teaching and Learning in the Professions*, Jossey-Bass, San Francisco.

Scott, D., Walker, L. and Gilmore, K., 1995, 'Counselling support for adults who have been sexually assaulted' in *Breaking the Silence: A Guide to Supporting Adult Victim/ Survivors of Sexual Assault*, 2nd edn, CASA House, Melbourne.

Seidman, S., 2013, *Contested Knowledge: Social Theory Today*, 5th edn, Blackwell Publishing, Carlton, Victoria.

Shankar, J. and Muthuswamy, S., 2007, 'Support needs of family caregivers of people who experience mental illness and the role of mental health services', *Families in Society*, 88 (2): 302–10.

Shier, M., Sinclair, C. and Gault, L., 2011, 'Challenging ableism and teaching about disability in a social work classroom: A training module for generalist social workers working with people disabled by the social environment', *Critical Social Work*, 12 (1).

Sire J., 2004, *Naming the Elephant: Worldview as a Concept*, InterVarsity Press, Westmont, Ill.

Sirin, S., 2005, 'Socio-economic status and academic achievement: A meta-analytic review of research', *Review of Educational Research*, 75 (3): 417–53.

Smith, L., 2005, 'On tricky ground: Researching the native in the age of uncertainty' in N. Denzin and Y. Lincoln, eds, *The SAGE Handbook of Qualitative Research'*, 3rd edn, Sage, Thousand Oaks.

Solomon, B., 1976, *Black Empowerment: Social Work in Oppressed Communities*, Columbia University Press, New York.

Soos, P., 2013, 'The truth behind our "dangerous" public debt levels', The Conversation, http://theconversation.com/the-truth-behind-our-dangerous-public-debt-levels-13245.

Soros, G., 1998, *The Crisis of Global Capitalism*, Public Affairs, New York.

Spicker, P., 2008, *British Social Policy 1601–1948*, Centre for Public Policy and Management, Robert Gordon University, Aberdeen.

Spratt, T. and Houston, S., 1999, 'Developing critical social work in theory and in practice: Child protection and communicative reason', *Child and Family Social Work*, 4: 315–24.

Stanton, B., 2005, 'School drug education in New South Wales: Moral panic and the individualisation of youth drug use', *Social Alternatives*, 24 (4): 50–4.

Stewart-Harawira, M., 2005, 'Cultural studies, Indigenous knowledge and pedagogies of hope', *Policy Futures in Education*, 3 (2): 153–63.

Stickley, T., 2006, 'Should service user involvement be consigned to history: A critical realist perspective', *Journal of Psychiatric and Mental Health Nursing*, 13: 570–7.

Stockton, E. and Nanson, G., 2004, 'Cranebrook Terrace Revisited', *Archaeology in Oceania*, 39 (1): 59–60.

Stringer, K., 2011, 'US spent $307 billion on prescription drugs in 2010', *Natural News*, http://www.naturalnews.com/032200_prescription_drugs_billions.html#.

Swain, P. A., 2002, 'Why social work and law?' in P. A. Swain and S. Rice, eds, *In the Shadow of the Law: The Legal Context of Social Work Practice*, 2nd edn, The Federation Press, Sydney.

Swain, P. A. and Rice, S., eds, 2009, *In the Shadow of the Law: The Legal Context of Social Work Practice*, 3rd edn, The Federation Press, Sydney.

Sydney University Settlement, 2008, 'Objectives', http://thesettlement.org.au/Objectives.

Tatem, A., Rogers, D. and Hay, S., 2006, 'Global transport networks and infectious disease spread', *Advances in Parasitology*, 62: 293–343.

Taylor, J., 2012, 'Queenslanders speak out against LNP job cuts', ABC News, http://www.abc.net.au/news/2012-09-17/queenslanders-speak-out-about-lnp-job-cuts/4264540.

Tew, J., 2005, 'Power relations, social order and mental distress' in J. Tew, ed, *Social Perspectives in Mental Health: Developing Social Models to Understand and Work with Mental Distress*, Jessica Kingsley Publishers, London and Philadelphia.

Thompson, N., 1992, *Anti-Discriminatory Practice*, Palgrave Macmillan, London.

— 1998, 'Discrimination and oppression' in N. Thompson, *Promoting Equality: Challenging Discrimination and Oppression in the Human Services*, Palgrave Macmillan, Basingstoke.

— 2001, *Anti-Discriminatory Practice*, 3rd edn, Palgrave Macmillan, Basingstoke.

— 2010, *Theorizing Social Work Practice*, Palgrave Macmillan, Basingstoke.

Thompson, S., De Bortoli, S., Nicholas, M., Hillman, K. and Buckley, S., 2011, *Challenges for Australian Education: Results from PISA 2009 Assessment of Students' Reading, Mathematical and Scientific Literacy*, ACER Press, Camberwell, Victoria.

Thorpe, R. and Petruchenia, J., eds, 1992, *Community Work or Social Change?: An Australian Perspective*, Hale & Iremonger, Sydney.

Throssell, H., ed, 1975, *Social Work: Radical Essays*, University of Queensland Press, St Lucia.

Tilley, C., 2003, *Contention and Democracy in Europe, 1650–2000*, Cambridge University Press, Cambridge.

Timberg, S., 2013, 'Jaron Lanier: The internet destroyed the middle class', Salon, 12 May, http://www.salon.com/2013/05/12/jaron_lanier_the_internet_destroyed_the_middle_class/.

Timimi, S., 2006, 'Critical child psychiatry' in D. Double, ed, *Critical Psychiatry: The Limits of Madness*, Palgrave Macmillan, Basingstoke.

Todd, N. and Wade, A. (with Renoux, M.), 2004, 'Coming to terms with violence and resistance' in T. Strong and D. Pare, eds, *Furthering Talk: Advances in Discursive Therapies*, Springer, New York.

Topsfield, J., 2012, 'Private school fees edge closer to minimum wage', *The Age*, 10 November.

Trevithick, P., 2005, *Social Work Skills: A Practice Handbook*, 2nd edn, Open University Press, Maidenhead.

Tucci, J. and Goddard, C., 2010, 'Kept in the dark on child protection', *The Age*, 3 November.

Turner, M. and Beresford, P., 2005, *User Controlled Research: Its Meanings and Potential – Final Report*, Shaping our Lives and the Centre for Citizen Participation, Brunel University.

UN Women, 2011, *Progress on the World's Women: In Pursuit of Justice*, United Nations, New York

United Nations Development Programme (UNDP), 1995, *Human Development Report 1995: Gender and Human Development*, United Nations, New York.

— 2006, *Human Development Report 2006: Beyond Scarcity: Power, Poverty and the Global Water Crisis*, United Nations, New York.

— 2011, *Fast Facts: United Nations Development Programme: Gender Equality and UNDP*, United Nations, New York

United Nations High Commission for Refugees, 1951, *Convention Relating to the Status of Refugees*, http://www.unhcr.org/3b66c2aa10.html.

United Nations Office on Drugs and Crime, 2013, 'Human trafficking', https://www.unodc.org/unodc/en/human-trafficking/what-is-human-trafficking.html?ref=menuside.

Universities Australia, 2008, *Participation and Equity: A Review of the Participation in Higher Education of People from Low Socioeconomic Backgrounds and Indigenous People*, Universities Australia and Centre for the Study of Higher Education, University of Melbourne, Melbourne.

Van Krieken, R., 1999, 'The "stolen generations" and cultural genocide: The forced removal of Australian Indigenous children from their families and its implications for the sociology of childhood', *Childhood*, 6 (3): 297–311.

Van Krieken, R., Habibas, D., Smith, P., Hutchins, B., Martin, G. and Maton, K., 2012, *Sociology*, 4th edn, Pearson Australia, Frenchs Forest, NSW.

Van Soest, D., 2012, 'Confronting our fears and finding hope in difficult times: Social work as a force for social justice', *Journal of Progressive Human Services*, 23 (2): 95–109.

Victorian Centres Against Sexual Assault (CASA) Forum, 2013, 'Fact sheet: Statistics about sexual assault', Victoria CASA Forum, Melbourne.

Victorian Health Promotion Foundation, 2005, *A Plan for Action 2005–2007: Promoting Mental Health and Wellbeing*, Mental Health and Wellbeing Unit, VicHealth, Melbourne.

Von Bertalanffy, L., 1968, *General System Theory: Foundations, Development, Applications*, George Braziller, New York.

Wachsler, S., 2007, 'The real quality of life issue for people with disabilities', *Journal of Progressive Human services*, 18 (2): 7–14.

Wadham, B., Pudsey, J. and Boyd, R., 2007, *Culture and Education*, Pearson Education, Frenchs Forest, NSW.

Wagner, D., 1990, *The Quest for a Radical Profession: Social Service Careers and Political Ideology*, University Press of America, California.

Waldegrave, C., 1990, 'Just therapy', *Dulwich Centre Newsletter*, no. 1: 5–25.

Walsh, D. and Weeks, W., 2004, *What a Smile Can Hide*, Royal Women's Hospital, Arena Printing Services, Melbourne.

Watkins, J., 1996, 'The journey of recovery: What workers need to know, do and be' in S. Rowland, ed, Recovery Conference Papers, VICSERV, Fitzroy, Victoria.

Webb, B., [1926] 1980, *My Apprenticeship: Beatrice Webb*, Cambridge University Press. Cambridge.

Webb, D., 2013, 'Pedagogies of hope', *Studies in Philosophy and Education*, 32 (4): 397–414.

Webb, S., 2006, *Social Work in a Risk Society*, Palgrave Macmillan, Basingstoke.

Weeks, W., 1994, *Women Working Together: Lessons from Feminist Women's Services*, Longman, Melbourne.

Wehbi, S., 2013, 'Challenging international social work placements: Critical questions, critical knowledge' in M. Gray, J. Coates, M. Yellow Bird and T. Hetherington, eds, *Decolonizing Social Work*, Ashgate, Surrey.

Wehbi, S. and Turcotte, P., 2007, 'Social work education: Neoliberalism's willing victim?', *Critical Social Work*, 8 (1): 1–9.

Weick, K., 1995, *Sensemaking in Organisations*, Sage, Thousand Oaks.

Weinocur, S. and Reisch, M., 1989, *From Charity to Enterprise: The Development of American Social Work in a Market Economy*, University of Illinois Press, Urbana.

Weinstein, J., 2011, '*Case Con*, and radical social work in the 1970s: The impatient revolutionaries' in M. Lavalette, ed, *Radical Social Work Today: Social Work at the Crossroads*, Policy Press, Bristol.

Wilkinson, R., 2011, 'How economic inequality harms societies', http://www.ted.com/talks/richard_wilkinson.

Wilkinson R. and Pickett, K., 2010, *The Spirit Level: Why Equality Is Better for Everyone*, Penguin, London.

Williams, J., 2005, 'Women's mental health: taking inequality into account' in J. Tew, ed, *Social Perspectives in Mental Health: Developing Social Models to Understand and Work with Mental Distress*, Jessica Kingsley Publishers, London and Philadelphia.

Willis, E., 1990, *Medical Dominance: Revised Edition*, Allen & Unwin, St Leonards, NSW.

Wilson, S., 2003, 'Progressing toward an Indigenous research paradigm in Canada and Australia', *Canadian Journal of Native Education*, 27 (2): 161–78.

Wong, Y., 2004, 'Knowing through discomfort: A mindfulness-based critical social work pedagogy', *Critical Social Work*, 5 (1).

Woodside, M. and McClam, T., 2011, *An Introduction to Human Services*, 7th edn, Brooks/Cole, Belmont, CA.

Workplace Gender Equality Agency (WGEA), 2013, *Gender Pay Gap Statistics*, http://www.wgea.gov.au.

Yang, X., 1997, 'Trying to do justice to the concept of justice in Confucian ethics', *Journal of Chinese Philosophy*, 24: 521–51.

Yates, J. and Berry, M., 2011, 'Housing and mortgage markets in turbulent times: Is Australia different?', *Housing Studies*, 26 (7/8): 1133–56.

Yuill, C. and Gibson, A., 2011, *Sociology for Social Work: An Introduction*, Sage, London.

Zastrow, C., 2010, *Introduction to Social Work and Social Welfare*, 10th edn, Cengage Learning, Belmont.

Zellmer, D., 2004–05, 'Teaching to prevent burnout in the helping professions', *Analytic Teaching*, 24 (1): 20–5.

Index